ENDING THE TOBACCO PROBLEM

A BLUEPRINT FOR THE NATION

Committee on Reducing Tobacco Use:
Strategies, Barriers, and Consequences
Board on Population Health and Public Health Practice

Richard J. Bonnie, Kathleen Stratton, and Robert B. Wallace, *Editors*

INSTITUTE OF MEDICINE
OF THE NATIONAL ACADEMIES

THE NATIONAL ACADEMIES PRESS
Washington, D.C.
www.nap.edu

THE NATIONAL ACADEMIES PRESS   500 Fifth Street, N.W.   Washington, DC 20001

NOTICE: The project that is the subject of this report was approved by the Governing Board of the National Research Council, whose members are drawn from the councils of the National Academy of Sciences, the National Academy of Engineering, and the Institute of Medicine. The members of the committee responsible for the report were chosen for their special competences and with regard for appropriate balance.

This study was supported by Grant ID Number 6210 between the National Academy of Sciences and the American Legacy Foundation. Any opinions, findings, conclusions, or recommendations expressed in this publication are those of the author(s) and do not necessarily reflect the view of the organizations or agencies that provided support for this project.

Library of Congress Cataloging-in-Publication Data

Institute of Medicine (U.S.). Committee on Reducing Tobacco Use: Strategies, Barriers, and Consequences.
   Ending the tobacco problem : a blueprint for the nation / Committee on Reducing Tobacco Use: Strategies, Barriers, and Consequences, Board on Population Health and Public Health Practice ; Richard J. Bonnie, Kathleen Stratton, and Robert B. Wallace, editors.
      p. ; cm.
   Includes bibliographical references and index.
   ISBN-13: 978-0-309-10382-4 (hardback : alk. paper)
   ISBN-10: 0-309-10382-7 (hardback : alk. paper) 1. Tobacco use—United States—Prevention. 2. Smoking—United States—Prevention. 3. Public health—United States. I. Bonnie, Richard J. II. Stratton, Kathleen R. III. Wallace, Robert B., 1942- IV. Title.
   [DNLM: 1. Tobacco Use Disorder—prevention & control—United States. 2. Health Policy—United States. 3. Smoking—legislation & jurisprudence—United States. 4. Smoking—prevention & control—United States. 5. Smoking Cessation—legislation & jurisprudence—United States. WM 290 I585e 2007]
   HV5763.I67 2007
   362.29'660973—dc22
                                   2007027676

Additional copies of this report are available from the National Academies Press, 500 Fifth Street, N.W., Lockbox 285, Washington, DC 20055; (800) 624-6242 or (202) 334-3313 (in the Washington metropolitan area); Internet, http://www.nap.edu.

For more information about the Institute of Medicine, visit the IOM home page at: **www. iom.edu.**

The serpent has been a symbol of long life, healing, and knowledge among almost all cultures and religions since the beginning of recorded history. The serpent adopted as a logotype by the Institute of Medicine is a relief carving from ancient Greece, now held by the Staatliche Museum in Berlin.

Suggested citation: IOM (Institute of Medicine). 2007. *Ending the tobacco problem: A blueprint for the nation.* Washington, DC: The National Academies Press.

"Knowing is not enough; we must apply.
Willing is not enough; we must do."

—Goethe

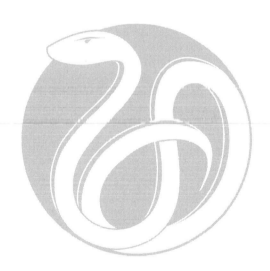

INSTITUTE OF MEDICINE
OF THE NATIONAL ACADEMIES

Advising the Nation. Improving Health.

THE NATIONAL ACADEMIES
Advisers to the Nation on Science, Engineering, and Medicine

The **National Academy of Sciences** is a private, nonprofit, self-perpetuating society of distinguished scholars engaged in scientific and engineering research, dedicated to the furtherance of science and technology and to their use for the general welfare. Upon the authority of the charter granted to it by the Congress in 1863, the Academy has a mandate that requires it to advise the federal government on scientific and technical matters. Dr. Ralph J. Cicerone is president of the National Academy of Sciences.

The **National Academy of Engineering** was established in 1964, under the charter of the National Academy of Sciences, as a parallel organization of outstanding engineers. It is autonomous in its administration and in the selection of its members, sharing with the National Academy of Sciences the responsibility for advising the federal government. The National Academy of Engineering also sponsors engineering programs aimed at meeting national needs, encourages education and research, and recognizes the superior achievements of engineers. Dr. Charles M. Vest is president of the National Academy of Engineering.

The **Institute of Medicine** was established in 1970 by the National Academy of Sciences to secure the services of eminent members of appropriate professions in the examination of policy matters pertaining to the health of the public. The Institute acts under the responsibility given to the National Academy of Sciences by its congressional charter to be an adviser to the federal government and, upon its own initiative, to identify issues of medical care, research, and education. Dr. Harvey V. Fineberg is president of the Institute of Medicine.

The **National Research Council** was organized by the National Academy of Sciences in 1916 to associate the broad community of science and technology with the Academy's purposes of furthering knowledge and advising the federal government. Functioning in accordance with general policies determined by the Academy, the Council has become the principal operating agency of both the National Academy of Sciences and the National Academy of Engineering in providing services to the government, the public, and the scientific and engineering communities. The Council is administered jointly by both Academies and the Institute of Medicine. Dr. Ralph J. Cicerone and Dr. Charles M. Vest are chair and vice chair, respectively, of the National Research Council.

www.national-academies.org

Reviewers

This report has been reviewed in draft form by individuals chosen for their diverse perspectives and technical expertise, in accordance with procedures approved by the National Research Council's Report Review Committee. The purpose of this independent review is to provide candid and critical comments that will assist the institution in making its published report as sound as possible and to ensure that the report meets institutional standards for objectivity, evidence, and responsiveness to the study charge. The review comments and draft manuscript remain confidential to protect the integrity of the deliberative process. We wish to thank the following individuals for their review of this report:

Lois Biener, Ph.D., University of Massachusetts, Boston
Richard Clayton, Ph.D., University of Kentucky
Phillip Cook, Ph.D., Duke University
Gordon DeFriese, Ph.D., University of North Carolina
Paul Fischer, M.D., Center for Primary Care
Gary Giovino, Ph.D., State University of New York, Buffalo
Jack Henningfield, Ph.D., Johns Hopkins University
Howard Koh, M.D., M.P.H., Harvard School of Public Health
Harold Pollack, Ph.D., University of Chicago
Eric A. Posner, J.D., University of Chicago Law School
Steven Schroeder, M.D., University of California, San Francisco

Although the reviewers listed above have provided many constructive comments and suggestions, they were not asked to endorse the conclusions or recommendations nor did they see the final draft of the report before its release. The review of this report was overseen by **Nancy E. Adler, Ph.D.,** University of California, San Francisco, and **Robert S. Lawrence, M.D.,** Johns Hopkins University. Appointed by the National Research Council and Institute of Medicine, they were responsible for making certain that an independent examination of this report was carried out in accordance with institutional procedures and that all review comments were carefully considered. Responsibility for the final content of this report rests entirely with the authoring committee and the institution.

Preface

"Cigarette smoking is a health hazard of sufficient importance in the United States to warrant appropriate remedial action." So stated the Advisory Committee to the Surgeon General of the Public Health Service in its seminal Report in 1964 (p. 33). Since then, the Surgeon General has issued 28 more reports on tobacco and health, most recently in 2005. The health effects of cigarette smoking and use of other tobacco products, including smokeless tobacco, are by now well-known.

Cigarette-smoking has decreased considerably in the United States since 1964 when about 52 million adults (representing 42 percent of the adult population) smoked, and public health leaders and tobacco control specialists deserve praise for what they have been able to accomplish over the past four decades. However, there are still approximately 44 million smokers in this country, and cigarette smoking is the "underlying cause" of more than 440,000 deaths a year in the United States.

Why has there not been greater progress in ending the tobacco problem? Although many social, economic, and political factors have played a role, perhaps the most important one is that the tobacco industry obscured the addictive properties and health risks of smoking, impeded and delayed many tobacco control interventions, and has so far successfully thwarted meaningful federal regulatory measures. As a result, more than forty years after the first Surgeon General's report, the necessary "remedial action" has not yet been taken. This report presents a two-prong strategic plan for intensifying and accelerating public health efforts, thereby taking long strides toward ending the tobacco problem in the United States. The first prong of the plan calls for making better use of tobacco control interventions known to be effective. These steps can be implemented immediately. The second prong of the committee's plan calls for federal legislative action to transform the current legal structure of tobacco control and for deploying innovative new regulatory approaches. Taken together, the blueprint outlines the strong measures that will be needed to reduce substantially the prevalence of cigarette-smoking and to assure that other forms of tobacco use are simultaneously contained or reduced. How quickly this can be done depends on how quickly the plan is implemented.

This is not the first time the Institute of Medicine (IOM) has addressed the need for strong remedial measures to control tobacco use. In 1994, the IOM issued *Growing Up Tobacco Free*, a report outlining a blueprint for reducing tobacco use among children and adolescents. The recommendations in that report figured prominently in the drafting of the FDA's Tobacco Rule—promulgated in 1996 but invalidated by the United States Supreme Court in 2000. In 2001, the IOM issued *Clearing the Smoke,* a report assessing the science base for reduced-risk tobacco products and specifying principles to guide federal legislative and administrative action. Although the IOM principles have provided a foundation for legislative proposals in both houses of Congress over the past 5 years, federal law remains unchanged.

The blueprint for action presented in this report is both comprehensive and specific. Although the recommendations are more detailed than those offered in most IOM reports, the committee followed the path plowed by the two previous IOM reports on tobacco policy, recognizing that the key elements of the blueprint require strong and unambiguous legislative and administrative action at all levels of government.

The committee commissioned 16 papers reviewing the literature in many of the areas of tobacco control covered in the report, and these papers are published in an appendix accompanying the committee's report (prepared as a CD). We asked the authors (most of whom also served as members of the committee) to draw conclusions from their work and, if indicated, to make policy recommendations. To avoid any confusion, it bears emphasis that the recommendations appearing in the committee's report represent the consensus judgment of the committee as a whole and are endorsed by all members of the committee except where otherwise indicated. In contrast, the recommendations appearing in the individually authored chapters in the Appendix should not be attributed to the committee itself.

The title of the committee's report warrants some explanation. What does the committee mean by "ending the tobacco problem"? We do not mean eliminating smoking and other forms of tobacco use altogether. That is both unrealistic and unnecessary. Instead, we have in mind reducing tobacco use so substantially that it no longer has a significant impact on public health.

The magnitude of tobacco's impact on the public health is inextricably linked to the highly addictive property of cigarettes and other tobacco products as they are currently designed and used. Four out of five current adult cigarette smokers are addicted to them, and the average length of a smoking career is several years. One strategy that should be explored, as the committee explains in Chapter 7, is gradually reducing the nicotine content of tobacco products so that they are no longer addictive. If that were accomplished, the residual use of tobacco decades from now might not amount to a significant public health problem.

Unless and until a nicotine reduction strategy is successfully implemented, however, the central aim for tobacco policy must continue to be reducing the number of tobacco users through a two-pronged strategy of reducing initiation and facilitating cessation. Harm reduction (reducing the risks of consumption) is, at best, an ancillary component of a comprehensive strategy for protecting the public health.

What levels of cigarette smoking, smokeless tobacco use, and cigar smoking would be "acceptable" from a public health perspective? Reducing the current adult prevalence of cigarette smoking in half (from about 21 percent to about 10 percent) would still leave more than 20 million adult smokers. That is not good enough. Is 5 percent good enough? 3 percent?

Ultimately, the committee concluded that answering this question has little practical significance at the present time. We see no reason to go through the hypothetical exercise of identifying particular initiation and prevalence rates that would signal "ultimate" success. Setting such targets requires delicate judgments based on data not now available and circumstances that cannot now be foreseen. There will be time enough for another committee to set these targets in the coming years. For the next decade or two, the aim must be to reduce initiation and increase cessation as much as possible without stimulating a substantial black market and its associated costs.

Speaking for the Committee on Reducing Tobacco Use, I hope that the recommendations outlined in this report are implemented with vigor, speed, and perseverance. Many components of the committee's plan can be implemented immediately without any federal action. However, if Congress moves quickly to empower FDA and the states to launch new regulatory initiatives recommended in this report, the nation will be on a promising course toward ending the tobacco problem by 2030.

Richard J. Bonnie, *Chair*
Committee on Reducing Tobacco Use

Contents

SUMMARY   1

INTRODUCTION   29

PART I: BACKGROUND

1   EPIDEMIOLOGY OF TOBACCO USE: HISTORY AND
    CURRENT TRENDS   41
    Growth of the Tobacco Problem, 41
    Decline in Tobacco Use: 1965–2005, 45
    Recent Trends: A Closer Look, 51
    Emerging Challenges, 68
    Summary, 70
    References, 71

2   FACTORS PERPETUATING THE TOBACCO PROBLEM   77
    Nature of Nicotine Addiction, 77
    Smoking Cessation, 82
    Smoking Initiation, 88
    Atypical Patterns of Tobacco Use, 93
    Populations at Greater Risk of Continuing Smoking, 95
    Conclusion, 97
    References, 99

3   CONTAINING THE TOBACCO PROBLEM   107
    Public Health Takes on the Tobacco Industry: 1964–1988, 109
    Advances in Tobacco Control: 1988–2005, 116

Tobacco Control in the Years Ahead: Will Progress Continue?, 128
Summary, 136
References, 137

PART II: A BLUEPRINT FOR REDUCING TOBACCO USE

4 REDUCING TOBACCO USE: A POLICY FRAMEWORK 145
Product Safety and Consumer Sovereignty, 145
The Policy Context, 146
The Ethical Context, 148
An Aside on the Paternalism Problem, 150
Tobacco Products Are Inherently Dangerous, 152
Blueprint Outline, 154
References, 154

5 STRENGTHENING TRADITIONAL TOBACCO CONTROL
MEASURES 157
Comprehensive State Programs, 158
Funding for Comprehensive State Programs, 172
Excise Tax, 182
Smoking Restrictions, 189
Youth Access, 203
Retail Shipments, 207
Prevention Interventions, 210
Media Campaigns to Prevent Smoking, 223
Cessation Interventions, 231
Community Mobilization, 241
Special Populations with Higher Rates of Cigarette Smoking, 247
Projected Impact of Strengthening Existing Tobacco Control
    Measures, 249
References, 253

6 CHANGING THE REGULATORY LANDSCAPE 271
Federal Regulatory Authority Is Needed, 272
Empowering FDA to Regulate Tobacco, 275
A Regulatory Philosophy, 277
Tobacco Product Characteristics Should Be Regulated, 279
Messages on Tobacco Packages Should Promote Health, 289
The Retail Environment for Tobacco Sales Should Be
    Transformed to Promote the Public Health, 299
The Federal Government Should Mandate Industry Payments for
    Tobacco Control and Should Support and Coordinate State
    Funding, 308

Tobacco Advertising Should Be Further Restricted, 319
Youth Exposure to Smoking in Movies and Other Media Should Be
     Reduced, 330
Surveillance and Evaluation Should Be Enhanced, 333
Summary, 335
References, 336

7   NEW FRONTIERS OF TOBACCO CONTROL   341
Tobacco Policy Analysis and Development, 341
Reducing the Nicotine Content of Cigarettes, 346
Conclusion, 353
References, 353

INDEX   355

APPENDIXES[1]

A   ABRAMS: COMPREHENSIVE SMOKING CESSATION
    FOR ALL SMOKERS

B   BONTÃ: CLEAN AIR LAWS

C   FERRENCE: WARNING LABELS AND PACKAGING

D   FLAY: THE LONG-TERM PROMISE OF EFFECTIVE SCHOOL-
    BASED SMOKING PREVENTION PROGRAMS

E   HALPERN–FELSHER: ADOLESCENTS' AND YOUNG
    ADULTS' PERCEPTIONS OF TOBACCO USE

F   HALPERN–FELSHER: INTERVENTIONS FOR CHILDREN
    AND YOUTH IN THE HEALTH CARE SETTING

G   HALPERN–FELSHER: REDUCING AND PREVENTING
    TOBACCO USE AMONG PREGNANT WOMEN, PARENTS,
    AND FAMILIES

H   HALPERN–FELSHER: SMOKING IN THE MOVIES

---

[1]All appendixes are available on a CD in the back of the report and at http://www.nap.
edu/catalog.php?record_ id=11795.

I   KINNEY: STATE STATUTES GOVERNING DIRECT
    SHIPMENT OF ALCHOLIC BEVERAGES TO CONSUMERS

J   LEVY: THE ROLE OF PUBLIC POLICIES IN REDUCING
    SMOKING PREVALENCE

K   MENDEZ: COMMISSIONED SIMULATION MODELING
    OF SMOKING PREVALENCE AS AN OUTCOME OF
    SELECTED TOBACCO CONTROL MEASURES

L   RABIN: CONTROLLING THE RETAIL SALES
    ENVIRONMENT

M   RIBISL: SALES AND MAREKTING OF CIGARETTES
    ON THE INTERNET

N   SLATER: MEDIA CAMPAIGNS AND TOBACCO CONTROL

O   SPARKS: ADVOCACY AS A TOBACCO CONTROL
    STRATEGY

P   WALLACE: SPECIAL POPULATIONS WITH HIGHER
    RATES OF CIGARETTE SMOKING

Summary

ABSTRACT *The ultimate goal of the committee is to end the tobacco problem; in other words, to reduce smoking so substantially that it is no longer a significant public health problem for our nation. While that objective is not likely to be achieved soon, the report aims to set the nation irreversibly on a course for doing so. After reviewing the ethical grounding of tobacco control, the committee sets forth a blueprint as a two-pronged strategy. The first prong envisions strengthening and fully implementing traditional tobacco control measures known to be effective. The second prong envisions changing the regulatory landscape to permit policy innovations that take into account the unique history and characteristics of tobacco use, such as strong federal regulation of tobacco products and their marketing and distribution. Aggressive policy initiatives will be necessary to end the tobacco problem. Any slackening of the public health response may reverse decades of progress in reducing tobacco-related disease and death.*

The substantial decline (58.2 percent) in the prevalence of smoking among adults since 1964 has been characterized as one of the 10 greatest achievements in public health in the 20th century, but today about 21 percent of U.S. adults smoke, despite clear evidence of the numerous health, economic, and social consequences associated with tobacco use.

Tobacco use causes 440,000 deaths in the United States every year (CDC 2005), with secondhand smoke responsible for 50,000 of those

1

deaths (DHHS 2006). All told, deaths associated with smoking account for more deaths than AIDS, alcohol use, cocaine use, heroin use, homicides, suicides, motor vehicle crashes, and fires combined.

The economic consequences of tobacco use are in the billions of dollars. Lost work productivity attributable to death from tobacco use amounts to more than $92 billion per year. Private and public health care expenditures for smoking-related health conditions are estimated to be $89 billion per year. In addition, the states and the federal government spend millions of dollars annually on tobacco use prevention and research efforts that could be directed to other needs.

Concerns about the waning momentum in tobacco control efforts and about declining public attention to what remains the nation's largest public health problem led the American Legacy Foundation to ask the Institute of Medicine (IOM) to conduct a major study of tobacco policy in the United States. The IOM appointed a 14-member committee and charged it to explore the benefits to society of fully implementing effective tobacco control interventions and policies, and to develop a blueprint for the nation in the struggle to reduce tobacco use. To carry out its charge, the committee conducted six meetings in which the committee members heard presentations from individuals representing academia, nonprofit organizations, and various state governments. The committee also reviewed an extensive literature from peer-reviewed journals, published reports, and news articles. The background information and supporting evidence for the committee's report are contained within 16 signed appendixes written by committee members and three commissioned papers written by outside researchers.

The committee found it useful to set some boundaries on its work concerning the goal ("reducing tobacco use") and the time frame within which it should be achieved. To make its task manageable and well-focused, the committee decided to focus its literature review and evidence gathering on reducing cigarette smoking, without meaning to overlook or dismiss the health consequences of other forms of tobacco use. However, the committee believes that its recommendations, although derived from the evidence regarding interventions to reduce cigarette smoking, are fully applicable to smoking of other tobacco products and that most of the recommendations are also applicable to smokeless tobacco products. First of all, trends in smokeless use and cigarette use tend to move in tandem, suggesting that the population-level factors at work at any given time are affecting all forms of tobacco use. Although some smokers may switch to smokeless tobacco as a "risk-reducing" tactic, thereby offsetting some of the gains from smoking cessation, successful efforts to curtail smoking initiation do not appear to be compromised by increased initiation of smokeless use. Second, the committee believes that most of the interventions shown to be effective for smoking (cessation, health-based interventions, school-based interventions, media efforts, sales restrictions, marketing restrictions) can be implemented in behavior-specific or product-specific manner, and that there is no apparent reason why their effectiveness would be weakened in relation to use of smokeless products if they were sensitively designed. Overall, therefore, the committee believes that it is reasonable to assume that implementation of its blueprint will, in the aggregate, lead to a reduction in all forms of tobacco use. Thus the committee refers throughout the report to the goal of "reducing tobacco use."

The overarching goal of reducing smoking subsumes three distinct goals: reducing the rate of initiation of smoking among youth (IOM 1994), reducing third-party environmental tobacco smoke exposure (NRC 1986), and helping people quit smoking. For the purposes of this report, the committee sets to one side additional strategies that might reduce the harm of smoking for smokers who cannot quit, a topic dealt with extensively in another recent IOM report (IOM 2001).

Another important question regarding the scope of the committee's work concerns the time frame. The committee wanted to design a blueprint for achieving substantial reductions in tobacco use, but to have a realistic opportunity for doing so, an ample period of time is needed. Yet, the target should not be so far in the distance as to lose its connection with current conditions or to outstrip the committee's collective capacity to imagine the future. The committee decided to set a 20-year horizon for its projections and for the policies that it recommends.

The common interest of all nations in reducing tobacco use has been declared and effectuated by the World-Health-Organization-sponsored Framework Convention for Tobacco Control, which went into effect in 2005 and has been ratified by 142 nations (unfortunately not including the United States). The United States has a direct stake in reducing smuggling of tobacco products into this country that could undermine domestic tobacco control efforts, and the committee also recognizes the compelling importance of international tobacco control efforts for world health. However, the committee's charge was to develop a tobacco control blueprint for the nation, not for the world. We hope, though, that some of the measures recommended in this report will provide useful models for other countries, just as the domestic interventions undertaken by other countries in recent years served as useful models for us.

In sum, the ultimate goal of the committee's blueprint is to reduce smoking so substantially that it is no longer a significant public health problem for our nation; this is what is meant by the phrase "ending the tobacco problem" used in the title of this report. While that objective is not likely to be achieved in 20 years, the report aims to set the nation irreversibly on a course for doing so.

REPORT OVERVIEW

The committee's report is divided into two parts. Part I, comprising Chapters 1 through 3, provides the context for the committee's proposed policy blueprint. Chapter 1 discusses the extraordinary growth of tobacco use during the first half of the 20th century and its subsequent reversal in 1965 in the wake of the 1964 Surgeon General's report. This chapter also closely examines recent trends in tobacco use. Chapter 2 summarizes the ways in which the addictive properties of nicotine make it so difficult for people to quit, thereby sustaining tobacco use at high levels, and the factors associated with smoking initiation, especially the failure of adolescents to appreciate the risks and consequences of addiction when they become smokers. Chapter 3 reviews the history of tobacco control and concludes by projecting the likely prevalence of smoking over the next 20 years if current trends remain unchanged or if tobacco control efforts are weakened.

Part II of the committee's report presents a blueprint for reducing tobacco use. After reviewing the ethical grounding of tobacco control in Chapter 4, the committee sets forth its blueprint as a two-pronged strategy. The first prong, presented in Chapter 5, envisions strengthening traditional tobacco control measures that are currently known to be effective. Chapter 5 closes with a projection of the likely effects over the next two decades of implementing the policies outlined in this part of the blueprint. The second prong, described in Chapter 6, envisions changing the regulatory landscape to permit new policy innovations that take into account the unique history and characteristics of tobacco use.

Building on the foundation laid in Chapter 6, Chapter 7 briefly explores new frontiers of tobacco control, and urges the federal government to establish the necessary capacity for long-term tobacco policy development. The committee specifically reviews a proposal for gradually reducing the nicotine content of cigarettes. Although the committee acknowledges that this proposal requires further investigation and careful assessment before it is implemented, carrying it out offers a reasonable prospect of substantially curtailing and eliminating the public health burden of tobacco use.

Tobacco Use Since 1965

Wide-angle comparisons of measures of smoking behavior between 1965 and 2005 clearly show that the rates of tobacco consumption and smoking prevalence have declined among adults, the rate of smoking initiation has declined among adolescents, and the rate of smoking cessation has increased. However, a closer look at the trends over the past two decades tells a somewhat more complex story of both modest progress and some backsliding. For instance, although smoking prevalence has continued to decline in the new millennium, it appears that progress in some areas may now be stalling.

Between 1965 and 2005, the percentage of adults who once smoked and who had quit more than doubled from 24.3 to 50.8 percent. Furthermore, the percentage of adults who had never smoked more than 100 lifetime cigarettes increased by approximately 23 percent from 1965 (44 percent) to 2005 (54 percent). Smoking initiation among adolescents and young adults has also declined since the mid-1960s. Among adolescents aged 12 to 17 years, 125.5 of every 1,000 smoked a cigarette for the first time in 1965. In 2003, 102.1 per 1,000 youths in the same age range had smoked a cigarette for the first time. The reduction in smoking initiation saved more than half a million adolescents from having a first cigarette between 1965 and 2004.

The steady decline in tobacco use since 1965 can be divided into two phases, the first running from 1965 to about 1980 and the second running from 1980 to the present. During the initial period, there was a sharp decline in smoking prevalence due to reduced initiation and increased cessation, accompanied by a modest increase in the average number of cigarettes smoked per day by smokers. However, since then, the continued decline in smoking prevalence has been accompanied by a substantial decline in cigarettes smoked per day among those who smoke. The committee believes that a substantial portion of the declines in smoking prevalence and smoking intensity over the past 25 years is attributable to tobacco control interventions, especially price increases and the emergence of a strong anti smoking social norm.

Current trends, however, suggest that the annual rate of cessation among smokers remains fairly low, that the decline in the initiation rate may have slowed, and that overall adult prevalence may be flattening out at around 20 percent. These trends suggest that substantial and sustained efforts will be required to further reduce the prevalence of tobacco use and thereby reduce tobacco-related morbidity and mortality.

Factors Perpetuating the Tobacco Problem

What factors are perpetuating the tobacco problem? First and foremost, tobacco products are highly addictive because they contain nicotine, one of the most addictive substances used by humans. Nicotine addiction stimulates and sustains long-term tobacco use, with all of its serious health hazards and social costs, and poses significant challenges to smoking cessation efforts at both the individual and the population levels. Although an overwhelming majority of smokers (90 percent) regret having begun to smoke, overcoming the grip of addiction and the associated withdrawal symptoms is difficult; most smokers must try quitting several times before they are successful. Progress in helping smokers who want to quit achieve successful and permanent cessation requires that a variety of cessation technologies—both clinical and population based—be readily available to the smoking population, and that they be used, and that they be effective.

Second, factors such as distorted risk and harm perceptions, which are associated with the initiation and maintenance of tobacco use among young smokers, pose a continuing obstacle for prevention and control strategies. Unfortunately, many youth view themselves as invulnerable to addiction and its associated harm. They are also sensitive to the social factors and norms that promote smoking, such as the influences exerted by peers, family members, and the exposure to smoking in the media. These influences tend to override the information about the risks of smoking. Therefore, to substantially reduce the rate of smoking initiation, it will be necessary to do a better job of counteracting the perceived benefits of smoking and to develop new tools that make the personal risks of starting to smoke more salient.

All new smokers are not young, however; some initiate smoking during their college years, which helps to explain why some new smokers have characteristics that differ from those of usual smokers. Specifically, they tend to have higher levels of education and income than other smokers. It is also noteworthy that some new smokers smoke at lower levels, and some never reach a level of dependence. It will be important for tobacco control experts to pay close attention to these emerging trends and to design appropriate interventions to respond to them.

On the other side of the ledger are smokers who have a more difficult time quitting, such as "hardcore" smokers with a long career of smoking and individuals with psychiatric comorbidities or special circumstances, including incarceration and homelessness. These groups have not been the primary targets of traditional cessation treatments or research studies. Achieving success in substantially reducing tobacco use will require taking stock of the progress made with current tobacco prevention and control strategies and identifying where they fall short in responding to emerging smoking trends and the characteristics and behaviors of subpopulations of smokers with particular vulnerabilities.

The Consequences of Unchanged or Weakened Tobacco Control

The committee has tried to project the likely public health consequences of intensified or weakened investments in tobacco control compared with those of the status quo. The good news is that even if tobacco control activities remain at present levels, smoking prevalence is likely to decline from about 21 percent in 2005 to a little less than 16 percent in 2025. This continued decline will occur because of the system's inertia: there are currently more middle-aged and older smokers than there would have been had their birth cohorts passed through the ages of tobacco initiation under higher tobacco prices and stronger tobacco controls. Over time, as those birth cohorts are replaced by aging younger cohorts who had lower rates of initiation, the prevalence of tobacco use will continue to decline. Shortly after 2025, however, the decline in prevalence appears likely to plateau at about 15 percent, well above the Healthy People 2010 target of 12 percent.

This steady-state scenario should be compared with a worst-case scenario, based on a weakening of tobacco control policies and programs. If a significant retrenchment occurred, the projected smoking prevalence in 2025 would be about 17 percent, resulting in approximately 4 million more people smoking than would otherwise occur. Although the momentum generated by the last four decades of tobacco control is unlikely to be erased altogether—the model does not take into account new smoking fads, other changes in demand, or industry innovations—these projections do show that a weakened commitment to tobacco control will affect millions of lives.

A BLUEPRINT FOR REDUCING TOBACCO USE

The committee believes that substantial and enduring reductions in tobacco use cannot be achieved simply by expecting past successes to continue. Continued progress will require the persistence and nimbleness needed to counteract industry innovations in marketing and product design as well as the larger cultural and economic forces that tend to promote and sustain tobacco use. The challenge is heightened by the fact that the customary tools of tobacco control may not be effective in reducing use among some tobacco users. Any slackening of the public health response not only will reduce forward progress but also may lead to backsliding.

Over the past 10 to 15 years, the operating assumptions of tobacco control policies in the United States and elsewhere in the world have fundamentally changed. The old paradigm that shaped public opinion and policymaking on tobacco control efforts tended to emphasize consumer freedom of choice and to decry all government intervention as paternalistic. In retrospect, however, the committee believes that these assumptions were rooted in the tobacco industry's successful efforts to deny and obscure the addictiveness and health consequences of tobacco use and on an array of resulting market failures, including information asymmetry between producers and users, distorted consumer choice due to information deficits, and product pricing that did not reflect the full social costs of tobacco use (especially the effects on nonsmokers). As the scientific evidence about addiction and initiation has grown and the tobacco industry's strategies have been exposed in the course of state lawsuits and other tobacco-related litigation, public understanding of tobacco addiction has quickly deepened and, as a result, the ethical and political context of tobacco policymaking has been transformed. A widespread popular consensus in favor of aggressive policy initiatives is now emerging, and this shift in popular sentiment has also been accompanied by support across most of the political spectrum.

From a policy standpoint, many analysts think of the tobacco problem as a product safety problem. In an economic and social system that values freedom of choice, consumers are generally permitted to select products and activities as they see fit. If they want to assume risks, they are permitted to do exactly that. Government does not guarantee absolute safety, nor should it. Of course, some dangers are too high to be acceptable. So long as consumers are properly informed, however, the presumption has traditionally been in favor of consumer sovereignty and freedom of choice. Yet, even most libertarians will admit that the tobacco market has been characterized by severe market failures, as noted above. They acknowledge the legitimacy of interventions aiming to prevent youth smoking, to disseminate accurate information and correct misinformation, and to assure that nonsmokers are protected from involuntary exposure to tobacco smoke if the market does not function properly. The residual issue concerns the legitimacy of interventions that burden the choices of the minority of smokers who do not want to quit.

The notion of consumer sovereignty—of unambivalent respect for private choices—runs into serious difficulty when the underlying product creates serious long-term harms and has addictive properties, when its use is usually initiated by young people who lack a full and vivid appreciation of the associated risks, and when most users want to quit. Even in such circumstances, consumer sovereignty should not be abandoned but must be rethought to take account of the unique characteristics of tobacco products.

Cigarettes and other tobacco products are not ordinary consumer products. For no other lawful consumer product can it be said that the acknowledged aim of national policy is to suppress consumption. The committee's major goal here is to set forth a framework for reducing tobacco use, and its associated morbidity and mortality, while being duly respectful of the interests of consumers who choose to smoke and do not want to quit.

The committee makes 42 recommendations in the report, 22 regarding ways to strengthen traditional tobacco control measures and 20 regarding the new regulatory landscape. This summary highlights 19 key recommendations that represent the major components of the committee's blueprint for ending the tobacco problem. A listing of all 42 recommendations organized by chapter can be found at the end of this summary.

Strengthening Traditional Tobacco Control Measures

The first prong of the committee's blueprint assumes that the existing legal structure of tobacco control remains unchanged. It envisions steps taken to strengthen traditional tobacco control measures that are known to be effective.

Support Comprehensive State Tobacco Control Programs

The committee finds compelling evidence that comprehensive state tobacco control programs can achieve substantial reductions in tobacco use. To effectively reduce tobacco use, states must maintain over time a comprehensive, integrated tobacco control strategy. However, large budget cutbacks in many states' tobacco control programs have seriously jeopardized further success. In the committee's view, states should adopt a funding strategy designed to provide stable support for the level of tobacco control funding recommended by the Centers for Disease Control and Prevention (CDC). The committee also finds that Master Settlement Agreement payments are not a reliable source of funds in most states. Tobacco excise tax revenues pose a potential funding stream for state tobacco control programs. Setting aside about one-third of the per-capita proceeds from tobacco excise taxes would help states fund programs at the level suggested by CDC.

> Recommendation 1: Each state should fund state tobacco control activities at the level recommended by the CDC. A reasonable target for each state is in the range of $15 to $20 per capita, depending on the state's population, demography, and prevalence of tobacco use. If it is constitutionally permissible, states should use a statutorily prescribed portion of their tobacco excise tax revenues to fund tobacco control programs.

Increase Excise Taxes

It is well established that an increase in price decreases cigarette use and that raising tobacco excise taxes is one of the most effective policies for reducing use, especially among adolescents. Many states have increased their tobacco excise taxes, but these increases vary widely and there is some evidence of cross-state smuggling. The committee believes that equalizing tobacco excise tax rates across the states would help remedy this problem. Furthermore, an increase in the federal excise tax would have the dual purposes of reducing consumption and making more funds available for tobacco control programs.

> Recommendation 2: States with excise tax rates below the level imposed by the top quintile of states should substantially increase their own rates to reduce consumption and to reduce smuggling and tax evasion. State excise tax rates should be indexed to inflation.

Recommendation 3: The federal government should substantially raise federal tobacco excise taxes, currently set at 39 cents a pack. Federal excise taxes should be indexed to inflation.

Strengthen Smoking Restrictions

The committee finds that smoking restrictions serve three purposes: (1) they protect nonsmokers from the health effects and the noxious odors of secondhand smoke; (2) they help smokers quit, cut down on their smoking, and avoid relapses; and (3) they reinforce a nonsmoking social norm. Clean air laws have done more to reduce tobacco consumption than any intervention other than cigarette price increases. The committee believes that smoking restrictions are a critical part of any tobacco control strategy. Smoking restrictions should be strengthened and should have broad coverage, including nonresidential indoor locations, health care facilities, correctional facilities, and residential complexes. The committee also believes that local government bans on indoor and outdoor smoking should not be preempted by state laws.

Recommendation 4: States and localities should enact complete bans on smoking in all nonresidential indoor locations, including workplaces, malls, restaurants, and bars. States should not preempt local governments from enacting bans more restrictive than the state ban.

Limit Youth Access to Tobacco Products

A reasonably enforced youth-access restriction is an essential element of modern tobacco control. Age verification, as contained in the 1996 FDA (Food and Drug Administration) Rule, as well as placing product displays behind the counter and banning self-service modes of access to tobacco work effectively to reduce youth access. Although a considerable number of states and localities currently license tobacco sales outlets and impose youth-access restrictions, weak enforcement in many states suggests that the potential deterrent threat of license suspension or revocation is not being realized.

Recommendation 11: All states should license retail sales outlets that sell tobacco products.

The number of Internet tobacco retailers has increased dramatically in recent years, generating concerns about minors accessing tobacco products and consumers evading excise tax payments. Given the inadequacy of current point-of-sale age verification for Internet transactions and the difficulty of policing Internet tobacco transactions, as well as constitutional barriers to additional, state-imposed delivery requirements, the only practical way to effectively regulate online tobacco retailers is through legislation prohibiting both online tobacco sales and direct shipment of tobacco products to consumers.

> Recommendation 12: All states should ban the sale of tobacco products directly to consumers through mail order or the Internet or other electronic systems. Shipments of tobacco products should be permitted only to licensed wholesale or retail outlets.

Intensify Prevention Interventions

The most fully developed programs for preventing tobacco use by youth have been implemented in school settings. School-based programs will and should remain the mainstay of group-oriented or individually-oriented tobacco use prevention activities. However, because teenage smoking initiation rates remain high, the committee also believes that investing in programs for families and health care providers is warranted, even though the evidence base remains thin. Furthermore the committee supports the funding of mass media campaigns, which a recent state-of-the-science panel of the National Institutes of Health identified as one of three effective approaches for reaching the general population and preventing tobacco use among adolescents and young adults.

> Recommendation 13: School boards should require all middle schools and high schools to adopt evidence-based smoking prevention programs and implement them with fidelity. They should coordinate these in-school programs with public activities or mass media programming, or both. Such prevention programs should be conducted annually. State funding for these programs should be supplemented with funding from the U.S. Department of Education under the Safe and Drug-Free School Act or by an independent body administering funds collected from the tobacco industry through excise taxes, court orders, or litigation agreements.

> Recommendation 15: A national, youth-oriented media campaign should be funded on an ongoing basis as a permanent component of the nation's strategy to reduce tobacco use. State and community tobacco control programs should supplement the national media campaign with coordinated youth prevention activities. The campaign should be implemented by an established public health organization with funds provided by the federal government, public-private partnerships, or

the tobacco industry (voluntarily or under litigation settlement agreements or court orders) for media development, testing, and purchases of advertising time and space.

Increase Smoking Cessation Interventions

Almost half of the estimated 44.5 million current adult smokers in the United States will die prematurely of a tobacco-related disease if nothing is done to help them stop smoking. A large number of randomized clinical trials and other research studies confirm the efficacy of smoking cessation interventions. Despite the availability of many successful interventions, only a small proportion of tobacco users receive any type of intervention. To enhance program utilization and smoking cessation rates among the general population, smokers must know that safe, effective, and accessible cessation programs, including medications, are available. The health care setting is an ideal venue in which individuals can be screened for their smoking behaviors and comprehensive smoking cessation services can be targeted to populations with a high prevalence of smoking. Ensuring the uptake of cessation interventions will require health insurance benefit packages to cover these services.

> **Recommendation 16: State tobacco control agencies should work with health care partners to increase the demand for effective cessation programs and activities through mass media and other general and targeted public education programs.**

> **Recommendation 20: All insurance, managed care, and employee benefit plans, including Medicaid and Medicare, should cover reimbursement for effective smoking cessation programs as a lifetime benefit.**

Projected Impact of Strengthening Traditional Tobacco Control Measures

What would be the impact on national tobacco use prevalence in 2025 of implementing these traditional tobacco control measures aggressively? In order to address this question, the committee modeled the effects of the following policies:

- Tax increases of $1 and $2 per pack
- Nationwide implementation of clean air laws for all work sites (including bars)
- Comprehensive media campaigns targeting youth and adults and funded at the levels recommended by the CDC (i.e., beyond the

levels that have been used in the past) to prevent initiation and to increase quit attempts, heighten consumer demand for proven cessation programs, and to increase smoker's health literacy about the value of using evidence-based treatments when trying to quit

- Comprehensive cessation policies (full coverage of pharmacotherapy and behavioral therapy, training and coverage for tobacco brief interventions, multisession quit lines, internet interventions, and free nicotine replacement therapy)
- Universal implementation of school-based prevention sufficient to cut the rate of smoking initiation by 10 percent
- Heavy enforcement of youth-access laws, accompanied by publicity and high penalties
- All of these things being done together with $1- or $2-per-pack tax increases

The committee's projections suggest that these individual policies, particularly the cessation interventions and tax increases, could have a substantial effect on tobacco use prevalence over time. Indeed, collectively they are projected to meet the Healthy People 2010 smoking prevalence target of 12 percent in about 2020, with a 10 percent prevalence reached in 2025.

Overall, however, the committee finds these model projections only modestly encouraging. On the positive side, the actions outlined in this chapter seem to be powerful and effective. Implementing this set of recommendations fully might allow the important goal of a 10 percent smoking prevalence to be achieved, albeit not until 2025. On the other hand, removing any single one of the comprehensive policy's components would prevent the modeled prevalence from hitting the 10 percent target in 2025. Hence the success of these strategies is, in some sense, fragile, requiring absolute commitment to full implementation. Given the recent retrenchment in tobacco control efforts, one might worry whether that level of commitment can be achieved and sustained.

Realistically, the committee is doubtful that the prevalence of smoking among adults will drop significantly below 15 percent or that the rate of smoking initiation will permanently fall below 15 percent if the basic legal structure of the tobacco market, and the tobacco control community's responses to that market, remain unchanged. Although achieving these levels would be a major improvement, they are not satisfactory from a public health standpoint simply because of the large numbers of premature deaths and other serious harmful consequences that would inevitably follow. The steps outlined so far are surely necessary in the short run, but the nation should be prepared to do more over the long run.

CHANGING THE REGULATORY LANDSCAPE

The second prong of the committee's blueprint envisions a much more substantial federal presence in antismoking efforts, characterized by a fundamentally transformed legal structure. The committee believes that the time has come for Congress to exercise its acknowledged authority to regulate tobacco products while freeing the states to supplement federal action with measures that serve the national objective of suppressing tobacco use and that are compatible with federal law. Under a transformed legal structure, a federal regulatory agency, most likely the FDA, would be given plenary regulatory authority and the states would be liberated to take aggressive actions against smoking now forbidden by federal law.

If Congress preempts direct state regulation of tobacco product characteristics and packaging, it should allow complementary state regulation in other domains of tobacco regulation, including marketing and distribution, and should make its intentions regarding the narrow scope of preemption clear in the legislative record.

> **Recommendation 23: Congress should repeal the existing statute preempting state tobacco regulation of advertising and promotion "based on smoking and health" and should enact a new provision that precludes direct state regulation only in relation to tobacco product characteristics and packaging while allowing complementary state regulation in all other domains of tobacco regulation, including marketing and distribution. Under this approach, federal regulation sets a floor while allowing states to be more restrictive.**

Empower FDA to Regulate Tobacco

Congress should confer broad authority on the FDA to regulate the manufacture, distribution, marketing, and use of tobacco products. Requiring tobacco products to be "safe" is not an available option, of course, and prohibition of the existing products is not a feasible regulatory strategy. Overall, the regulatory standard should be to "protect the public health" by reducing initiation, promoting cessation, preventing relapse, reducing consumption, and reducing product hazards. This standard incorporates its own limitation because it will require the agency to evaluate the likely consumer responses to any proposed regulation, including the likelihood of product substitution and the creation of black markets that could nullify the anticipated public health benefits of the regulation.

> **Recommendation 24: Congress should confer upon the FDA broad regulatory authority over the manufacture, distribution, marketing, and use of tobacco products.**

Recommendation 25: Congress should empower the FDA to regulate the design and characteristics of tobacco products to promote the public health. Specific authority should be conferred

- to require tobacco manufacturers to disclose to the agency all chemical compounds found in both product and the product's smoke, whether added or occurring naturally, by quantity; to disclose to the public the amount of nicotine in the product and the amount delivered to the consumer based on standards established by the agency; to disclose to the pubic research on their product, as well as behavioral aspects of its use; and to notify the agency whenever there is a change in a product;
- to prescribe cigarette testing methods, including how the cigarettes are tested and which smoke constituents must be measured;
- to promulgate tobacco product standards, including reduction of nicotine yields and reduction or elimination of other constituents, wherever such a standard is found to be appropriate for protection of the public health, taking into consideration the risks and benefits to the population as a whole, including users and non-users of tobacco products; and
- to develop specific standards for evaluating novel products that companies intend to promote as reduced-exposure or reduced-risk products, and to regulate reduced-exposure and reduced-risk health claims, assuring that there is a scientific basis for claims that are permitted

Strengthen Health Warnings on Tobacco Packages

Tobacco packages can be an effective channel for health communications. The currently mandated federal health warnings are inadequate and should be strengthened to promote greater understanding of the health risks of tobacco use and to discourage consumption. Aside from printed health warnings, regulatory authorities can convey other health-related information on or with tobacco packages, including information about quitting. Congress should empower FDA to update warnings and other package-based health communications on a regular basis. In addition, the agency should be empowered to ban such terms as "light" as well as other descriptors, signals, or practices that have the purpose or effect of leading consumers to believe that smoking the cigarette brand with that descriptor may result in a lower risk of disease or may be less hazardous to their health than smoking other brands of cigarettes.

Recommendation 26: Congress should strengthen the federally mandated warning labels for tobacco products immediately and should delegate authority to the FDA to update and revise these warnings on a regular basis upon finding that doing so would promote greater public understanding of the risks of using tobacco products or reduce tobacco consumption. Congress should require or authorize the FDA to require rotating color graphic warnings covering 50 percent of the package equivalent to those required in Canada.

Recommendation 28: Congress should ban, or empower the FDA to ban, terms such as "mild," "lights," "ultra-lights," and other misleading terms mistakenly interpreted by consumers to imply reduced risk, as well as other techniques, such as color codes, that have the purpose or effect of conveying false or misleading impressions about the relative harmfulness of the product.

Transform the Retail Environment

Effective measures for restricting the commercial distribution of tobacco products to youth are only a starting point. Tobacco is not an ordinary consumer product and should not be treated as such. The sale of tobacco products to adults, although permitted, is disfavored as a matter of public policy. The retail environment should be designed to effectuate the public health goals of discouraging tobacco use and reducing the numbers of people with tobacco-related diseases.

Recommendation 30: Congress and state legislatures should enact legislation regulating the retail point of sale of tobacco products for the purpose of discouraging consumption of these products and encouraging cessation. Specifically:

- All retail outlets choosing to carry tobacco products should be licensed and monitored. (See also youth access section in Chapter 5.)
- Commercial displays or other activity promoting tobacco use by or in retail outlets should be banned, although text-only informational displays (e.g., price or health-related product characteristics) may be permitted within prescribed regulatory constraints.
- Retail outlets choosing to carry tobacco products should be required to display and distribute prescribed warnings about the health consequences of tobacco use, information regarding products and services for cessation, and corrective messages designed to offset misstatements or implied claims regarding the health effects of tobacco use (e.g., that "light" cigarettes are less harmful than other cigarettes).

- Retail outlets choosing to carry tobacco products should be required to allocate a proportionate amount of space to cessation aids and nicotine replacement products and, after regulatory clearance by the FDA or a designated state agency, to "qualifying" exposure-reduction products. (The FDA or a suitable state health agency should promulgate a list of "qualifying" exposure-reducing products.)

Recommendation 32: State governments should develop and, if feasible, implement and evaluate legal mechanisms for restructuring retail tobacco sales and restricting the number of tobacco outlets.

Recommendation 33: Congress should empower the FDA to restrict outlets in order to limit access and facilitate regulation of the retail environment, and thereby protect the public health.

Coordinate State Tobacco Control Through a Federal Assessment on Tobacco Companies

In Recommendation 2, the committee urges the low-tax states to raise their excise taxes to what is now the upper quintile of state tax rates. If that recommendation were implemented by all the states, it would substantially decrease, if not eliminate, the incentive for cross-state smuggling. However, if the states do not deal successfully with this problem on their own, the increasing variation in state tobacco excise taxes should be addressed by the federal government. The committee offers a new federal funding scheme (the National Tobacco Control Funding Plan, described below) as a back-up plan to support and coordinate state tobacco control programs while giving the states with low tobacco excise taxes the incentive to raise them.

Recommendation 34: If most states fail to increase tobacco control funding and reduce variations in tobacco excise tax rates as proposed in Recommendations 1 and 2, Congress should enact a National Tobacco Control Funding Plan raising funds through a per-pack remedial assessment on cigarettes sold in the United States. Part of the proceeds should be used to support national tobacco control programs and the remainder of the funds should be distributed to the states to subsidize state tobacco control programs according to a formula based on the level of state tobacco control expenditures and state tobacco excise rates. The plan should be designed to give states an incentive, not only to increase state spending on tobacco control, but also to raise cigarette taxes, especially in low-tax states. Congress should assure that any federal coordination mechanism affecting the coverage and collection of state tobacco excise taxes applies to Indian tribes.

Restrict Advertising and Promotion by Manufacturers

The scientific evidence documenting the relationship between exposure to tobacco advertising and tobacco consumption has accumulated, and prevailing scientific opinion is that the relationship is a causal one.

Recommendation 35: Congress and state legislatures should enact legislation limiting visually displayed tobacco advertising in all venues, including mass media and at the point-of-sale, to a text-only, black-and-white format.

Recommendation 36: Congress and state legislatures should prohibit tobacco companies from targeting youth under 18 for any purpose, including dissemination of messages about smoking (whether ostensibly to promote or discourage it) or to survey youth opinions, attitudes and behaviors of any kind. If a tobacco company wishes to support youth prevention programs, the company should contribute funds to an independent non-profit organization with expertise in the prevention field. The independent organization should have exclusive responsibility for designing, executing, and evaluating the program.

CONCLUSION

The committee recognizes that important advances in reducing tobacco use have been made over the past two decades. Accordingly, the recommendations offered in Chapter 5 of the report seek to emphasize and strengthen tobacco control interventions that have proven effective over time. If this part of the blueprint is successfully implemented and sustained, it could have a significant impact on tobacco use; but even an optimistic projection leaves prevalence at 10 percent in 2025, and a more realistic projection might be 15 percent. The main argument presented in Chapter 6 is that a more substantial long-term impact requires a change in the current legal framework of tobacco control and the adoption of regulatory innovations that take into account the unique history and characteristics of tobacco. It is too soon to project the effects of such new regulatory initiatives, but the committee believes that a concerted effort to transform the regulatory environment is a necessary condition for ending the tobacco problem in the United States.

COMPLETE LIST OF RECOMMENDATIONS

Strengthening Traditional Tobacco Control Measures

Recommendation 1: Each state should fund state tobacco control activities at the level recommended by the CDC. A reasonable target for each state is in the range of $15 to $20 per capita, depending on the state's population, demography, and prevalence of tobacco use. If it is constitutionally permissible, states should use a statutorily prescribed portion of their tobacco excise tax revenues to fund tobacco control programs.

Recommendation 2: States with excise tax rates below the level imposed by the top quintile of states should also substantially increase their own rates to reduce smuggling and tax evasion. State excise tax rates should be indexed to inflation.

Recommendation 3: The federal government should substantially raise federal tobacco excise taxes, currently set at 39 cents a pack. Federal excise tax rates should be indexed to inflation.

Recommendation 4: States and localities should enact complete bans on smoking in all nonresidential indoor locations, including workplaces, malls, restaurants, and bars. States should not preempt local governments from enacting bans more restrictive than the state ban.

Recommendation 5: All health care facilities, including nursing homes, psychiatric hospitals, and medical units in correctional facilities, should meet or exceed JCAHO standards in banning smoking in all indoor areas.

Recommendation 6: The American Correctional Association should require through its accreditation standards that all correctional facilities (prisons, jails, and juvenile detention facilities) implement bans on indoor smoking.

Recommendation 7: States should enact legislation requiring leases for multiunit apartment buildings and condominium sales agreements to include the terms governing smoking in common areas and residential units. States and localities should also encourage the owners of multiunit apartment buildings and condominium developers to include nonsmoking clauses in these leases and sales agreements and to enforce them.

Recommendation 8: Colleges and universities should ban smoking in indoor locations, including dormitories, and should consider setting a smoke-free campus as a goal. Further, colleges and universities should ban the promotion of tobacco products on campus and at all campus-sponsored events. Such policies should be monitored and evaluated by oversight committees, such as those associated with the American College Health Association.

Recommendation 9: State health agencies, health care professionals, and other interested organizations should undertake strong efforts to encourage parents to make their homes and vehicles smoke free.

Recommendation 10: States should not preempt local governments from restricting smoking in outdoor public spaces, such as parks and beaches.

Recommendation 11: All states should license retail sales outlets that sell tobacco products. Licensees should be required to (1) verify the date of birth, by means of photographic identification, of any purchaser appearing to be 25 years of age or younger; (2) place cigarettes exclusively behind the counter and sell cigarettes only in a direct face-to-face exchange; and (3) ban the use of self-service displays and vending machines. Repeat violations of laws restricting youth access should be subject to license suspension or revocation. States should not preempt local governments from licensing retail outlets that sell tobacco products.

Recommendation 12: All states should ban the sale and shipment of tobacco products directly to consumers through mail order or the Internet or other electronic systems. Shipments of tobacco products should be permitted only to licensed wholesale or retail outlets.

Recommendation 13: School boards should require all middle schools and high schools to adopt evidence-based smoking prevention programs and implement them with fidelity. They should coordinate these in-school programs with public activities or mass media programming, or both. Such prevention programs should be conducted annually. State funding for these programs should be supplemented with funding from the U.S. Department of Education under the Safe and Drug-Free School Act or by an independent body administering funds collected from the tobacco industry through excise taxes, court orders, or litigation agreements.

Recommendation 14: All physicians, dentists, and other health care providers should screen and educate youth about tobacco use during their annual health care visits and any other visit in which a health screening occurs. Physicians should refer youth who smoke to counseling services or smoking cessation programs available in the community. Physicians should also urge parents to keep a smoke-free home and vehicles, to discuss tobacco use with their children, to convey that they expect their children to not use tobacco, and to monitor their children's tobacco use. Professional societies, including the American Medical Association, the American Nursing Association, the American Academy of Family Physicians, the American College of Physicians, and the American Academy of Pediatrics, should encourage physicians to adopt these practices.

Recommendation 15: A national, youth-oriented media campaign should be funded on an ongoing basis as a permanent component of the nation's strategy to reduce tobacco use. State and community tobacco control programs should supplement the national media campaign with coordinated youth prevention activities. The campaign should be implemented by an established public health organization with funds provided by the federal government, public-private partnerships, or the tobacco industry (voluntarily or under litigation settlement agreements or court orders) for media development, testing, and purchases of advertising time and space.

Recommendation 16. State tobacco control agencies should work with health care partners to increase the demand for effective cessation programs and activities through mass media and other general and targeted public education programs.

Recommendation 17: Congress should ensure that stable funding is continuously provided to the national quitline network.

Recommendation 18: The Secretary of the U.S. Department of Health and Human Services, through the National Cancer Institute, the Centers for Disease Control and Prevention, and other relevant federal health agencies, should fund a program of developmental research and demonstration projects combining media techniques, other social marketing methods, and innovative approaches to disseminating smoking cessation technologies.

Recommendation 19: Public and private health care systems should organize and provide access to comprehensive smoking cessation programs by using a variety of successful cessation methods and a staged disease management model (i.e. stepped care), and should specify the successful delivery of these programs as one criterion for quality assurance within those systems.

Recommendation 20: All insurance, managed care, and employee benefit plans, including Medicaid and Medicare, should cover reimbursement for effective smoking cessation programs as a lifetime benefit.

Recommendation 21: While sustaining their own valuable tobacco control activities, state tobacco control programs, CDC, philanthropic foundations, and voluntary organizations should continue to support the efforts of community coalitions promoting, disseminating, and advocating for tobacco use prevention and cessation, smoke-free environments, and other policies and programs for reducing tobacco use.

Recommendation 22: Tobacco control programs should consider populations disproportionately affected by tobacco addiction and tobacco-related morbidity and mortality when designing and implementing prevention and treatment programs. Particular attention should be paid to ensuring that health communications and other materials are culturally-appropriate and that special outreach efforts target all high-risk populations. Standard prevention or treatment programs that are modified to reach high-risk populations should be evaluated for effectiveness.

Changing the Regulatory Landscape

Recommendation 23: Congress should repeal the existing statute preempting state tobacco regulation of advertising and promotion "based on smoking and health" and should enact a new provision that precludes all direct state regulation only in relation to tobacco product characteristics and packaging while allowing complementary state regulation in all other domains of tobacco regulation, including marketing and distribution. Under this approach, federal regulation sets a floor while allowing states to be more restrictive.

Recommendation 24: Congress should confer upon the FDA broad regulatory authority over the manufacture, distribution, marketing, and use of tobacco products.

Recommendation 25: Congress should empower the FDA to regulate the design and characteristics of tobacco products to promote the public health. Specific authority should be conferred

- to require tobacco manufacturers to disclose to the agency all chemical compounds found in both product and the product's smoke, whether added or occurring naturally, by quantity; to disclose to the public the amount of nicotine in the product and the amount delivered to the consumer based on standards established by the agency; to disclose to the pubic research on their product, as well as behavioral aspects of its use; and to notify the agency whenever there is a change in a product;
- to prescribe cigarette testing methods, including how the cigarettes are tested and which smoke constituents must be measured;
- to promulgate tobacco product standards, including reduction of nicotine yields and reduction or elimination of other constituents, wherever such a standard is found to be appropriate for protection of the public health, taking into consideration the risks and benefits to the population as a whole, including users and non-users of tobacco products; and
- to develop specific standards for evaluating novel products that companies intend to promote as reduced-exposure or reduced-risk products, and to regulate reduced-exposure and reduced-risk health claims, assuring that there is a scientific basis for claims that are permitted.

Recommendation 26: Congress should strengthen the federally mandated warning labels for tobacco products immediately and should delegate authority to the FDA to update and revise these warnings on a regular basis upon finding that doing so would promote greater public understanding of the risks of using tobacco products or reduce tobacco consumption. Congress should require or authorize the FDA to require rotating color graphic warnings covering 50 percent of the package equivalent to those required in Canada.

Recommendation 27: Congress should empower the FDA to require manufacturers to include in or on tobacco packages information about the health effects of tobacco use and about products that can be used to help people quit.

Recommendation 28: Congress should ban, or empower the FDA to ban, terms such as "mild," "lights," "ultra-lights," and other misleading terms mistakenly interpreted by consumers to imply reduced risk, as well as other techniques, such as color codes, that have the purpose or effect of conveying false or misleading impressions about the relative harmfulness of the product.

Recommendation 29: Whenever a court or administrative agency has found that a tobacco company has made false or misleading communications regarding the effects of tobacco products, or has engaged in conduct promoting tobacco use among youth or discouraging cessation by tobacco users of any age, the court or agency should consider using its remedial authority to require manufacturers to include corrective communications on or with the tobacco package as well as at the point of sale.

Recommendation 30: Congress and state legislatures should enact legislation regulating the retail point of sale of tobacco products for the purpose of discouraging consumption of these products and encouraging cessation. Specifically:

- All retail outlets choosing to carry tobacco products should be licensed and monitored. (See also youth access section in Chapter 5.)
- Commercial displays or other activity promoting tobacco use by or in retail outlets should be banned, although text-only informational displays (e.g., price or health-related product characteristics) may be permitted within prescribed regulatory constraints.
- Retail outlets choosing to carry tobacco products should be required to display and distribute prescribed warnings about the health consequences of tobacco use, information regarding products and services for cessation, and corrective messages designed to offset misstatements or implied claims regarding the health effects of tobacco use (e.g., that "light" cigarettes are less harmful than other cigarettes).
- Retail outlets choosing to carry tobacco products should be required to allocate a proportionate amount of space to cessation aids and nicotine replacement products and, after regulatory clearance by the FDA or a designated state agency, to "qualifying" exposure-reduction products. (The FDA or a suitable state health agency should promulgate a list of "qualifying" exposure-reducing products.)

Recommendation 31: Congress should explicitly and unmistakably include production, marketing, and distribution of tobacco products on Indian reservations by Indian tribes within the regulatory jurisdiction of FDA. Authority to investigate and enforce the Jenkins Act should be transferred to the Bureau of Alcohol, Tobacco, Firearms and Explosives. State restrictions on retail outlets should apply to all outlets on Indian reservations.

Recommendation 32: State governments should develop and, if feasible, implement and evaluate legal mechanisms for restructuring retail tobacco sales and restricting the number of tobacco outlets.

Recommendation 33: Congress should empower the FDA to restrict outlets in order to limit access and facilitate regulation of the retail environment, and thereby protect the public health.

Recommendation 34: If most states fail to increase tobacco control funding and reduce variations in tobacco excise tax rates as proposed in Recommendations 1 and 2, Congress should enact a National Tobacco Control Funding Plan raising funds through a per-pack remedial assessment on cigarettes sold in the United States. Part of the proceeds should be used to support national tobacco control programs and the remainder of the funds should be distributed to the states to subsidize state tobacco control programs according to a formula based on the level of state tobacco control expenditures and state tobacco excise rates. The plan should be designed to give states an incentive, not only to increase state spending on tobacco control, but also to raise cigarette taxes, especially in low-tax states. Congress should assure that any federal coordination mechanism affecting the coverage and collection of state tobacco excise taxes applies to Indian tribes.

Recommendation 35: Congress and state legislatures should enact legislation limiting visually displayed tobacco advertising in all venues, including mass media and at the point-of-sale, to a text-only, black-and-white format.

Recommendation 36: Congress and state legislatures should prohibit tobacco companies from targeting youth under 18 for any purpose, including dissemination of messages about smoking (whether ostensibly to promote or discourage it) or to survey youth opinions, attitudes and behaviors of any kind. If a tobacco company wishes to support youth prevention programs, the company should contribute funds to an independent non-profit organization with expertise in the prevention field. The independent organization should have exclusive responsibility for designing, executing, and evaluating the program.

Recommendation 37: The Motion Picture Association of America (MPAA) should encourage and facilitate the showing of anti-smoking advertisements before any film in which smoking is depicted in more than an incidental manner. The film rating board of the MPAA should consider the use of tobacco in the movies as a factor in assigning mature film ratings (e.g., an R rating indicating Restricted: no one under age 17 admitted without parent or guardian) to films that depict tobacco use.

Recommendation 38: Congress should appropriate the necessary funds to enable the U.S. Department of Health and Human Services to conduct a periodic review of a representative sample of movies, television programs, and videos that are offered at times or in venues in which there is likely to be a significant youth audience (e.g., 15 percent) in order to ascertain the nature and frequency of images portraying tobacco use. The results of these reviews should be reported to Congress and to the public.

Recommendation 39: State tobacco control agencies should conduct surveillance of tobacco sales and use and the effects of tobacco control interventions in order to assess local trends in usage patterns; identify special groups at high risk for tobacco use; determine compliance with state and local tobacco-related laws, policies, and ordinances; and evaluate overall programmatic success.

Recommendation 40: The Secretary of HHS, through FDA or other agencies, should establish a national comprehensive tobacco surveillance system to collect information on a broad range of elements needed to understand and track the population impact of all tobacco products and the effects of national interventions (such as attitudes, beliefs, product characteristics, product distribution and usage patterns, and marketing messages and exposures to them).

New Frontiers in Tobacco Control

Recommendation 41: Congress should direct the Centers for Disease Control and Prevention to undertake a major program of tobacco control policy analysis and development and should provide sufficient funding to support the program. This program should develop the next generation of macro-level simulation models to project the likely effects of various policy innovations, taking into account the possible initiatives and responses of the tobacco industry as well as the impacts of the innovations on consumers.

Recommendation 42: Upon being empowered to regulate tobacco products, the FDA should give priority to exploring the potential effectiveness of a long-term strategy for reducing the amount of nicotine in cigarettes and should commission the studies needed to assess the feasibility of implementing such an approach. If such a strategy appears to be feasible, the agency should develop a long-term plan for implementing the strategy as part of a comprehensive plan for reducing tobacco use.

REFERENCES

CDC (Centers for Disease Control and Prevention). 2005. Annual smoking-attributable mortality, years of potential life lost, and productivity losses—United States, 1997–2001. *MMWR (Morbidity and Mortality Weekly Report)* 54(25):625-628.

DHHS (U.S. Department of Health and Human Services). 2006. *The Health Consequences of Involuntary Exposure to Tobacco Smoke: A Report of the Surgeon General.* Atlanta, GA: U.S. Department of Health and Human Services, Centers for Disease Control and Prevention, Coordinating Center for Health Promotion, National Center for Chronic Disease Prevention and Health Promotion, Office on Smoking and Health.

IOM (Institute of Medicine). 1994. *Growing Up Tobacco Free: Preventing Nicotine Addiction in Children and Youth.* Washington, DC: National Academy Press.

IOM. 2001. *Clearing the Smoke: Assessing the Science Base for Tobacco Harm Reduction.* Washington, DC: National Academy Press.

NRC (National Research Council). 1986. *Environmental Tobacco Smoke: Measuring Exposures and Assessing Health Effects.* Washington, DC: National Academy Press.

Introduction

In 1964, almost half of the adults in the United States smoked cigarettes. Today, the prevalence of cigarette smoking among adults is 20.9 percent (CDC 2006). This substantial decline led the Centers for Disease Control and Prevention to characterize the reduction of smoking as one of the 10 greatest achievements in public health in the 20th century (CDC 1999). It was a great achievement, but the mission remains unfinished. Tobacco use still causes 440,000 deaths in the United States every year (CDC 2005), with secondhand smoke responsible for 50,000 of those deaths (DHHS 2006). All told, approximately one in every five deaths is smoking-related, accounting for more deaths than those from AIDS, alcohol use, cocaine use, heroin use, homicides, suicides, motor vehicle crashes, and fires combined (Healthy People 2010 2005).

The health consequences of tobacco use are numerous (CDC 2005). Each year between 1997 and 2001, smoking caused 160,000 deaths from cancer that affect the lips, mouth, throat, stomach, pancreas, lungs, cervix, kidney, and bladder. Smoking caused 140,000 deaths annually from hypertension, stroke, heart disease, and other cardiovascular problems. The third largest specific cause of smoking-related death is respiratory diseases, comprising 100,000 deaths annually. Smoking is a major cause of morbidity and mortality from infectious diseases, including influenza, pneumococcal pneumonia, tuberculosis, and others (Arcavi and Benowitz 2004). Smoking during pregnancy and infant exposure to tobacco smoke also causes poor birth outcomes such as prematurity, low birth weight, respiratory problems in the newborn, and sudden infant death syndrome (CDC 2004; DHHS 2006).

Although cigarette smoking is often referred to as the single leading preventable cause of death in the United States, other forms of tobacco are also dangerous. For example, men who report moderate inhalation and smoke at least five cigars a day experience lung cancer deaths at about two-thirds the rate of men who smoke one pack of cigarettes a day. Cigar smokers experience higher rates of lung cancer, heart disease, and chronic obstructive lung disease than nonsmokers. Cigar smokers who inhale are 6 times more likely to die from oral cancer and 39 times more likely to die from laryngeal cancers than nonsmokers (NCI 1998). Bidis and Kreteks are associated with increased risks of cancers in the gastrointestinal and respiratory systems as well as other respiratory problems. Smokeless tobacco contains 28 carcinogens and is associated with the risk of oral cancer. It is also associated with gum recession and a condition called leukoplakia, a precancerous change in buccal and gingival mucosa (CDC 2004).

The health consequences of tobacco use have substantial economic effects. Because of smoking-related mortality, more than 3.3 million years of potential life among men and 2.2 million years of potential life among women are lost annually (compared with the life expectancies among nonsmokers). The lost productivity attributable to these years of life lost amounts to more than $92 billion annually (CDC 2005).[1] Other economic costs of tobacco use amount to more than $155 billion every year. Private and public health care expenditures for smoking related health conditions are an estimated $89 billion, including $28.4 billion in federal and state payments to Medicaid. Health care expenditures for secondhand smoke alone are approximately $5 billion per year (Lindblom and McMahon 2005).

Other social costs associated with tobacco use include the costs associated with smoking-related fires and casualties and degradation of the environment. Smoking is the fifth most frequent cause of residential fires—the leading cause of fire deaths. In addition, states and the federal government spend millions of dollars annually on prevention and research efforts relating to tobacco use. In FY 2002, for instance, state and federal funding for tobacco control programs totaled $861.9 million, or $3.16 per capita (CDC 2002). In FY 2005, state spending alone totaled $538.4 million, or $2.76 per capita (data for state and national funding combined since FY 2002 are not available).

Tobacco use will not disappear in the United States simply because of the momentum of past achievements. The decline in tobacco use achieved over the last several decades is likely to flatten out in the coming decade, and strong measures are likely to be needed to maintain continued progress

---

[1]This estimate of years of potential life lost and its associated productivity losses does not include deaths from burns or deaths from secondhand smoke.

thereafter. One problem is that the annual rate of cessation, never very high, has been flat since 2002. In addition, a major impediment to achieving a permanent long-term reduction in the prevalence of tobacco use is the high smoking initiation rate among teenagers. Notwithstanding substantial investment in tobacco control efforts in recent years, prevalence of current smoking among high school seniors remains at about 20 percent, and most of these individuals will remain smokers as adults. Approximately 90 percent of adult smokers began smoking as teenagers (SAMHSA 2006).

THE COMMITTEE'S CHARGE

Concerns about the waning momentum of tobacco control efforts and about declining public attention to what remains the nation's largest public health problem led the American Legacy Foundation to ask the Institute of Medicine (IOM) to conduct a major study of tobacco policy in the United States. The IOM appointed a 14-member committee and charged it to assess past progress and future prospects in tobacco control and to develop a blueprint for reducing tobacco use in the United States. The study's statement of task is presented in Box I-1.

To carry out its charge, the committee conducted six meetings between May 2004 and June 2005 at which the members heard presentations from individuals representing academia, nonprofit organizations, and various state governments. The committee also reviewed an extensive literature from peer-reviewed journals, published reports, and news articles. The background information and supporting evidence for the committee's report are contained in 12 signed appendixes written by committee members and three commissioned papers written by outside researchers.

The committee found it useful to set some boundaries on its work concerning the goal ("reducing tobacco use") and the time frame within which it should be achieved. To make its task manageable and well-focused, the committee decided to focus its literature review and evidence gathering on reducing cigarette smoking, without meaning to overlook or dismiss the health consequences of other forms of tobacco use. However, the committee believes that its recommendations, although derived from the evidence regarding interventions to reduce cigarette smoking, are fully applicable to smoking of other tobacco products and that most of the recommendations are also applicable to smokeless tobacco products. First of all, trends in smokeless use and cigarette use tend to move in tandem, suggesting that the population-level factors at work at any given time are affecting all forms of tobacco use. Although some smokers may switch to smokeless tobacco as a "risk-reducing" tactic, thereby offsetting some of the gains from smoking cessation, successful efforts to curtail smoking initiation do not appear to be compromised by increased initiation of smokeless use. Second, the

> **BOX I-1 Statement of Task**
>
> The nation has made tremendous progress in reducing tobacco use over the past 40 years. Despite extensive knowledge about successful interventions to reduce tobacco use, approximately one-quarter of American adults still smokes. Tobacco-related illnesses and death place a huge burden on our society. A committee at the Institute of Medicine will examine which prevention and treatment interventions are most promising to reduce tobacco use further, the barriers to action, and which policies need to be changed or adopted. The committee will also explore the benefits to society of fully implementing effective tobacco control interventions and policies. The committee's recommendations will be broad reaching, targeting federal, state, local, non-profit, and for-profit entities. The purpose of this committee is to generate a blueprint for the nation in the struggle to reduce tobacco use.

committee believes that most of the interventions shown to be effective for smoking (cessation, health-based interventions, school-based interventions, media efforts, sales restrictions, marketing restrictions) can be implemented in behavior-specific or product-specific manner, and that there is no apparent reason why their effectiveness would be weakened in relation to use of smokeless products if they were sensitively designed. Overall, therefore, the committee believes that it is reasonable to assume that implementation of its blueprint will, in the aggregate, lead to a reduction in all forms of tobacco use. Thus the committee refers throughout the report to the goal of "reducing tobacco use."

The overarching goal of reducing smoking subsumes three distinct goals: reducing the rate of initiation of smoking among youth (IOM 1994), reducing third-party environmental tobacco smoke (ETS) exposure (NRC 1986), and helping people quit smoking. For the purposes of this report, the committee sets to one side additional strategies that might reduce the harm of smoking for smokers who cannot quit, a topic dealt with extensively in another recent IOM report (IOM 2001).

Another important question regarding the scope of the committee's work concerns the time frame. The committee wanted to design a blueprint for achieving substantial reductions in tobacco use, but to have a realistic opportunity for doing so, an ample period of time is needed. Yet, the target should not be so far in the distance as to lose its connection with current conditions or to outstrip the collective capacity to imagine the future. The committee decided to set a 20-year horizon for its projections and for the policies that it recommends.

In sum, the ultimate goal of the committee's blueprint is to reduce tobacco use so substantially that it is no longer a significant public health problem; this is what is meant by the phrase "ending the tobacco problem" used in the title of this report. While that objective is not likely to be achieved in 20 years, the report aims to set the nation irreversibly on a course for doing so.

The committee also needed to decide what it means to formulate a "blueprint." One possible approach was for the committee to regard its task as a purely scientific one—simply to offer technical advice to policymakers. Under this approach, the committee would confine itself to the task of evaluating the effectiveness (and perhaps the costs) of various policy tools for reducing smoking, leaving it to policymakers to take individual liberty, justice, and other values into account in deciding which policies to implement. However, such a restrained approach struck the committee as incompatible with the specific, direct, and emphatic nature of the instruction we had been given "to generate a blueprint for the nation in the struggle to reduce tobacco use." Accordingly, the committee's recommendations are direct and specific.

The Policy Context

For many years, a policy paradigm emphasizing consumer freedom of choice and decrying unwarranted "paternalism" dominated public opinion and policymaking on tobacco. In retrospect, however, the committee believes that predominant emphasis on consumer choice in public opinion during this period was largely shaped by the tobacco industry's successful efforts to deny and obscure the addictiveness and health consequences of tobacco use, and on an array of resulting market failures, including information asymmetry between producers and users, distorted consumer choice due to information deficits, and product pricing that did not reflect the full social costs (especially the effects on nonsmokers). As the scientific evidence about addiction and the health effects of tobacco use has grown, and the industry's deceptive strategies have been exposed in the course of state lawsuits and other tobacco-related litigation, public understanding of tobacco addiction has quickly deepened and the ethical and political context of tobacco policymaking has been transformed.

Consequently, over the past 10–15 years, the operating assumptions of tobacco policy in the United States and elsewhere in the world have fundamentally changed. As shown in Chapters 3 and 5, a widespread popular consensus is now emerging in favor of aggressive policy initiatives, and this shift in popular sentiment has also been accompanied by support across most of the political spectrum.

In this context, it is worth pausing to take note of the ethical foundation for taking strong steps to reduce tobacco use. From a traditional public health perspective, the legitimacy and importance of reducing tobacco use lies in the enormous social costs attributable to tobacco-related disease; reducing tobacco use increases overall population health. Further, even within a libertarian paradigm, each of the subsidiary goals of tobacco policy is clearly justified: reducing exposure to ETS prevents harm to nonsmokers; preventing initiation by youth is justified by the recognized shortcomings of adolescent judgment; and promoting cessation helps to restore the liberty of smokers who are able to quit. Ethically speaking, the most controversial interventions are those aimed exclusively at reducing use by the minority of adult smokers who do not want to quit. This is the nub of the so-called paternalism problem.

However, since every intervention aimed at current smokers serves the interests and express wishes of the subset who want to quit, interventions designed to protect the health of adult smokers do not necessarily rest on a paternalistic foundation. Instead, they entail both liberty-enhancing effects (achieved by assisting addicted smokers to quit) and liberty-restricting effects (insofar as they also "burden" the choices of smokers who do not want to quit or object to the restrictions and costs imposed on them). Thus ethical analysis of tobacco control interventions within the libertarian paradigm requires a weighing of liberty-reducing effects of particular intervention against the liberty-enhancing effects of these interventions for nonsmokers whose freedom to avoid ETS exposure is protected, youths whose long-run autonomy is preserved, and adult smokers whose ability to quit is enhanced (and therefore regard the intervention as a benefit rather than a cost). This problem is addressed further in Chapter 4.

Limits of the Charge

Reducing tobacco use is, of course, a global challenge. According to a recent World Health Organization (WHO) study, tobacco-related diseases will kill 6.4 million people a year by 2015, accounting for 10 percent of all deaths worldwide. There are now many millions of smokers in the world, served by increasingly aggressive transnational tobacco companies. The common interest of all nations in reducing tobacco use has been declared and effectuated by the WHO-sponsored Framework Convention for Tobacco Control, which went into effect in 2005 and has been ratified by 142 nations (unfortunately not including the United States). The United States has a direct stake in reducing smuggling of tobacco products into this country that could undermine domestic tobacco control efforts, and the committee also recognizes the compelling importance of international tobacco control efforts for world health. However, the committee's charge was to develop a tobacco control blueprint for the nation, not for the world. We hope, though, that some of the measures recommended in this report will provide useful models for other countries, just as the domestic interventions undertaken by other countries in recent years served as useful models for us.

This is not a report about a research agenda. Many gaps in current knowledge were noted in our deliberations, and the committee is concerned that current National Institutes of Health expenditures on tobacco use (including both initiation and cessation) are not commensurate with the disease burden of smoking and other forms of tobacco use. However, our charge was to propose a blueprint for tobacco control, not for research.

OUTLINE OF REPORT

The committee's report is divided into two parts. Part I, comprising Chapters 1 through 3, provides the context for the committee's proposed policy blueprint. Chapter 1 discusses the extraordinary growth of tobacco use during the first half of the 20th century and its subsequent reversal in 1965 in the wake of the 1964 Surgeon General's report on the harmful health effects of smoking. Chapter 1 also examines closely recent trends in tobacco use. Chapter 2 summarizes the ways in which the addictive properties of nicotine make it so difficult for people to quit, thereby sustaining tobacco use at high levels. Chapter 2 also reviews the salient factors associated with smoking initiation, especially the failure of adolescents to appreciate the risk and consequences of addiction when they become smokers. The chapter concludes by discussing several recent trends in smoking epidemiology that may pose problems for tobacco control in the future.

Chapter 3 reviews the history of tobacco control. After the 1964 Surgeon General's report, the public's opinion toward smoking changed dramatically. However, until the mid 1980s, antismoking efforts had little success in combating the financial and political power of the tobacco industry. Tobacco control efforts began to make progress when grassroots initiatives galvanized public concern about the health effects of environmental tobacco smoke and began to erode pro-smoking social norms. The tobacco policy debate became transformed in the late 1980s and 1990s, when the public recognized the addictive nature of nicotine, the continued importance of teenage initiation in sustaining the public health burden of tobacco use, and the tobacco industry's extensive efforts to manipulate and deceive the public. Chapter 3 concludes by projecting the likely prevalence of smoking over the next 20 years if current trends remain unchanged or if tobacco control efforts are weakened.

Part II of the committee's report presents a blueprint for reducing tobacco use. After reviewing the ethical grounding of tobacco control in Chapter 4, the committee sets forth its blueprint as a two-pronged strategy and offers a vast array of recommendations. The first prong, presented in Chapter 5, envisions strengthening traditional tobacco control measures.

The committee summarizes the evidence regarding the effectiveness of the tobacco control methods now being deployed and makes recommendations for broadening and strengthening them. For the most part, the chapter emphasizes state and local initiatives supported by public health partnerships and community advocacy programs. The two pillars of the blueprint are substantial increases in excise taxes on tobacco and smoke-free-air laws with broad coverage. In addition, the blueprint includes other elements of comprehensive state programs, such as youth access restrictions, school-based prevention programs, programs aimed at families and health care systems, media campaigns, smoking cessation programs, and grassroots community advocacy. Chapter 5 closes with a projection of the likely effects over the next two decades of implementing the policies outlined.

The premise of Chapter 6 is that a more substantial long-term impact on reducing tobacco use requires a change in the current legal framework of tobacco control. The second prong of the blueprint envisions changing the regulatory landscape to permit new policy innovations that take into account the unique history and characteristics of tobacco. Under the proposed approach, federal power would enhance and support state efforts in the traditional domains of tobacco control while taking aggressive steps in the currently under-regulated areas of tobacco marketing, distribution, and product design. A key feature of the federal program would be the exercise of regulatory jurisdiction by the Food and Drug Administration. In addition, the federal government would also play a more substantial role in funding and coordinating state tobacco control activities.

One of the most important aims of the plan outlined in Chapter 6 is to establish a platform for major innovations in tobacco control. However, any major innovations will have to be formulated with great care, based on thorough analysis of the possible consequences. It will be essential, therefore, for the federal government to create a capacity for tobacco policy research and development. In Chapter 7 the committee recommends that a new policy development office undertake a major program of policy analysis, based on improved statistical models, and that it explore new frontiers of tobacco control, including proposals to gradually reduce the nicotine content of cigarettes.

REFERENCES

Arcavi L, Benowitz NL. 2004. Cigarette Smoking and Infection. *Archives of Internal Medicine* 165:2206-2216.
CDC (Centers for Disease Control and Prevention). 1999. Ten great public health achievements—United States, 1900–1999. *MMWR (Morbidity and Mortality Weekly Report)* 48(12):241-243.
CDC. 2002. *Tobacco Control State Highlights 2002: Impact and Opportunity.* Albuquerque M, Kelly A, Schooley M, Fellows JL, Pechacek TF. Atlanta, GA.

CDC. 2004. *The Health Consequences of Smoking: A Report of the Surgeon General.* Web Page. Available at: http://www.cdc.gov/tobacco/data_statistics/sgr/sgr_2004/index.htm; accessed May 25, 2007.

CDC. 2005. Annual smoking attributable mortality, years of potential life lost, and productivity losses—United States, 1997-2001. *MMWR (Morbidity and Mortality Weekly Report)* 54(25):625-628.

CDC. 2006. Tobacco use among adults—United States, 2005. *(MMWR Morbidity and Mortality Weekly Report)* 55(42):1145-1148.

DHHS (U.S. Department of Health and Human Services). 2006. *The Health Consequences of Involuntary Exposure to Tobacco Smoke: A Report of the Surgeon General.* Atlanta, GA: U.S. Department of Health and Human Services, Centers for Disease Control and Prevention, Coordinating Center for Health Promotion, National Center for Chronic Disease Prevention and Health Promotion, Office on Smoking and Health.

Healthy People 2010. 2005. *Leading Health Indicators.* Web Page. Available at: http://www.healthypeople.gov/document/html/uih/uih_4.htm; accessed May 7, 2007.

IOM (Institute of Medicine). 1994. *Growing Up Tobacco Free: Preventing Nicotine Addiction in Children and Youth.* Editors Lynch BJ, Bonnie RJ. Washington, DC: National Academy Press.

IOM. 2001. *Clearing the Smoke: Assessing the Science Base for Tobacco Harm Reduction.* Washington, DC: National Academy Press.

Lindblom E, McMahon K. 2005. *Toll of Tobacco in the United States of America.* Web Page. Available at: http://www.tobaccofreekids.org/research/factsheets/pdf/0072.pdf; accessed August 11, 2006.

NCI (National Cancer Institute). *Cigars: Health Effects and Trends. Smoking and Tobacco Control Monograph No. 9* ed. 1998.

NRC (National Research Council). 1986. *Environmental Tobacco Smoke: Measuring Exposures and Assessing Health Effects.* Washington, DC: National Academy Press.

SAMHSA (Substance Abuse and Mental Health Services Administration). 2006. *Results from the 2005 National Survey on Drug Use and Health: National Findings.* Web Page. Available at: http://oas.samhsa.gov/nsduh/2k5nsduh/2k5results.pdf; accessed November 28, 2006

PART I

BACKGROUND

1

Epidemiology of Tobacco Use: History and Current Trends

Since at least the colonial era, tobacco has been a popular commodity in the United States, with tobacco use increasing almost exponentially from the 1800s to the mid-1960s (DHHS 2000a). The invention of the cigarette fueled this dramatic rise in tobacco consumption, and cigarette smoking quickly outpaced the use of any other form of tobacco product (Brandt 2007). When tobacco use peaked in the mid-1960s, more than 40 percent of the U.S. adult population smoked cigarettes (National Center for Health Statistics 2005). This chapter reviews the growth of tobacco use over the 20th century, and the dramatic reversal of that trend beginning in 1965. The chapter examines recent trends in the epidemiology of smoking over the past four decades, takes a close look at the characteristics of smokers and those who have quit smoking, and discusses variations in the prevalence rate of smoking by sociodemographic characteristics and state of residence. Finally, the chapter highlights some possible threats to continued progress in reducing smoking in the United States.

GROWTH OF THE TOBACCO PROBLEM

In the late 19th and early 20th centuries, Americans consumed tobacco primarily in the form of chewing tobacco and cigars. According to Giovino, the per-capita consumption of tobacco products in the early 1880s was approximately 6 pounds of tobacco per person aged 18 and older; 56 percent of that tobacco was in the form of chewing tobacco, whereas only 1 percent took the form of manufactured cigarettes (Giovino 2002). For several reasons, cigarettes became the preferred tobacco product of Americans over the 20th century; in particular, cigarettes served as a more efficient vehicle for the absorption of nicotine and a less expensive form of tobacco. Also, by the 1880s, cigarette production had been mechanized with the advent of the Bonsack machine, which made it possible to produce additional units for little or no additional cost, and the prices of cigarettes were cut in half (Chaloupka et al. 2002; Giovino 2002). The lower price made cigarettes more accessible to a wider clientele (DHHS 2000b). By the 1950s, manufactured cigarettes represented 80 percent of per-person tobacco consumption (Giovino 2002).

In 1900, on a per-capita basis, American adults smoked approximately 54 cigarettes per year. That number increased almost exponentially until its peak in 1963, when an estimated 4,345 cigarettes were consumed per adult in that year alone, as shown in Figure 1-1 (ALA 2006). This growth in consumption occurred for many reasons, but was driven largely by the mass production of cigarettes; the mildness, packaging, addictiveness, and convenience of the product; glamorization of smoking in movies and on television; and persuasive advertising campaigns (Chaloupka et al. 2002; DHHS 2000a; Giovino 2002).

The milder flavor of the Turkish and domestic blended tobacco products also increased the appeal of cigarettes to a wider clientele. In the early twentieth century, cigarette manufacturers developed new blends using American-grown tobacco, such as sugared burley tobaccos (Giovino 2002). Manufacturers also used new methods of curing the tobacco, including flue

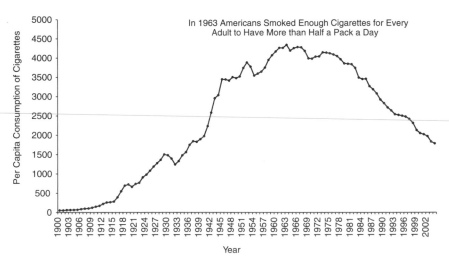

FIGURE 1-1 Per capita consumption of cigarettes among adults ages 18 years and older from 1900 to 2004.
SOURCES: (ALA 2004, 2006; Capehart 2004).

curing. This process results in a product called "bright tobacco," which has a high sugar content and a medium nicotine content (IOM 2001). These production changes created cigarettes that were milder and less alkaline than other forms of tobacco. The more acidic nature of these cigarettes allowed the nicotine in their smoke to be efficiently absorbed by the lungs. This feature provided cigarettes an advantage over cigars, as cigar smoke is absorbed in the mouth rather than in the lungs. More nicotine is absorbed with cigarettes compared to cigars due to the much larger surface area of the lung compared to the mouth. In addition, nicotine more quickly gets into the brain via the carotid artery following pulmonary absorption compared to buccal absorption, in which it travels through the liver before getting to the brain. Furthermore, as cigarettes are inhalable, they require less skill to use than cigars (DHHS 2000b; Giovino 2002). Thus people who may have abstained from smoking because they were intimidated by the cigar were drawn to the ease of smoking a cigarette (DHHS 2000b). The efficient absorption of nicotine has the added effect of making cigarettes more addictive than other forms of tobacco (Giovino 2002). These two features combined in order to drive high addiction rates among soldiers in World War I, to whom cigarettes were distributed without charge (Burns et al. 1997; DHHS 2000a; Schoenberg 1933).

Intensity and innovation in advertising have been hallmark features of the cigarette industry throughout its history. In 1913, Camel became the first cigarette brand to gain nationwide popularity, following a mass marketing campaign by the R. J. Reynolds Company that introduced this "American blend" cigarette to the American public through a teaser advertisement (R.J. Reynolds 2006). Other companies followed suit, especially after World War I, as heavy advertising propelled the demand for cigarettes on a national scale (Schoenberg 1933). Ernster reported that Lucky Strike drew women's attention with the diet slogan "Reach for a Lucky Instead of a Sweet" (Ernster 1985). Throughout the 1930s and 1940s, meanwhile, the Brown and Williamson Company included health claims in its ads for Kool, the first menthol cigarette distributed nationwide, claiming that smoking menthol cigarettes could protect against colds and soothe the throat (IOM 2001; R.J. Reynolds 2006).

The boom period of tobacco consumption occurred between the 1920s and the mid-1960s (DHHS 2000b). During this period, tobacco users shifted from the traditional practices of using chewing tobacco, inhaling snuff, and smoking cigars and pipes, to smoking cigarettes, and the number of tobacco users increased as the rising number of initiates, including many women, became cigarette smokers (DHHS 2000b; Giovino 2002). The manufactured cigarette was convenient because it was already rolled and, along with the safety match, it provided an easy, portable, and disposable indulgence (DHHS 2000b).

Over the 20th century, cigarette consumption fell only a few times before 1965: during the Great Depression, at the end World War II, and in 1953 and 1954 (Giovino 2002). The drop in consumption during the Great Depression was directly related to the decline in real disposable income,[1] whereas the declines in the early 1950s followed the first real claims of tobacco's harmful effects on health, which linked smoking to the development of cancer (Giovino 2002; Hamilton 1972; Havrilesky and Barth 1969). Hamilton (1972) showed that the reduction in consumption in the mid-1950s was attributable to the health scare associated with the use of tobacco products and that the effect of this public concern negated any market boost that might have come from advertising. Other studies suggest that the positive health claims in cigarette advertising made during this period might have had an indirect negative effect on tobacco consumption by giving the impression that protection was needed, thereby reinforcing the health scare (IOM 2001).

To mollify the public's growing concern about the health effects of smoking, tobacco companies introduced filtered cigarettes in the 1950s and the so-called low-tar cigarettes in the 1960s. Filters reduce tar and nicotine yields on government test machines. The market share of filtered cigarettes jumped from less than 5 percent in 1953 to almost 20 percent 2 years later. By 1960, more than half of all cigarettes consumed had filters (Giovino 2002). In 2004 and 2005, 99 percent of cigarettes on the market had filters (FTC 2007). The market share of low-tar cigarettes, those purportedly yielding less than or equal to 15 milligrams of tar, increased from 2 percent to more than 55 percent in the 20 years between 1967 and 1987. By 2003, almost 85 percent of cigarettes distributed within the United States were low-tar products (FTC 2005; Giovino 2002).

Some manufacturers added chemicals to cigarettes to improve their flavor and aroma. One such chemical was menthol, an additive with an anesthetizing effect that was claimed to sooth the throat (Gardiner 2004; IOM 2001). Because menthol did indeed make the passage of tobacco smoke into the throat a smoother experience, consumers inhaled more deeply. In 1963, 16 percent of cigarettes sold in the United States contained menthol. The market share of menthol cigarettes peaked at slightly under 30 percent in the 1980s (FTC 2005; Giovino 2002; Giovino et al. 2004).

---

[1]Historical records show that per capita cigarette consumption rises and falls in tandem with changes in price and in real incomes (DHHS 2000b). Although demand for cigarettes is what economists call "relatively inelastic" because of their addictiveness, that just means that consumption responds less than proportionally to changes in price, not that consumption is unresponsive to price. Several studies have estimated the price elasticity of the demand of cigarettes at approximately –0.40, which implies that a 10 percent increase in the price would result in a 4 percent decrease in consumption (Chaloupka et al. 2002; Hamilton 1972).

DECLINE IN TOBACCO USE, 1965–2005[2]

Despite the development of new products purportedly reducing smokers' exposure to tobacco toxins, Americans have greatly reduced their tobacco consumption since the publication of the first Surgeon General's report on the harmful effects of cigarette smoking in 1964. In fact, cigarette consumption has declined substantially since the mid-1960s (see Figure 1-1 for annual trends). By 1983, the annual per-capita consumption of cigarettes had declined approximately 20 percent from the 1963 level to 3,494 cigarettes per adult; by 2004, it had declined an additional 49 percent to 1,791 cigarettes, its lowest level in 67 years (ALA 2006; Capehart 2005). The halving of per-capita consumption of cigarettes over the last 20 years stems from a decline in smoking prevalence coupled with a decline in the number of cigarettes smoked per day among those who smoke.[3]

The percentage of adults who currently smoke (see Box 1-2 for a definition of this and other terms) has also declined in the past 40 years, as indicated in Figure 1-2. In 1965, 41.9 percent of Americans ages 18 years and over, or approximately 52.2 million adults, smoked either every day or on some days (National Center for Health Statistics 2005). The percentage of adults who are current smokers declined steeply between 1965 and 1991, with an estimated 39 percent drop in the prevalence of cigarette smoking. By 2005, the prevalence of adult cigarette smoking had declined to half the 1965 rate. An estimated 20.9 percent of American adults, or 45.1 million people, were current smokers in 2005 (CDC 2006b).

The reduction in the prevalence of current smokers was driven by an increase in the rate of smoking cessation as well as a decrease in the rate of smoking initiation. Between 1965 and 2005, the percentage of adults who once smoked and who had quit more than doubled from 24.3 to 50.8 percent, as shown in Figure 1-3 (CDC 2006b; TIPS 2005a). Furthermore, the percentage of adults who have never smoked more than 100 lifetime cigarettes increased by approximately 23 percent from 1965 (44 percent) to 2005 (54 percent) (CDC 2005c; TIPS 2005b).

Smoking initiation among adolescents and young adults has also declined since the mid-1960s, as estimated by the National Survey on Drug Use and Health (NSDUH) (SAMHSA 2005). In 1965, among adolescents aged 12 to 17 years, 125.5 of every 1,000 smoked a cigarette for the first time. In 2003, 102.1 per 1,000 youths in the same age range had smoked a cigarette for the first time (Figure 1-4). The reduction in smoking initiation saved more than half a million adolescents from having a first cigarette between 1965 and 2004. Young adults (individuals ages 18 to 25 years) have

---

[2]See Box 1-1 for a list of commonly used data sets regarding tobacco use.

[3]As discussed in a subsequent section, mean number of cigarettes per day consumed by current smokers rose steadily until 1979, when the trend reversed.

BOX 1-1 Commonly Used Data Sets

BRFSS Behavior Risk Factor Surveillance Survey.
State-level prevalence of current tobacco use and cessation among adults (ages 18 years and older). All 50 states have participated since 1996.

CPS Current Population Survey Tobacco Use Supplement.
National- and state-level prevalence of tobacco use and cessation behavior among individuals ages 15 years and older.

MTF Monitoring the Future.
National-level prevalence of cigarette use, age at initiation, and cessation behavior among students in the 8th, 10th, and 12th grades, as well as young adults.

NHIS National Health Interview Survey.
National-level prevalence of tobacco use and cessation behavior among adults. Surveillance data have been collected since 1965, with changes in the definitions of current and former smoker made in 1991.

NSDUH National Survey on Drug Use and Health.
Formerly the National Household Survey on Drug Abuse. National-level prevalence of tobacco use by specific form, including bedes and kreteks among individuals ages 12 years and older. Surveillance since 2002.

YBRSS Youth Behavior Risk Surveillance System.

traditionally been less likely to initiate smoking behavior than adolescents, but their initiation rates also declined, from an annual level of 89.4 first-time smokers per 1,000 people in 1965 to one of 67.5 per 1,000 in 2003 (SAMHSA 2005). It should be noted, however, that despite this overall decline in initiation since 1965, trends over the past twenty years are not entirely encouraging. Developments in youth and young adult initiation over the past two decades are discussed in further detail later in the chapter when the committee more closely reviews recent developments.

Industry Response

These reductions in smoking over the past half century represent hard-won successes for tobacco control programs, because efforts to reduce tobacco consumption have frequently been countered by the tobacco industry in ways designed to maintain its customer base. Just as it did in the early part of the 20th century, the tobacco industry has recently attempted to use pricing, new product development, and advertising to counteract health-driven declines in tobacco consumption (Chaloupka et al. 2002).

BOX 1-2 Definition of Terms

Smoker
Adult:[a] person aged 18 years or over who has smoked at least 100 cigarettes in his or her lifetime.
Adolescent: (a) a person between the ages of 12 and 17 years who has smoked even once or twice,[b] (b) a person between the ages of 12 and 17 years who has ever smoked, even one or two puffs.[c]

Current Smoker
Adult (1965 to 1991): a person who was ever a smoker who reported smoking now.
Adult: (1992 to present): a person who was ever a smoker who reported that he or she currently smokes either every day or on some days.
Adolescent: a person between the ages of 12 and 17 who smokes on one or more days in the past 30 days.

Former Smoker
Adult (1965 to 1991): a person who was ever a smoker who no longer smokes.
Adult (1991 to present): a person who was ever a smoker who no longer smokes every day or on some days.

Heavy Smoker
Adult: a current smoker who smokes at least 25 cigarettes in one day.
Adolescent: a high school senior who smoked in the past 30 days and smoked at least one-half pack of cigarettes per day.[d]

---

[a]Definitions for adults come from the National Health Interview Survey.
[b]Monitoring the Future.
[c]Youth Behavior Risk Surveillance System and Youth Tobacco Survey.
[d]Monitoring the Future.
SOURCE: Adapted from text in Giovino (2002).

The tobacco industry has dramatically increased its investment in advertising and promotional expenditures since the 1960s. From 1963 to 2003, total advertising and promotional expenditures by the five largest tobacco manufacturers increased from $1.5 billion (indexed for inflation) to $15.15 billion, the largest amount ever reported to the Federal Trade Commission (FTC 2005). Expenditures have risen particularly dramatically in recent years; the $15.15 billion spent in 2003 represents a 48 percent increase over the $10.25 billion spent in 2000, and an increase of 170 percent over the $5.62 billion spent in 1990 (FTC 2005).

It should be noted, however, that the allocation of these advertising and promotional expenditures has changed substantially in recent years. As

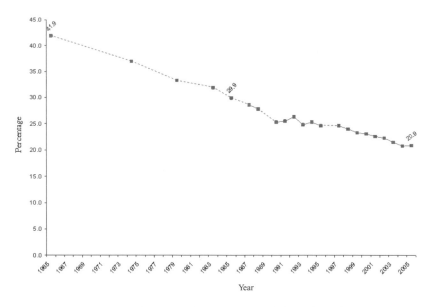

FIGURE 1-2 Current smoking prevalence among adults, selected years from 1965 to 2005 (all years for which NHIS data on annual smoking prevalence are available are included). Solid lines represent changes in smoking prevalence between consecutive years. Dotted lines represent approximate changes in smoking prevalence between nonconsecutive years. For years 1965 to 2004, age-adjusted data are provided. For 2005, crude data are provided.

SOURCES: (CDC 2006b; National Center for Health Statistics 2006).

the industry's advertising opportunities have become increasingly limited, tobacco companies have dedicated significant portions of their marketing budgets to price discounts and other promotions at the retail level (Chaloupka et al. 2002; White et al. 2006). As discussed further below, the main target of these price-oriented promotions is current smokers.

Manufacturers have also developed new products with the hopes of countering prevalent health concerns. Marketing campaigns have promoted purportedly low-tar, low-nicotine, and low-yield products, catering to perceptions that such cigarettes are safer or less harmful than the alternatives (Giovino et al. 1996). Taking advantage of the increasing popularity of these purportedly low-yield products, the R.J. Reynolds Company repositioned the Winston brand in 1997, claiming that its product was made with "100 percent tobacco" and "no additives" (Arnett 1999). Manufacturers have also promoted menthol-containing products, in response to consumer perceptions that such cigarettes were less harmful than nonmenthol brands (Gardiner 2004; IOM 2001; Pollay and Dewhirst 2002).

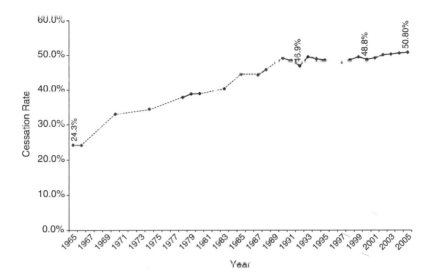

FIGURE 1-3 Cessation rate among adult EVER smokers selected years from 1965 to 2005 (all years for which NHIS data on annual cessation prevalence are available are included). Solid lines represent changes in cessation prevalence between consecutive years. Dotted lines represent approximate changes in cessation prevalence between nonconsecutive years.
SOURCES: (TIPS 2005a; CDC 2003, 2004b, 2005a,b, 2006b).

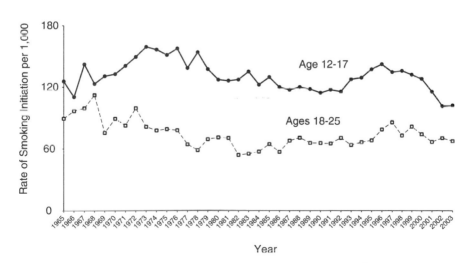

FIGURE 1-4 Smoking initiation rates among adolescents and young adults, 1965 to 2003.
SOURCE: (SAMHSA 2005).

Cigarette manufacturers also sought to expand the market for their products by recruiting women and youth smokers. Marketing efforts toward women increased dramatically in the late 1960s and early 1970s (Ernster 1985; Pierce et al. 1994). Products such as Virginia Slims grew popular through campaigns that depicted stylish, independent, and healthy women. In the 1980s and 1990s, manufacturers also turned increasingly to advertising directed toward youth to grow their market. For example, in 1988 R.J. Reynolds introduced the Joe Camel cartoon character, which quickly proved to be powerfully appealing to adolescents (DiFranza et al. 1991; Pierce et al. 1999). Between 1989 and 1993, Camel's market share among adolescents increased by 64 percent (CDC 1994). Moreover, although advertising in magazines with high youth readership has declined since tobacco companies committed to avoid targeting youth as a condition of the Master Settlement Agreement, cigarette companies continue to promote their products in magazines that reach high percentages and numbers of young readers (FTC 2005; Krugman et al. 2005).

In addition to the techniques mentioned above, the tobacco industry has frequently turned to pricing strategies to increase tobacco consumption. The real price of cigarettes declined between 1955 and 1980 (Gruber 2001; IOM 1994). A doubling of the federal excise tax between 1982 and 1983 and an increase in the wholesale price of cigarettes preceded an estimated 5 percent decline in per-capita consumption between 1983 and 1984 (Chaloupka et al. 2002; Gruber 2001; IOM 1994). The tobacco industry responded by offering "branded generics," discounted cigarettes marketed specifically at young adults who were more likely to quit smoking in response to the price increase. Many smokers switched to discounted generic brands, and the decline in consumption slowed by the early 1990s as the market share of discounted brands rose to nearly 40 percent (Chaloupka et al. 2002; Gruber 2001).

On April 2, 1993, a day referred to as Marlboro Friday, Philip Morris, Inc., led the industry in cutting the prices of premium brand cigarettes by offering Marlboros for a 40-cent-per-pack discount (Chaloupka et al. 2002; Gruber 2001; IOM 1994). The wholesale price of Marlboro's premium cigarettes dropped from 123 cents per pack to 84 cents per pack to compete with discounted brands, which cost only 83 cents per pack, and deeply discounted brands, listed at 57 cents (Bulow and Klemperer 1998). That price cut helped to recapture the market for premium brands and to boost Philip Morris's profits, as more than 80 percent of the company's sales were in premium brands in 1997 (Bulow and Klemperer 1998).

After the Master Settlement Agreement in November 1998, the price of all brands was increased, in large part to cover the cost of the settlement. As a result, the price of premiums returned to their pre-Marlboro Friday nominal price (Bulow and Klemperer 1998). Premium brands have maintained their dominance in the market over the past decade, actually gaining market share throughout the 1990s (Bulow and Klemperer 1998). Part of the reason for this increase in market share is the effect of discounting (Bulow and Klemperer 1998). In 2003, of the $15.15 billion reportedly spent on adverting and promotion, $10.8 billion (approximately 71 percent) was allocated to price discounts paid to retailers or wholesalers. These discounts allowed for reduced prices for consumers (FTC 2005). The percentage of disposable income that smokers spent on cigarettes fell from 1993 through 1998 but rose consistently through 2002 (Capehart 2004). The effect of price on consumption is discussed in more detail in Chapter 5.

RECENT TRENDS: A CLOSER LOOK

Wide-angle comparisons of measures of smoking behavior between 1965 and 2005 clearly show that the rates of tobacco consumption and smoking prevalence have declined among adults, the rate of smoking initiation has declined among adolescents, and the rate of smoking cessation has increased. However, a closer look at the trends over the past two decades tells a somewhat more complex story of both modest progress and some backsliding. For instance, although smoking prevalence has continued to decline in the new millennium, it appears that progress in some areas may now be stalling. These recent trends are examined more closely in this section.

Adult Prevalence

In 1985, nearly 30 of every 100 American adults were current smokers; by 2005, that figure had fallen to approximately 21 in 100 adults (CDC 2006b; National Center for Health Statistics 2005). That said, a closer look at the trend reveals a steep decline in the number of adults who were current smokers from 1985 through 1990, a slight increase in 1991-1992, and a relatively flat, although downward-sloping, curve from 1992 through 2005, as illustrated in Figure 1-2 (CDC 2006b; Mendez and Warner 2004; National Center for Health Statistics 2005). Moreover, although a reduction in the prevalence of adults who are current smokers occurred each year during the first half of this decade, data for 2005 reveals no change in adult prevalence from the previous year (CDC 2006b; TIPS 2006).

Data on the prevalence of smoking among men ages 25 to 64 years and women ages 35 to 64 each display a flattening of this downward-trending curve from the early 1990s through the mid-2000s for both genders (see Figures 1-5 and 1-6). Mendez and Warner were optimistic that smoking prevalence would continue to fall on course, as it had in the early 2000s, but they concluded that major reductions, such as those presented in the

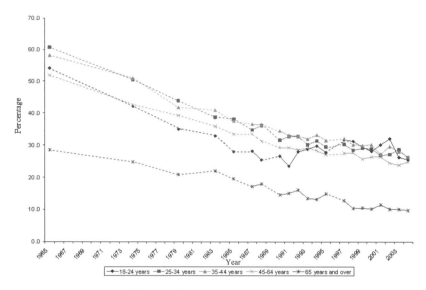

FIGURE 1-5 Age-specific prevalence rates among adult males, selected years, 1965 to 2003 (all years for which NHIS data on annual smoking prevalence are available are included). Solid lines represent changes in smoking prevalence between consecutive years. Dotted lines represent approximate changes in smoking prevalence between nonconsecutive years.
SOURCE: (National Center for Health Statistics 2006).

Healthy People 2010 target, were unrealistic (Mendez and Warner 2004). Predictive models of smoking prevalence reduction are presented and discussed further in Chapters 3 and 5 of this report.

Prevalence of Smoking Among Youth

From 1999 to 2006, the prevalence of daily smoking[4] among 12th graders decreased dramatically, according to data from the Monitoring the Future survey. In 1999, the prevalence of daily smoking among 12th graders (23.1 percent) was roughly equal to that among adults (23.3 percent); by 2006, the rate of daily smoking for 12th graders had fallen to 12.2 percent[5] (Johnston et al. 2006). This is a genuinely noteworthy decline. However, because trends in youth smoking behavior tend to fluctuate substantially, it is important to view this recent trend within a broader time frame. When

---

[4]Daily smoking is defined as an average of one or more cigarettes per day.

[5]Prevalence of daily smoking in 10th graders dropped from 15.9 percent in 1999 to 7.6 percent in 2006. Prevalence of daily smoking in 8th graders dropped from 8.1 percent to 4 percent over that time period as well.

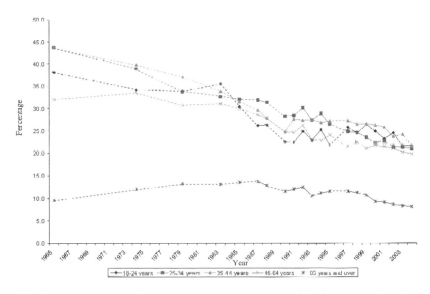

FIGURE 1-6 Age-specific prevalence rates among adult females, selected years, 1965 to 2003 (all years for which NHIS data on annual smoking prevalence are available are included). Solid lines represent changes in smoking prevalence between consecutive years. Dotted lines represent approximate changes in smoking prevalence between nonconsecutive years.
SOURCE: (National Center for Health Statistics 2006).

the decline in the prevalence of daily smoking among youth is viewed over a 15-year perspective, the long-term decline can be seen to be more modest. Comparison of the rates of daily smoking among 12th graders in 2006 with those in 1992, for example, reveals that daily smoking prevalence has dropped from 17.2 to 12.2, a 5 percentage point net decrease (Johnston et al. 2006), showing that much of the decline in youth prevalence rates in this century has simply offset the significant increase in youth smoking that had occurred in the 1990s. A similar pattern is shown by trends in 30-day prevalence (current smoking) among high school youth (see Figure 1-7 for the 12th grade data).

Not all indicators show a continuing downward trend, however. Daily smoking did not decline at all among 8th graders and 10th graders in 2006 (Johnston et al. 2007). Moreover, 2005 data from a separate source, the Centers for Disease Control and Prevention's Youth Behavior Risk Surveillance System (YRBSS), show a slight rise in the prevalence of use among high school youth (combining grades 9 through 12) between 2003 and 2005, from 21.9 to 23 percent (CDC 2006a).

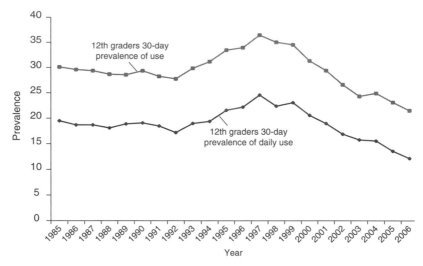

FIGURE 1-7 Smoking prevalence among 12th graders for selected years, 1985 to 2005.
SOURCE: (Johnston 2005, 2006, 2007).

In sum, there has been an impressive decline in the prevalence of youth smoking in the 21st century. However, trends of various measures of youth cigarette smoking from the last 15 years indicate that youth smoking rates tend to fluctuate considerably more than adult rates, and that it is likely that this recent decline will flatten out, or even turn upward again. In any case, the endemic level of youth smoking remains disturbingly high.

Intensity of Consumption

On average, smokers are smoking less than they did three decades ago; daily consumption among smokers began falling in 1979 (see Figure 1-8). Decreased daily consumption among smokers appears to be attributable largely to reduced smoking among heavy smokers; specifically, as shown in Figure 1-9, the percentage of smokers consuming more than 25 cigarettes per day was significantly smaller in 2004 than it was in 1993. Meanwhile, the percentage of smokers consuming between 5 and 14 cigarettes per day has increased since 1993, and the percentage of smokers consuming between 15 and 24 cigarettes per day has remained relatively flat over this time period (CDC 2005b).

The combined effect of the declining prevalence of adult smokers and the declining quantity smoked has led to a substantial decline in per-capita consumption over the last 20 years. Overall, per-capita consumption among

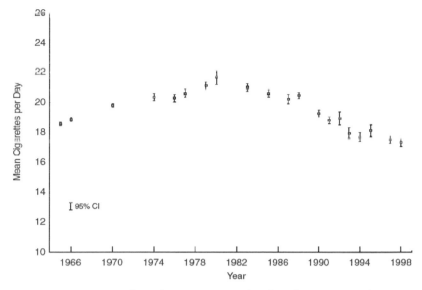

FIGURE 1-8 Mean number of cigarettes per day for all current smokers in each NHIS Survey Year. NOTE: Average number of cigarettes per day standardized to the age and race distribution of NHIS 1965. Brackets indicate 9 percent confidence intervals on the estimates.
SOURCE: (Burns et al. 2003).

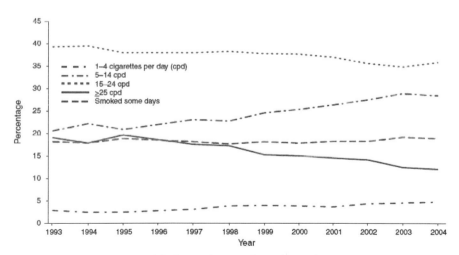

FIGURE 1-9 Percentage of daily smokers and smokers who smoked some days by number of cigarettes smoked, 1993 to 2004.
SOURCE: (CDC 2005b).

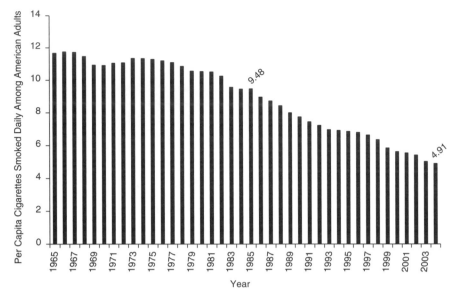

FIGURE 1-10 Daily per capita consumption of cigarettes among adults ages 18 and over, 1985 to 2004.
SOURCE: Calculations based on figures from ALA, 2006.

adults has decreased more than 48 percent since 1985, although it has declined unevenly from year to year, with annual changes ranging from 0.75 percent between 1994 and 1995 to 7.9 percent between 1998 and 1999 (following the Master Settlement Agreement and price increases) (ALA 2006) (see Figure 1-10).

Initiation

Recent data from the National Survey on Drug Use and Health (NSDUH) on smoking initiation rates[6] among adolescents (ages 12–17 years) reveal a striking decline from 1996 through 2005. As suggested earlier, however, this recent decline must be seen in the context of the significant increases in initiation rates among youth that occurred in the early 1990s (see Figure 1-4). Thus, what might initially appear to be a sign of dramatic recent progress merely signals only slight reductions in smoking initiation rates among youth over the past decade. In 2001, for example, the smoking initiation rate was 115.3 per 1,000 youth, almost equal to the rate in 1992.

---

[6]NSDUH defines initiation as the percentage of nonsmokers who initiated cigarette use (sometimes referred to as "first use") within the past 12 months.

Moreover, the modest successes in reducing smoking initiation rates among adolescents during the past two decades have been offset by net increases in initiation among young adults (between 18 and 25 years of age) during the same time period. Figure 1-4 reveals that between 1985 and 2003, smoking initiation rates among young adults increased 4.3 percent, from 64.7 per 1,000 individuals to 67.5 per 1000 (SAMHSA 2005). The reduction in smoking initiation among adolescents and the increase in smoking initiation among young adults thus indicate delayed smoking initiation rather than pure abstinence, which could signify a moving target for antismoking campaigns. This conclusion is supported by prevalence data as well (Johnston et al. 2006).

Smoking Cessation

The rate at which smoking cessation increased in the 1960s and 1970s has slowed over time, as evidenced by the flattening of Figure 1-3. A comparison of the annual smoking cessation rates[7] between 1992 and 2005 reveals that the largest annual increase occurred between 1992 and 1993, at 5.32 percent. During four periods (1993–1994, 1994–1995, 1995–1996, and 1999–2000), the smoking cessation rate actually declined from the previous year. The rates of cessation increased approximately 4 percent in the first five years of the 2000s. In 2000, 48.8 percent of adult ever smokers had quit smoking (TIPS 2005a). In 2005, 50.8 percent of adults who had ever smoked had quit smoking (CDC 2006b). Cessation seems to be approaching an asymptote, however, because the rate has increased an average of only 0.50 annually since 2002 (CDC 2004b, 2005a, 2005b, 2006b).

Correlates of Current Smoking

Tobacco use varies among individuals according to socioeconomic and demographic characteristics as well as by geography. Although smoking prevalence has declined overall since the 1960s, large disparities in rates of tobacco use among racial and ethnic groups and by socioeconomic status persist. The most vulnerable subpopulations—young people who start smoking early, individuals who are poor or uneducated, and some racial and ethnic minorities—are at the highest risk of being lifelong smokers. This section compares the differences in the prevalence of current smoking compared by age, race, sex, educational attainment, poverty status, and

---

[7]The percentage of ever smokers who are former smokers. Although this term technically refers to results from a cohort study, it is used in this chapter more generally to refer to results from any study design.

geographic location. This section also highlights the subpopulations most in need of targeted efforts.

Age

Figures 1-5 and 1-6 show the trends in age-specific smoking prevalence among males and females, respectively (National Center for Health Statistics 2005). Older individuals (ages 65 years and older) are much less likely than young adults to be current smokers. This trend has been consistent for four decades. However, prevalence rates among adults younger than age 65 years have tended to converge. According to NSDUH data, young adults ages 18 to 25 years had the highest rate of current use of any tobacco product (44.3 percent) (SAMHSA 2006).

The oldest age group (those ages 65 years and older) comprises people who were in their youth when smoking prevalence and consumption were highest. The low prevalence of current smoking among individuals in this age group reflects the combined effect of smoking cessation efforts and smoking-related mortality. Figure 1-11 shows the trends in smoking cessation rates[8] among four age groups. Individuals age 65 years and older are most likely to have been former smokers, and the cessation rate among individuals in that group has risen dramatically since 1965. However, quit rates have actually declined among adults ages 25 to 44 years since the mid-1990s and have flattened among those ages 18 to 24 years.

Understanding the natural history of smoking (also referred to as the "smoking career") would help tobacco control programs identify the critical ages to be targeted for interventions. Unfortunately, few studies have followed the trajectory of the natural history of smoking from initiation to cessation. Compared with the careers of users of illegal drugs, which peak in the 20s and then trail off by the mid-30s, careers of cigarette smokers follow a different trajectory. This is partly because tobacco is more addictive than most other drugs, and smokers do not mature out of consuming tobacco, possibly because tobacco use doesn't interfere with adult functioning, such as employment (Bachman et al. 2001; Kandel 2002). Unlike age-specific prevalence rates for illegal drug use, those for tobacco use remain elevated and flat beyond the late 20s (Chassin et al. 2000; 1996; Kandel 2002). Chen and Kandel (1995) monitored a cohort of adolescents and found that more than half of males and just under half of females were still smoking at ages 34 and 35, whereas 25.3 percent of males and 14.3 percent of females were using marijuana and 18.2 percent of males and 12.7 percent of females were using other illicit drugs at that same age.

---

[8]Percentage of ever smokers who are former smokers.

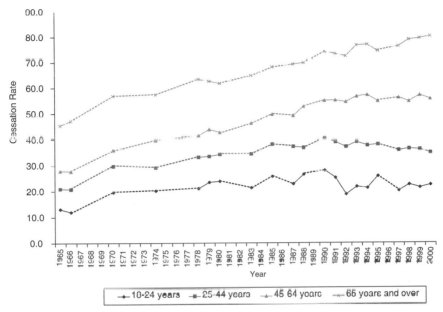

FIGURE 1-11 Age-specific cessation rates of ever smokers, selected years, 1965 to 2000 (all years for which NHIS data on prevalence of cessation are available are included). Solid lines represent changes in cessation prevalence between consecutive years. Dotted lines represent approximate changes in cessation prevalence between nonconsecutive years.
SOURCE: (TIPS 2005a).

It is difficult to predict how long a middle-aged smoker, for example, will continue before quitting, because smoking careers are highly dependent on the age at initiation, the quantity smoked, and the presence of nicotine dependence. Moreover, the quantity smoked, as well as the presence of nicotine dependence, is correlated with the age at initiation. With all else being equal, the older that a person is when he or she starts smoking, the likelihood that he or she will quit is higher and the probability that he or she will become dependent is lower (Hyland et al. 2004; Kandel 2002). Those who are dependent are more than twice as likely as nondependent smokers to continue smoking (Breslau et al. 2001). Hyland and colleagues (2004) found that there was a gradient in the cessation rate by age of initiation: 37.3 percent of those who started smoking when they were age 15 or younger had quit, 41.3 percent of those who started smoking when they were ages 16 to 19 years had quit, and 47.6 percent of those who started smoking when they were older than age 19 years had quit.

Race and Ethnicity

For the majority of years that smoking prevalence has been tracked by race, only African Americans and whites were compared. During many of those years, African American adults were reportedly more likely to be current smokers than were whites. Data from the National Health Interview Survey (NHIS) indicate that this differential may be reversing, starting with a convergence of the rates in the late 1990s and slightly lower rates among African Americans than among whites in the early 2000s. This is likely due to a drop in African American adolescent smoking, which continued into young adult years (CDC 1998). Race-specific smoking rates among adults are presented in Table 1-1. In 2004, approximately 22 percent of non-Hispanic whites and 20 percent of non-Hispanic African Americans were current smokers.

Data collected over the past decade and a half allow the rates of smoking among additional racial and ethnic groups to be identified and compared. Hispanics are less likely to be current smokers than non-Hispanic whites and non-Hispanic African Americans. An estimated 15.0 percent of Hispanic adults were current smokers in 2004, an 11 percent reduction in prevalence since 2002 (CDC 2004b, 2005b). Although Hispanics are less likely than non-Hispanics to be current smokers, Hispanic smokers are less likely to quit. In 2000, the rate of Hispanic smokers who had quit was 42.9 percent, whereas the rate was 49.2 percent among non-Hispanic smokers of all races (ALA 2006).

American Indian and Alaska Natives have the highest prevalence of current smoking in the United States. According to the 2004 NHIS, more than one-third of American Indian and Alaska Native adults currently smoke cigarettes. (Note that the estimates of the prevalence for the American Indian and Alaska Native population are based on small sample sizes and have wide variances. They should be interpreted with some caution.)

Asians have the lowest prevalence of current smoking among adults compared with those for all other racial and ethnic groups. In 2004, 11.3 percent of Asians were current smokers. Asians were 85 percent less likely than the general population of adults to be smokers. Asian women have

TABLE 1-1 Current Smoking Prevalence (Percent) by Race, 2002–2004

	2004	2003	2002
Non-Hispanic white	22.2	22.7	23.6
Non-Hispanic African American	20.2	21.3	22.6
Hispanic	15	16.4	16.7
American Indian or Alaska Native	33.4	39.7	40.8
Asian	11.3	11.7	13.3

SOURCE: (CDC 2004a, 2005b, 2005c).

the lowest prevalence of smoking of any group highlighted in the data: less than 5 percent in 2004 (CDC 2004b, 2005b).

Ethnic differences in smoking behavior are subsumed within the broad racial categories, concealing important differentials that could reflect a negative effect of American acculturation (Shelley et al. 2004). Data from the NSDUH reveal disparities in the rates of smoking among some Asian and Hispanic subgroups (CDC 2004a). In 1999 and 2000, Korean Americans were more likely to smoke than the general population (27.2 versus 26.5 percent), and the prevalence of smoking among Vietnamese-Americans was equal to the overall rate. Among Hispanics, Puerto Ricans were the most likely to smoke, with a prevalence rate of 30.4 percent. Puerto Ricans were the only group of Hispanics to be more likely to smoke than non-Hispanic whites or African Americans (CDC 2004a). Chinese American men were reported to have high rates of smoking in regional studies but not in the national survey (Shelley et al. 2004).

Racial differences in smoking status tend to obscure the depth of racial disparities in health that stem from tobacco smoking. Even though African Americans are no more likely to smoke than whites, they are more likely to from suffer smoking-related mortality than whites (CDC 1998; Gadgeel et al. 2001). Some have suggested that the smoking-related mortality differential between African Americans and whites is because African Americans overwhelmingly smoke menthol cigarettes, which are potentially more addictive (e.g., [IOM 2001]). In 2000, 68.9 percent of African American smokers aged 12 years and older smoked menthol cigarettes, whereas 22.4 percent of white smokers and 29.2 percent of Hispanic smokers smoked menthol cigarettes (Giovino et al. 2004).

Smoking cessation rates for African Americans are lower than those for whites (37.4 percent versus 50.3 percent in 2000) (ALA 2006), although these data might reflect the lag in smoking cessation among African Americans compared to whites. A recent study shows that promotional offers from the tobacco industry may be working to keep African American smokers from quitting. White and colleagues (2006) found that 43.0 percent of African American smokers reported that they used a promotional offer "every time I saw one," whereas the rates were 39.1 percent for whites, 24.3 percent for Hispanics, 31.9 percent for Asian/Pacific Islanders, and 39.6 percent for other groups. Also, African Americans who smoked menthol brands (Newport or Kool) were more than twice as likely to use the promotional coupons as African Americans who smoked other brands (White et al. 2006).

Gender

Men are more likely to smoke than women. On average, men are also more likely to be heavy smokers and to smoke more cigarettes per day

(Giovino 2004). The greater prevalence of smoking among men is evident among groups subdivided by race and ethnicity and has persisted for decades. The gender gap in smoking has narrowed considerably since the 1970s, however (Giovino 2004). Since the mid-1980s, the prevalence of smoking among men and women has declined at similar rates. The difference in quit rates between men and women has also narrowed over time, particularly since the mid-1990s, and the rates are converging (Giovino 2004).

In 2004, 23.4 percent of men and 18.5 percent of women were current smokers.[9] The gender difference is even larger within racial subgroups. Among Hispanics, for example, men are almost twice as likely as women to be smokers (prevalences of 18.9 percent among men and 10.9 percent among women). The rate of smoking among Asian men is almost four times higher than that among Asian women: 17.8 versus 4.8 percent. Differences in current smoking prevalence by gender are smaller among non-Hispanic whites, African Americans, and American Indians and Alaska Natives than among Asians or Hispanics, but are still evident (CDC 2005b).

Educational Attainment and Income

Smokers are increasingly likely to be poor and uneducated. As a result, smoking has contributed significantly to the disparity in the rates of mortality between those with lower levels and those with higher levels of educational attainment (Wong et al. 2002). According to NHIS, adults aged 25 years and over with a general educational development (GED) diploma were more likely to be current smokers than those with any other level of education (CDC 2004b). More than 40 percent of adults with a GED were current smokers in 2005. This group was followed by those who have completed 9 to 11 years of schooling, just under one-third of whom were current smokers. In general, current smoking prevalence decreased with increasing years of education (CDC 2006b).

Individuals whose household incomes are below the poverty threshold are significantly more likely to be smokers than those with incomes at or above the poverty level. In 2005, an estimated 29.9 percent of individuals living below the poverty level reported being a current smoker whereas 20.6 percent of those who had income levels at or above the threshold reported being a current smoker (CDC 2006b).

Dichotomous measures of socioeconomic status (SES) conceal the gradient effect of SES on smoking that has persisted over decades. Gilman and

---

[9]Although data for 2005 has been published by CDC breaking down adult smoking prevalence by gender (23.9 percent of men and 18.1 percent of women were current smokers in 2005), 2005 data on the gender difference among racial subgroups is still unavailable (CDC 2006b).

colleagues (2003) found graduated rates of smoking behavior measures by several indicators of adult and childhood SES,[10] showing that the smoking risk decreased and the rate of cessation increased among those at successively higher levels of SES. They also found that those with lower SES were more likely to initiate smoking, progress to become regular smokers, and sustain a smoking career than those with higher SES.

Figure 1-12 shows the smoking prevalence by four levels of income among the five major racial/ethnicity groups in the United States and among the total population, as estimated by Barbeau and colleagues (2004). The researchers based their findings on data from the 2000 NHIS, which revealed an overall weighted smoking prevalence rate of 25.9 percent. They found that when the smoking rates among all races and ethnicities are taken into account, smoking is the most prevalent among those who are poor (34.7 percent) and nearly poor (34.2 percent), lower among the middle income group (31.4 percent), and the lowest among the higher income sub-population (20.7 percent). Within the total population and among whites and African Americans, there is a clear gradient in smoking prevalence level of income. Those in the higher income classification (representing individuals with annual incomes at 300 percent of the poverty level or higher and comprising 45 percent of the total sample) were significantly less likely to smoke than those at lower income levels. The gradient effect was much less pronounced among the lower-income classifications, although individuals in the middle (those with annual incomes between 200 and 299 percent of the poverty level) income category were less likely to be current smokers than those in the poor and near-poor categories. This phenomenon held true across the total population and among whites and African Americans (Barbeau et al. 2004).

The gradient effect is not evident among other racial/ethnic groups, however. Higher income was not protective against smoking for American Indians and Alaska Natives or Hispanics. For Asians, those in the highest and lowest income categories demonstrated a significantly reduced prevalence of smoking, whereas those in the middle-income category had the highest smoking rates of all groups divided by income levels (Barbeau et al. 2004).

The effects of income and education on smoking behavior are not clear-cut. Data from the 1999 and 2000 National Household Survey on Drug Abuse (NHSDA; NHSDA was renamed the National Survey on Drug Use and Health [NSDUH] in 2002) indicate an interaction between income and educational attainment and their effects on smoking prevalence. Figure 1-13 shows the difference in the ranking of smoking prevalence by educational attainment and various family income levels (SAMHSA 2002). College

---

[10]As indicated by maternal education, parental occupation, and household poverty status.

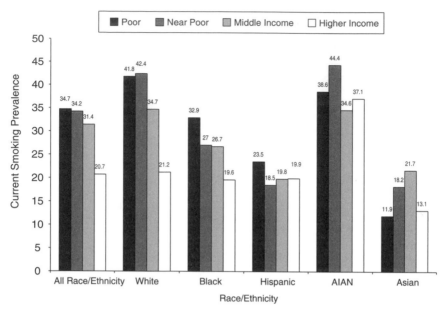

FIGURE 1-12 Adult smoking prevalence rates by race/ethnicity and poverty status.
SOURCE: (Barbeau et al. 2004).

graduates at all income levels are less likely to smoke. People with some college education with the lowest levels of family income (less than $20,000 annually) are the most likely to be smokers, but at higher levels of income, their smoking rates are below those of people with no college education (high school graduates and those who did not graduate from high school). Those who did not graduate from high school with lower income levels are less likely to be smokers than high school graduates and people with some college education. At the high levels of income, however, those who did not graduate from high school are the most likely to smoke.

State of Residence

Smoking prevalence and cessation vary widely by region and state. Regional smoking prevalence rates range from approximately 17 percent in the West to more than 23 percent in the Midwest, according to data from the Tobacco Use Supplement of the Current Population Survey for 2001–2002 (Hartman et al. 2004). Among the four regions defined here, the South has the second highest prevalence of smoking, but it contains three of the six states where smoking is the most prevalent (Kaiser Family Foundation 2006). The West had the highest quit rate according to these data: 39.5 percent of

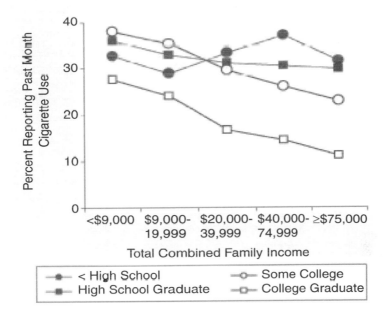

FIGURE 1-13 Prevalence of current cigarette use by family income and educational attainment.

people who have ever smoked reported having some cessation activity[11] in the past year, including quitting. The least cessation activity occurred in the South, where 31.2 percent of ever smokers had cessation activity in the past year. Figures 1-14 and 1-15 provide trends in smoking prevalence and smoking cessation by U.S. state and territory in 2004, respectively.

In 2004, the prevalence of current smoking among adults in 49 states, the District of Columbia, Puerto Rico, and the Virgin Islands was estimated by using data from the Behavior Risk Factor Surveillance Survey (CDC 2005c). Hawaii was excluded from the analysis because of insufficient data. Among the 52 locations for which smoking behavior was described, the current smoking rates varied widely. In the states ranking the highest among current smokers, more than a quarter of the adult population currently smokes. Those states include Kentucky (27.6 percent), West Virginia (26.9

---

[11]Defined as a) daily smokers having one or more (24 hour or longer) quit attempts in the past year, b) current some day smokers who had previously smoked daily about 12 months ago, c) former smokers who quit less than 3 months prior to the interview, and d) former smokers who quit 3 or more months prior to interview.

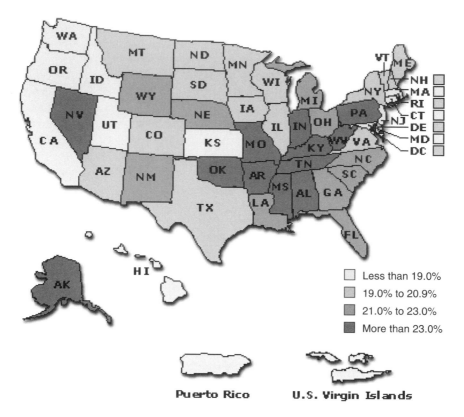

FIGURE 1-14 Smoking prevalence among adults by state or territory, 2005.
SOURCE: (Kaiser Family Foundation 2006). Located at: *http://www.statehealth
facts.org/cgi-bin/healthfacts.cgi?previewid=292&action=compare&category=
Health+Status&subcategory=Smoking&topic=Adult+Smoking+Rate.*

percent), Oklahoma (26.1 percent), Tennessee (26.1 percent), Ohio (25.9 percent), and Arkansas (25.7 percent). The states that ranked the lowest in current smoking had prevalence rates of less than 15 percent. Only two of the contiguous 48 states met this criterion: California with 14.9 percent and Utah with 10.5 percent. Puerto Rico and the Virgin Islands also had very low current smoking prevalence rates: 12.7 and 9.5 percent, respectively.

State-level cessation rates ranged from 42.5 percent in Kentucky to 62.5 percent in Connecticut. Kentucky, the state with the highest smoking prevalence rate, also had the lowest quit rate (CDC 2005c). Of the six states with the lowest quit rates, three (Tennessee with 45.9 percent, Ohio with 49.0 percent, and Kentucky with 46.1 percent) also ranked in the top six in smoking prevalence. All six of the states ranking the highest among current

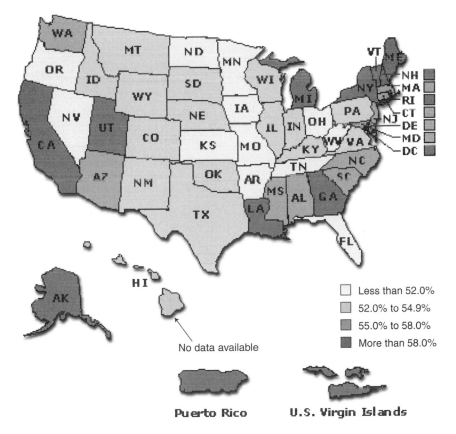

FIGURE 1-15 Smoking cessation prevalence among adults by state or territory, 2004.
SOURCE: (Kaiser Family Foundation 2006). Located at: *http://www.statehealth facts.org/cgi-bin/healthfacts.cgi?previewid=3&action=compare&category=Health+ Status&subcategory=Smoking&topic=Attempts+to+Quit+Smoking.*

smokers had quit rates of less than 50 percent. In the states with the highest quit rates, 60 percent or more of individuals who had ever smoked had quit. These included Utah (60.1 percent), Vermont (60.5 percent), California (62.0 percent), and Connecticut (62.5 percent). All four of these states had smoking prevalence rates at or below 20.0 percent.

Many factors contribute to the differences in the smoking cessation prevalence and smoking cessation rates among states, including the demographic and social characteristics of the state populations. The communities with large percentages of poor populations and populations with low levels of education tend to have the highest prevalence of smoking (Dell et al.

2005). As discussed in Chapter 5, it is likely that variations in the levels of tobacco control activities among the states also account for some of these variations in smoking prevalence. It is widely accepted that California's lower prevalence is attributable at least in part to the intensity of tobacco control efforts in that state (CDC 1996). Kuiper and colleagues (2005) present evidence that comprehensive state programs reduce the prevalence of smoking among adults and adolescents at the state and national levels. Jemal and colleagues (2003) examined comprehensive smoking cessation programs among 33 states and found that the intensity of the program had a very large negative correlation with the prevalence of current smoking ($r = -0.81$, $p < 0.0001$) and a large positive correlation with the quit rate ($r = 0.82$, $p < 0.0001$) among adults ages 30 to 39 years. The impact of comprehensive state tobacco control programs is discussed in more detail in Chapter 5 of this report.

States with a high prevalence of smoking among adults also have high rates of smokers who made no attempt to change their behavior in the last year (Burns and Warner 2003), suggesting that environment plays a role in sustaining smoking behavior or promoting cessation efforts.

Comorbidity

Several recent studies have documented a relationship between mental illness and smoking among adults and adolescents (Black et al. 1999; Lasser et al. 2000; Upadhyaya et al. 2002). As used by Lasser and colleagues (2000), the term "mental illness" in this context is defined very broadly to include major depression, bipolar disorder, dysthymia, panic disorder, agoraphobia, social phobia, simple phobia, generalized anxiety disorder, alcohol abuse, alcohol dependence, drug abuse, drug dependence, antisocial personality, conduct disorder, or nonaffective psychosis (Lasser et al. 2000). Adults who currently experience symptoms of these disorders smoke more than 44 percent of the cigarettes consumed in the United States (Lasser et al. 2000). Lasser and colleagues also found that adults with a lifetime history of mental illness (broadly defined as above) were more likely to be current smokers than adults with no history of mental illness. Adults with mental illnesses manifesting within the past month were the most likely to smoke and the least likely to quit. Figure 1-16 compares the smoking prevalence and cessation rates by mental illness status. The study also revealed that those with a larger number of mental illness comorbidities have a greater likelihood of smoking and a greater tendency to smoke heavily.

EMERGING CHALLENGES

Although the prevalence of smoking among adults continues a 40-year decline, some recent trends suggestive of a flattening in rates of adult smok-

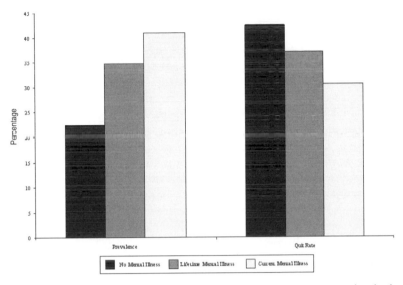

FIGURE 1-16 Current smoking prevalence and quit rates among individuals ages 15 to 54 years by mental illness status.
SOURCE: (Lasser et al. 2000).

ing and cessation raise an important question: Are tobacco control programs confronting a hardening target? The term "hardening" is used in this context to refer to the residual smokers who either resist cessation efforts or who have more difficulty quitting than former smokers (Burns and Warner 2003). For the purposes of this report, the key question is the one posed by a recent National Cancer Institute monograph: Is achieving abstinence harder, and do changes to interventions need to be made? This chapter has identified several subpopulations that appear to pose an elevated risk of lifelong smoking. Because these groups are more likely to continue to smoke despite cessation efforts, it seems likely that more aggressive efforts may be needed to reach them and to change their behavior.

Another potentially worrisome trend is the increase in initiation by young adults (18–24) and a possible increase in occasional smoking that may be associated with it. Such an increase was shown in one national survey (CDC 2005b), but not in another, (see Figure 1-9). Occasional smokers differ from heavier or hard-core smokers in many ways: occasional smokers are more highly educated whereas hard-core smokers have lower levels of education; occasional smokers are more likely to be racial and ethnic minorities whereas hard-core smokers are more likely to be white; and hard-core smokers tend to begin smoking at an earlier age (Augustson and Marcus 2004). Whether an increase in occasional smoking, if it is occurring, signals a more difficult challenge for tobacco control is not altogether clear.

SUMMARY

The phenomenal increase in tobacco use over the course of the 20th century was finally reversed in the wake of the publication of the Surgeon General's important report in 1964. The data reviewed in this chapter suggest that the gradual decline in tobacco use since 1965 can be divided into two phases, the first running from 1965 to about 1980 and the second running from 1980 to the present. During the initial period, there was a sharp decline in smoking prevalence, accompanied by a modest increase in the average number of cigarettes smoked per day by smokers. Since then, however, the continued decline in smoking prevalence has been accompanied by a substantial decline in cigarettes smoked per day among those who smoke. As will be explained in Chapters 3 and 5, the committee believes that a substantial portion of the declines in smoking prevalence and smoking intensity over the past 25 years is attributable to tobacco control interventions, especially price increases and the emergence of a strong antismoking social norm.

In the committee's opinion, the data suggest that the Surgeon General's 1964 report and the dissemination of information on the adverse health effects of smoking had a strong impact on smoking prevalence. However, industry efforts to respond to the health threat of smoking by promoting filtered and so-called "light" cigarettes tended to counteract the effects of antismoking messages and to sustain smoking by those who smoked the most heavily. This interpretation would explain the increase in smoking intensity during this initial phase of tobacco control activity. During the second phase of tobacco control efforts, however, the tobacco industry's dominance of the playing field was finally challenged by strong advocacy at the local and state levels and by significant increases in price. These efforts not only sustained the downward trend in prevalence but also helped to cut down on the intensity of smoking among a significant portion of smokers.

If this overall interpretation is correct, it suggests that continued implementation of strong tobacco control interventions will be needed to sustain progress. However, it also tends to highlight some important warning signs. First, tobacco control efforts will need to address the needs of a residual population of smokers who are particularly difficult to influence (e.g., smokers with mental illness). Second, a disturbing increase in later-onset, less frequent smoking by 18- to 25-year-olds could portend a growing cohort of new smokers who may be overlooked by traditional prevention programs for teens and by traditional cessation programs developed for older smokers. Finally, the volatile and frequently high rate of initiation of smoking among teens poses a continuing obstacle to society's long-term goal of reducing the public health burden of tobacco use.

REFERENCES

ALA (American Lung Association). 2004. Trends in Tobacco Use. New York: American Lung Association.

ALA. 2006. Trends in Tobacco Use. New York: American Lung Association.

Arnett JJ. 1999. Winston's "No Additives" campaign: "straight up"? "No bull"? *Public Health Reports* 114(6):522-527.

Augustson E, Marcus S. 2004. Use of the current population survey to characterize subpopulations of continued smokers: a national perspective on the "hardcore" smoker phenomenon. *Nicotine and Tobacco Research* 6(4):621-629.

Bachman JG, O'Malley PM, Johnston LD, Schulenberg JE, Ludden AB, Merline AC. 2001. *The Decline of Substance Use in Young Adulthood: Changes in Social Activities, Roles, and Beliefs.* Research Monographs in Adolescence. Mahwah, NJ: Lawrence Erlbaum Associates, Inc.

Barbeau EM, Krieger N, Soobader MJ. 2004. Working class matters: socioeconomic disadvantage, race/ethnicity, gender, and smoking in NHIS 2000. *American Journal of Public Health* 94(2):269-278.

Black DW, Zimmerman M, Coryell WH. 1999. Cigarette smoking and psychiatric disorder in a community sample. *Annals of Clinical Psychiatry* 11(3):129-136.

Brandt AM. 2007. *The Cigarette Century: The Rise, Fall, and Deadly Persistence of the Product That Defined America.* New York: Basic Books.

Breslau N, Johnson EO, Hiripi E, Kessler R. 2001. Nicotine dependence in the United States: prevalence, trends, and smoking persistence. *Archives of General Psychiatry* 58(9):810-816.

Bulow J, Klemperer P. 1998. The tobacco deal. Brookings Papers on Economic Activity. *Microeconomics* 1998:323-394.

Burns DM, Lee L, Shen LZ, Gilpin E, Tolley HD, Vaughn J, Shanks TG. 1997. *Cigarette smoking behavior in the United States. Changes in Cigarette Related Disease Risks and Their Implication for Prevention and Control. Smoking and Tobacco Control Monograph No. 8.* Bethesda, MD: DHHS, National Institutes of Health, National Cancer Institute. Pp. 13-112.

Burns DM, Major JM, Shanks TG. 2003. *Changes in Number of Cigarettes Smoked per Day: Cross-Sectional and Birth Cohort Analyses Using NHIS. Those Who Continue to Smoke: Is Achieving Abstinence Harder and Do We Need to Change Our Approach? Smoking and Tobacco Control Monograph 15.* Bethesda, MD: U.S. Department of Health and Human Services, National Institutes of Health, National Cancer Institute. Pp. 83-99.

Burns DM, Warner KE. 2003. *Smokers who have not quit: is cessation more difficult and should we change our strategies? Those Who Continue to Smoke: Is Achieving Abstinence Harder and Do We Need to Change Our Approach? Smoking and Tobacco Control Monograph 15.* Bethesda, MD: U.S. Department of Health and Human Services, National Institutes of Health, National Cancer Institute. Pp. 11–32.

Capehart T. 2004. *The Changing Tobacco User's Dollar.* Washington, DC: Economic Research Service, U.S. Department of Agriculture.

Capehart T. 2005. *Tobacco Outlook: Tobacco Acreage Plunges for 2005 Crop Year.* Washington, DC: Economic Research Service, U.S. Department of Agriculture.

CDC (Centers for Disease Control and Prevention). 1994. Changes in the cigarette brand preferences of adolescent smokers—United States, 1989–1993. *MMWR (Morbidity and Mortality Weekly Report)* 43(32):577-581.

CDC. 1996. Cigarette smoking before and after an excise tax increase and an antismoking campaign—Massachusetts, 1990–1996. *MMWR (Morbidity and Mortality Weekly Report)* 45(44):966-970.

CDC. 1998. Tobacco use among US racial/ethnic minority groups, A report of the Surgeon General, 1998, Executive Summary. *Tobacco Control* 7:198–209.

CDC. 2003. Cigarette smoking among adults—United States, 2001. *MMWR. (Morbidity and Mortality Weekly Report)* 52(40):953–980.

CDC. 2004a. Prevalence of cigarette use among 14 racial/ethnic populations—United States, 1999–2001. *MMWR. (Morbidity and Mortality Weekly Report)* 53(3):49–52.

CDC. 2004b. Cigarette smoking among adults—United States, 2002. *Journal of the American Osteopathic Association* 104(8):324–327.

CDC. 2005a. Cigarette smoking among adults—United States, 2003. *MMWR (Morbidity and Mortality Weekly Report)* 54(20):509–528.

CDC. 2005b. Cigarette smoking among adults—United States, 2004. *MMWR (Morbidity and Mortality Weekly Report)* 54(44):1121-1124.

CDC. 2005c. State-specific prevalence of cigarette smoking and quitting among adults—United States, 2004. *MMWR (Morbidity and Mortality Weekly Report)* 54(44):1124-1127.

CDC. 2006a. Cigarette use among high school students—United States, 1991–2005. *MMWR (Morbidity and Mortality Weekly Report)* 55(26):724-726.

CDC. 2006b. Tobacco use among adults—United States, 2005. *MMWR (Morbidity and Mortality Weekly Report)* 55(42):1145-1148.

Chaloupka FJ, Cummings KM, Morley CP, Horan JK. 2002. Tax, price and cigarette smoking: evidence from the tobacco documents and implications for tobacco company marketing strategies. *Tobacco Control* 11(Suppl 1):I62-I72.

Chassin L, Presson CC, Pitts SC, Sherman SJ. 2000. The natural history of cigarette smoking from adolescence to adulthood in a midwestern community sample: multiple trajectories and their psychosocial correlates. *Health Psychology* 19(3):223-231.

Chassin L, Presson CC, Rose JS, Sherman SJ. 1996. The natural history of cigarette smoking from adolescence to adulthood: demographic predictors of continuity and change. *Health Psychology* 15(6):478-484.

Chen K, Kandel DB. 1995. The natural history of drug use from adolescence to the mid-thirties in a general population sample. *American Journal of Public Health* 85(1):41-47.

Dell JL, Whitman S, Shah AM, Silva A, Ansell D. 2005. Smoking in 6 diverse Chicago communities—a population study. *American Journal of Public Health* 95(6):1036-1042.

DHHS (U.S. Department of Health and Human Services). 2000a. *Reducing Tobacco Use: A Report of the Surgeon General.* Atlanta, GA: DHHS, CDC, National Center for Chronic Disease Prevention and Health Promotion, Office on Smoking and Health.

DHHS. 2000b. *Reducing Tobacco Use: A Report of the Surgeon General.* Atlanta, GA DHHS.

DiFranza JR, Richards JW, Paulman PM, Wolf-Gillespie N, Fletcher C, Jaffe RD, Murray D. 1991. RJR Nabisco's cartoon camel promotes camel cigarettes to children. *Journal of the American Medical Association* 266(22):3149-3153.

Ernster VL. 1985. Mixed messages for women. A social history of cigarette smoking and advertising. *New York State Journal of Medicine* 85(7):335-340.

FTC (Federal Trade Commission). 2005. *Cigarette Report for 2003.* Washington, DC: FTC.

FTC. 2007. *Cigarette Report for 2004 and 2005.* Washington, DC: FTC.

Gadgeel SM, Severson RK, Kau Y, Graff J, Weiss LK, Kalemkerian GP. 2001. Impact of race in lung cancer: analysis of temporal trends from a surveillance, epidemiology, and end results database. *Chest* 120(1):55-63.

Gardiner PS. 2004. The African Americanization of menthol cigarette use in the United States. *Nicotine and Tobacco Research* 6(Suppl 1):S55-S65.

Gilman SE, Abrams DB, Buka SL. 2003. Socioeconomic status over the life course and stages of cigarette use: initiation, regular use, and cessation. *Journal of Epidemiology and Community Health* 57(10):802-808.

Giovino GA. 2002. Epidemiology of tobacco use in the United States. *Oncogene* 21(48): 7326-7340.

Giovino GA. 2004. *Epidemiology of Tobacco Use in the United States*. PowerPoint Presentation presented to the IOM meeting Reducing Tobacco Use.

Giovino GA, Sidney S, Gfroerer JC, O'Malley PM, Allen JA, Richter PA, Cummings KM. 2004. Epidemiology of menthol cigarette use. *Nicotine and Tobacco Research* 6(Suppl 1):S67-S81.

Giovino GA, Tomar SL, Reddy MN, Peddicord JP, Zhu B-P, Escobedo LG, Friksen MP. 1996. *Attitudes, knowledge, and beliefs about low-yield cigarettes among adolescents*. National Cancer Institute. The FTC Cigarette Test Method for Determining Tar, Nicotine, and Carbon Monoxide Yields of U.S. Cigarettes (Smoking and Tobacco Control, Monograph 7). Bethesda, MD: National Institutes of Health. Pp. 39-57.

Gruber J. 2001. Tobacco at the crossroads: the past and future of smoking regulation in the United States. *The Journal of Economic Perspectives* 15(2):193-212.

Hamilton JL. 1972. The demand for cigarettes: advertising, health scare, and the cigarette advertising ban. *Review of Economics and Statistics* 54:401-411.

Hartman A, Willis G, Lawrence D, Gibson JT. 2004. *The 2001–2002 Tobacco Use Supplement to the Current Population Survey (TUS-CPS): Representative Survey Findings*. Web Page. Available at: http://riskfactor.cancer.gov/studies/tus-cps/results/data9899/cps_results.pdf.

Havrilesky T, Barth R. 1969. Tests of market share stability in the cigarette industry 1950–1966. *The Journal of Industrial Economics* 17(2):145-150.

Hyland A, Li Q, Bauer JE, Giovino GA, Steger C, Cummings KM. 2004. Predictors of cessation in a cohort of current and former smokers followed over 13 years. *Nicotine and Tobacco Research* 6(Suppl 3):S363-S369.

IOM (Institute of Medicine). 1994. *Growing Up Tobacco Free: Preventing Nicotine Addiction in Children and Youth*. Washington, DC: National Academy Press.

IOM. 2001. *Clearing the Smoke: Assessing the Science Base for Tobacco Harm Reduction*. Washington, DC: National Academy Press.

Jemal A, Cokkinides VE, Shafey O, Thun MJ. 2003. Lung cancer trends in young adults: an early indicator of progress in tobacco control (United States). *Cancer Causes and Control* 14(6):579-585.

Johnston LD, O'Malley PM, Bachman JG, Schulenberg JE. 2006. *Monitoring the Future: National Results on Adolescent Drug Use: Overview of Key Findings, 2005*. (NIH Publication No. 07-6202). Bethesda, MD: National Institute on Drug Abuse. P. 71.

Johnston LD, O'Malley PM, Bachman JG, Schulenberg JE. 2007. *Monitoring the Future: National Results on Adolescent Drug Use: Overview of Key Findings, 2006*. (NIH Publication No. 07-6202). Bethesda, MD: National Institute on Drug Abuse.

Kaiser Family Foundation. 2006. *Percent of Adults Who Are Smokers, 2004*. Web Page. Available at: http://www.statehealthfacts.kff.org/cgi-binhealthfacts.cgi?action=compare&category=Health+Status&subcategory=Smoking&topic=Smoking+Rate; accessed April 3, 2006.

Kandel DB. 2002. *Natural History of Smoking and Nicotine Dependence*. In The Royal Society of Canada, ed. Proceedings of the Royal Society of Canada 2002 Symposium on Addictions: Impact on Canada. Ottawa, Ontario: Royal Society of Canada.

Krugman DM, Quinn WH, Sung Y, Morrison M. 2005. Understanding the role of cigarette promotion and youth smoking in a changing marketing environment. *Journal of Health Communication* 10(3):261-278.

Kuiper NM, Nelson DE, Schooley M. 2005. *Evidence of Effectiveness: A Summary of State Tobacco Control Program Evaluation Literature*. Atlanta, GA: DHHS, CDC, National Center for Chronic Disease Prevention and Health Promotion, Office on Smoking and Health.

74   ENDING THE TOBACCO PROBLEM

Lasser K, Boyd JW, Woolhandler S, Himmelstein DU, McCormick D, Bor DH. 2000. Smoking and mental illness: a population-based prevalence study. *Journal of the American Medical Association* 284(20):2606-2610.

Mendez D, Warner KE. 2004. Adult cigarette smoking prevalence: declining as expected (not as desired). *American Journal of Public Health* 94(2):251-252.

National Center for Health Statistics. 2005. *Health, United States, 2005.* Hyattsville, MD: U.S. Government Printing Office.

National Center for Health Statistics. 2006. *Health, United States, 2006.* Hyattsville, MD: U.S. Government Printing Office.

Pierce JP, Gilpin EA, Choi WS. 1999. Sharing the blame: smoking experimentation and future smoking-attributable mortality due to Joe Camel and Marlboro advertising and promotions. *Tobacco Control* 8(1):37-44.

Pierce JP, Lee L, Gilpin EA. 1994. Smoking initiation by adolescent girls, 1944 through 1988. An association with targeted advertising. *Journal of the American Medical Association* 271(8):608-611.

Pollay RW, Dewhirst T. 2002. The dark side of marketing seemingly "Light" cigarettes: successful images and failed fact. *Tobacco Control* 11(Suppl 1):I18-I131.

R.J. Reynolds. 2006. *R.J. Reynolds Tobacco Company History.* Web Page. Available at: http://www.brownandwilliamson.com/company/profileHistory.aspx; accessed April 5, 2006.

SAMHSA (Substance Abuse and Mental Health Services Administration). 2002. *The NHSDA Report: Tobacco Use, Income, and Educational Level.* Web Page. Available at: http://oas.samhsa.gov/2k2/Tob/tob.pdf; accessed May 19, 2006.

SAMHSA. 2005. *Table 4.18A Numbers (in Thousands) of Persons Who Initiated Cigarette Use in the United States, Their Mean Age at First Use, and Rates at First Use (Per 1,000 Person-Years of Exposure): 1965-2003, Based on 2002-2004 NSDUHs.* Web Page. Available at: http://oas.samhsa.gov/NSDUH/2k4nsduh/2k4tabs/Sect4peTabs1to50.htm#tab4.18a; accessed May 18, 2006.

SAMHSA. 2006. *Results from the 2005 National Survey on Drug Use and Health: National Findings.* Web Page. Available at: http://oas.samhsa.gov/nsduh/2k5nsduh/2k5results.pdf; accessed November 28, 2006.

Schoenberg EH. 1933. The demand curve for cigarettes. *The Journal of Business of the University of Chicago* 6(1):15-35.

Shelley D, Fahs M, Scheinmann R, Swain S, Qu J, Burton D. 2004. Acculturation and tobacco use among Chinese Americans. *American Journal of Public Health* 94(2):300-307.

TIPS (Tobacco Information and Prevention Source). 2005a. *Percentage of Adult Ever Smokers Who Are Former Smokers (Prevalence of Cessation), Overall and by Sex, Race, Hispanic Origin, Age, and Education, National Health Interview Surveys, Selected Years-United States, 1965–2000.* Web Page. Available at: http://www.cdc.gov/tobacco/research_data/adults_prev/adstat4print.htm; accessed October 26, 2006.

TIPS. 2005b. *Percentage of Adults Who Were Current, Former, or Never Smokers, Overall and by Sex, Race, Hispanic Origin, Age, and Education, Ever Smokers Who Are Former Smokers (Prevalence of Cessation), Overall and by Sex, Race, Hispanic Origin, Age, and Education, National Health Interview Surveys, Selected Years-United States, 1965–2000.* Web Page. Available at: http://www.cdc.gov/TOBACCO/research_data/adults_prev/adstat1.htm; accessed December 1, 2006.

TIPS. 2006. *Smoking Prevalence Among U.S. Adults.* Web Page. Available at: http://www.cdc.gov/tobacco/research_data/adults_prev/prevali.htm; accessed December 7, 2006.

Upadhyaya HP, Deas D, Brady KT, Kruesi M. 2002. Cigarette smoking and psychiatric co-morbidity in children and adolescents. *Journal of the American Academy of Child and Adolescent Psychiatry* 41(11):1294-1305.

White VM, White MM, Freeman K, Gilpin EA, Pierce JP. 2006. Cigarette promotional offers who takes advantage? *American Journal of Preventive Medicine* 30(3):225-231.

Wong MD, Shapiro MF, Boscardin WJ, Ettner SL. 2002. Contribution of major diseases to disparities in mortality. *New England Journal of Medicine* 347(20):1585 1592.

2

Factors Perpetuating the Tobacco Problem

Over the past 40 years, much progress has been made in reducing the number of individuals who initiate tobacco use and in increasing the percentage of tobacco users who have quit. Current trends, however, indicate that reductions in the initiation of tobacco use have slowed and that the annual rate of cessation among smokers remains fairly low. This chapter provides an overview of the factors that impede additional progress and suggests that substantial and sustained efforts will be required to further reduce the prevalence of tobacco use and thereby reduce tobacco-related morbidity and mortality summarized in the introduction of this report and in numerous Surgeon General reports (see Box 2-1). First and foremost, tobacco products are highly addictive because they contain nicotine, one of the most addictive substances used by humans. Nicotine's addictive power thus poses significant challenges to smoking cessation efforts at both the individual and the population levels. Second, factors such as distorted risk and harm perceptions, which are associated with the initiation and maintenance of tobacco use among young smokers, pose a continuing obstacle for prevention and control strategies. Finally, the apparent concentration of heavy smoking among populations with particular vulnerabilities and a possible emerging trend toward the later onset of less frequent smoking suggest that new approaches and strategies may be needed to reduce the prevalence of tobacco use on a permanent basis.

NATURE OF NICOTINE ADDICTION

Nicotine is considered a highly addictive substance (DHHS 1988; Royal College of Physicians 2000; WHO 2003). The science base supporting this

BOX 2-1 Surgeon General's Reports on Tobacco Use 1964–2006

1964 Smoking and Health: Report of the Advisory Committee to the Surgeon General of the Public Health Service

1967 The Health Consequences of Smoking: A Public Health Service Review

1968 The Health Consequences of Smoking: 1968 Supplement to the 1967 Public Health Service Review

1969 The Health Consequences of Smoking: 1969 Supplement to the 1967 Public Health Service Review

1971 The Health Consequences of Smoking: A Report of the Surgeon General

1972 The Health Consequences of Smoking: A Report of the Surgeon General

1973 The Health Consequences of Smoking

1974 The Health Consequences of Smoking

1975 The Health Consequences of Smoking

1976 The Health Consequences of Smoking: Selected Chapters from 1971 through 1975

1978 The Health Consequences of Smoking, 1977–1978

1979 Smoking and Health: A Report of the Surgeon General

1980 The Health Consequences of Smoking for Women: A Report of the Surgeon General

1981 The Health Consequences of Smoking—The Changing Cigarette: A Report of the Surgeon General

1982 The Health Consequences of Smoking—Cancer: A Report of the Surgeon General

1983 The Health Consequences of Smoking—Cardiovascular Disease: A Report of the Surgeon General

1984 The Health Consequences of Smoking—Chronic Obstructive Lung Disease: A Report of the Surgeon General

1985 The Health Consequences of Smoking—Cancer and Chronic Lung Disease in the Workplace: A Report of the Surgeon General

1986 The Health Consequences of Involuntary Smoking: A Report of the Surgeon General

1988 The Health Consequences of Smoking—Nicotine Addiction: A Report of the Surgeon General

1989 Reducing the Health Consequences of Smoking—25 Years of Progress: A Report of the Surgeon General

1990 The Health Benefits of Smoking Cessation: A Report of the Surgeon General

1992 Smoking and Health in the Americas: A Report of the Surgeon General

1994 Preventing Tobacco Use Among Young People: A Report of the Surgeon General

1998 Tobacco Use Among U.S. Racial/Ethnic Minority Groups

2000 Reducing Tobacco Use: A Report of the Surgeon General

2001 Women and Smoking: A Report of the Surgeon General

2004 The Health Consequences of Smoking: A Report of the Surgeon General

2006 The Health Consequences of Involuntary Exposure to Tobacco Smoke: A Report of the Surgeon General

SOURCE: (CDC 2006).

claim has been reviewed in-depth by the Institute of Medicine (IOM) in its 2001 report, Clearing the Smoke: Assessing the Science Base for Tobacco Harm Reduction (IOM 2001), and by the U.S. Department of Health and Human Services in the 1988 Surgeon General's report, The Health Consequences of Smoking: Nicotine Addiction (DHHS 1988). These reports highlight the research literature showing that nicotine, through a complex set of mechanisms and actions that affect the neurochemistry of the brain, establishes and maintains dependence on tobacco use. The evidence derives from animal and human studies, from molecular biology and neurochemistry to behavioral studies. The evidence, in fact, is overwhelming. One of the main implications of addiction is the loss of control of drug (nicotine) use. This means that when a person would like to stop or reduce the level of consumption of an addictive drug, like nicotine, it is difficult to do so.

Physical dependence on nicotine is associated with psychoactive as well as positive and negative reinforcing effects, the development of tolerance, and the experience of withdrawal symptoms. Dependence is associated with direct and indirect effects of nicotine on brain neurotransmitters, which are directly related to the behaviors associated with addiction and withdrawal. In addition, behavioral factors, including conditioning, play an important role along with the neurochemical effects. Finally, there are some physiological effects of cigarette smoke independent of the nicotine that might contribute to the overall pleasure and addictive properties of nicotine.

Nicotine from cigarette smoke is rapidly absorbed in the lungs, from which it is quickly passed into the brain. Nicotine exerts its actions by binding to nicotinic cholinergic receptors (nAChRs) in the brain (Dani and De Biasi 2001). Composed of five subunits, the main receptor mediating nicotine dependence is believed to be the $\alpha 4\beta 2$ nicotinic cholinergic receptor. Mice lacking the $\beta 2$ subunit gene do not self-administer nicotine, nor do they exhibit other behavioral effects associated with nicotine exposure. The $\alpha 4$ subunit is associated with nicotine sensitivity. Mutations of that subunit lead to increased sensitivity to nicotine-induced reward behaviors as well as to effects on tolerance and sensitization (Tapper et al. 2004).

Nicotine affects many neurotransmitter systems: dopamine, norepinephrine, acetylcholine, serotonin, γ-aminobutyric acid, glutamate, and endorphins. The major effect of nicotine is to stimulate release of these transmitters. The result of dopamine release is critical to the reinforcing effects of nicotine and occur in the mesolimbic area, the corpus striatum, and the frontal cortex. A pathway of particular importance to drug-induced reward involves the dopaminergic neurons in the ventral tegmental area of the midbrain and the release of dopamine in the shell of the nucleus accumbens. Dopamine release signals a pleasurable experience. For example, the threshold for intracranial self-stimulation in rats, a model for brain reward, is lowered acutely with nicotine exposure, indicating greater reward.

As would be expected with substances associated with tolerance and addictive properties, neuroadaptation occurs with chronic nicotine exposure. A suspected biological correlate of this is an increase in nAChRs in the brain. This increase is thought to reflect nicotine-mediated desensitization, meaning that more nicotine is required to deliver the same neurochemical effect. For example, nicotine withdrawal in rodent models is associated with increased threshold for intracranial self-stimulation, indicating reduced reward due to inadequate dopamine release. Independent of nicotine effects, cigarette smoking is associated with decreased activity of monoamine oxidase enzymes in the brain, which are associated with the degradation of dopamine. Inhibition of monoamine oxidase activity would augment nicotine effects of increasing dopamine levels and contribute to positive reinforcement, tolerance, and addiction.

As most smokers report, stopping smoking is acutely associated with withdrawal symptoms of irritability, restlessness, anxiety, problems getting along with friends and family, difficulties concentrating, increased hunger and eating, and cravings for tobacco. Another symptom is the lack of pleasure or enjoyment, known as anhedonia. These symptoms are believed to be due to the relative deficiency in dopamine release, related to nicotine-mediated changes in receptor function and structure. Nicotine addiction is thus sustained by a combination of positive effects of nicotine on neurotransmitter levels related to pleasure and arousal, the dampening effect of those pleasure or reward mechanisms over time, and the need for continued nicotine exposure to avoid the negative affects related to the decreased neurotransmitter levels, particularly that of dopamine, that would occur without nicotine. However, in addition to the pharmacological mechanisms of nicotine, conditioning is also thought to play an important role in tobacco addiction.

With regular drug use, specific moods or other environmental factors, known as "cues," become associated with the pleasurable or rewarding effects of the drug. This association between the cues and the anticipated pleasure associated with the drug, known as conditioning, is a powerful contributor to addiction (O'Brien 2001). Smoking is maintained in part by conditioning. For example, smoking becomes associated with specific behaviors, such as drinking a cup of coffee or alcohol. Repetition of these coexisting behaviors over time leads to the behavior becoming a cue the person to want to smoke. Behaviors can be conditioned to either the positive or negative reinforcing effects of nicotine. For example, because smoking becomes associated with relieving the negative affects of nicotine withdrawal, the smoker can associate smoking with relieving other negative feelings, such as stress. Managing conditioned behaviors is often an important factor in the success of nicotine cessation.

Smoking also facilitates nicotine dependence through sensorimotor factors associated with the act of smoking. Several studies have found that sensorimotor factors play an important role in maintaining smoking behavior in some smokers (Brauer et al. 2001; Naqvi and Bechara 2005; Rose 2006; Rose et al. 2000, 2003). A number of researchers, including Rose and colleagues, have used nicotinized and denicotinized cigarettes to study the separate roles of pharmacological actions of nicotine and the sensory/behavioral aspects of cigarette smoking on smoking withdrawal and smoking behavior (Rose et al. 2000). The results of those studies indicate that smoking denicotinized cigarettes can produce satisfaction as well as psychological rewards and can reduce the craving sensations. This finding is consistent with reports from smokers who described positive feelings as they inhale cigarette smoke but who do not experience these feelings when these sensory effects are blocked (Rose 1988; Rose et al. 1999). It has been suggested that the stimulation of nicotinic receptors on vagal nerve endings in the respiratory tract plays a role in mediating the immediate subjective effects of cigarette smoking (Rose et al. 1999).

The findings from this body of work thus suggest that airway sensory replacement may be an important aspect to be considered when determining the smoking cessation strategies to be used for some smokers (Rose et al. 1999; Westman et al. 1995).

In recent years, a body of research literature on the genetics of tobacco use has emerged. Over the past decade, researchers have cast some light on the role of genetic factors in tobacco use and dependence (Hall et al. 2002; Kendler et al. 1999; Lerman and Berrettini 2003; Li 2003, 2006; Madden et al. 1999; Sullivan and Kendler 1999). A review of a number of studies with twins suggests a significant genetic component in the initiation and maintenance of tobacco use (Kendler et al. 1999; Sullivan and Kendler 1999). On the basis of findings from studies of families, adopted children, and twins, Sullivan and Kendler estimate that a genetic influence may contribute approximately 60 percent to the possibility of smoking initiation, with environmental and personal influences contributing the remainder (Sullivan and Kendler 1999). Genetic influences are also estimated to contribute significantly (about 70 percent) to nicotine dependence.

Tyndale (2003), meanwhile, has reported on differences in the estimates of genetic influences on smoking initiation by gender, with rates ranging from 32 to 70 percent among females and 31 to 61 percent among males (Tyndale 2003). Estimates of the genetic influence on smoking persistence range from 4 to 49 percent among females and from 50 to 71 percent among males. Additional studies indicate that the age of smoking onset, the amount smoked, and smoking persistence are also influenced by genetics (Heath et al. 1999; Koopmans et al. 1999; Madden et al. 1999).

The number of studies that have assessed the role of specific genes in smoking behavior continues to grow. The work of Malaiyandi and colleagues (2005), for example, suggests that cytochrome P450 (CYP) 2A6, the liver enzyme which mediates the conversion of nicotine to cotinine, may play an important role in smoking (Malaiyandi et al. 2005). In a review of recent genetic studies of nicotine dependence, Li (2006) presents evidence that several genes may be implicated in nicotine dependence (Li 2006). Some of these genes include gamma-aminobutyric acid 2, which modulates neuronal excitability; nicotinic acetylcholine receptor alpha4, (CHRNA4), which modulates tolerance to nicotine; decarboxylase and brain-derived neurotropic factor, which influence dopamine and serotonin, which play important roles in the reward system of addiction; and the catechol-O-methyltransferase gene, which plays a role in the dopaminergic circuits central to the reward system. These and future studies of the role of genetic influences on smoking have the potential to further the understanding of nicotine addiction and its treatment.

The role of genetics in identifying the best treatment strategies for subgroups of smokers is another important emerging area of research. Pharmacogenetics researchers have examined a variety of polymorphisms and gene variances in smokers and their response to a number of current and widely used cessation pharmacotherapies for nicotine dependence. The results of these studies suggest that specific subgroups of smokers have a significantly higher probability of abstinence when they use nicotine patches, nicotine nasal spray, and bupropion treatment (Lerman et al. 2002, 2004; Swan et al. 2005). However, these studies generally involve small numbers of subjects and the genetic associations need to be replicated. It is expected that continuing research in this area will provide results that can better guide clinicians in selecting the best treatment options for individuals who want to quit smoking and will aid the in development of new drug targets that will help in cessation (Lee and Tyndale 2006).

SMOKING CESSATION

Once the grip of nicotine addiction has taken hold, quitting is hard. Epidemiological data from the 2004 National Health Interview Survey (NHIS) suggest that of the 44.5 million U.S. adults who were current smokers, about 40.5 percent (or 14.6 million) of smokers reported that they had stopped smoking for at least 1 day in the preceding 12 months in an effort to quit (CDC 2005b). Although the number of smokers who attempt to quit is significant, actual quit rates are about 5 percent, and in studies that include biochemical verification of abstention, the actual quit rate is about 3 percent (Shiffman 2004). Some researchers suggest that each year only about 2 percent of smokers will quit permanently (Hughes 2003;

Shiffman 2004). Eventually, however, 50 percent of individuals who have ever smoked will quit (CDC 2005a).

Many smokers regret having engaged in smoking behavior. One major study of smokers in four countries (the United States, Canada, the United Kingdom, and Australia) found an overwhelming high level of regret among adult smokers (about 90 percent). This finding was consistent across the four countries (Fong et al. 2004). Regret was defined as responses of strong agreement and agreement with the statement "If you had to do it over again, you would not have started smoking." Although the overall level of regret was high, it was more likely to be experienced by older smokers, women, and those who had tried to quit more often.

With such high levels of regret, it is not surprising that 70 percent of smokers report an interest in quitting (Fiore et al. 2000; Hughes 1999; Hymowitz et al. 1997). Interest in quitting, however, does not translate into immediate plans or actions to quit (Larabie 2005). When smokers interested in quitting are queried about their specific plans to quit, only 10 to 20 percent report a plan to quit in the next month (Etter et al. 1997). Eventually, however, about 70 percent of smokers will make at least one quit attempt (Fiore et al. 2000).

Individuals who contemplate taking steps to quit often engage in a process of weighing the pros and cons of smoking (Velicer et al. 1999). In a comprehensive review of the literature spanning five decades, McCaul and colleagues found that the primary factor motivating smokers to quit is a health concern (McCaul et al. 2006). This finding was robust across retrospective studies of former smokers, cross-sectional studies of current smokers, and prospective studies of smokers in cessation studies. Health concerns were also reported as a primary motivating factor among smokers in the Community Intervention Trial for Smoking Cessation (COMMIT) cohort study of smokers monitored for 13 years. Smokers who had made one serious attempt to quit in the period from 1993 to 2001 reported the most common reasons for quitting were concerns for current and future health (92 percent), expense (59 percent), concern for effects on others (56 percent), and setting a good example for children (52 percent) (Hyland et al. 2004). These results are similar to those found in an early COMMIT survey (1988 to 1993) (Hymowitz et al. 1997).

Physicians are in a unique position to encourage smoking cessation by their patients (Fiore et al. 2000; Russell et al. 1979; Schroeder 2005). Physician counseling and intervention are estimated to double the likelihood of quitting (Goldstein et al. 1997). Many physicians, however, miss clinical opportunities to counsel patients. Schroeder (2005) notes that only a minority of physicians are aware of and implement the 5 A's (ask, advise, assess, assist, and arrange) of cessation treatment.

A number of factors may contribute to physicians' limited participation in encouraging patients to stop smoking. External factors such as time constraints, lack of financial incentives, or reimbursement for cessation services can be a hindrance (Schroeder 2005), as can the lack of smoking cessation educational resources in the practice setting or in the community (Tremblay M et al. 2001). Physicians' lack of knowledge, expertise, or skill in smoking cessation, as well as their negative beliefs and perceptions regarding their role in getting patients to quit have also been noted (Schroeder 2005; Tremblay et al. 2001). Physicians, for example, may believe that patients can't quit or do not fully understand that patients may try and fail a number of times before they are successful at quitting. Physicians may also fear a negative response from a patient if quitting smoking is addressed in the clinical visit (Schroeder 2005). Strategies to support physicians in engaging patients to quit smoking need to be identified and tested. Schroeder (2005), for example suggests a shortcut option encouraging physicians to ask, advise, and refer. Such strategies, however, will require enhanced support for community resources available for referral, such as quitlines.

Stages of Change

The desire or intention to quit smoking, along with an eventual attempt to quit smoking, has been viewed by many researchers as a series of transitional change stages by proponents of the transtheoretical model of change. The stages of change include precontemplation, contemplation, preparation, action, and maintenance (Prochaska and DiClemente 1983). Early studies that used the model found that cessation activity differed substantially by stage of change and that stages of change were, in turn, predictive of quit attempts and the success of quitting at 1 and 6 months (DiClemente et al. 1991).

Wewers and colleagues (using data from Current Populations Surveys conducted in 1992–1993, 1995–1996, and 1998–1999) used the Stages-of-Change Model to study movement in the readiness to quit among Americans in the 1990s (Wewers et al. 2003). The percentage of individuals in each stage of change over the three survey periods ranged from 63.7 to 59.1 in the precontemplation stage (not seriously thinking of stopping within the next 6 months), 33.2 to 28.7 percent in the contemplation stage (planning on quitting in the next 6 months but not in the next 30 days or planning on quitting in the next 30 days but making no quitting attempts in the past 12 months), and 9.3 to 7.7 percent in the preparation stage (planning on quitting in the next 30 days and making a quit attempt of at least 24 hours duration in the past 12 months). Overall, the study results indicated very little movement in the stages of readiness to change among the U.S. population in the 1990s.

Some surveys examining the stages of change and quitting have described mixed results. Etter (2004) reported an association between smoking prevalence and stages of change: a higher prevalence of smoking was associated with a lower motivation to quit, as were fewer quit attempts and higher levels of cigarette consumption (Etter 2004). These findings were reported on the basis of data from all 50 U.S. states; these results were seen in the 1996 and 1999 Behavioral Risk Factor Surveillance System surveys but not in the 1993 survey.

Although the Stages-of-Change Model has been useful in moving cessation research from a focus on smoking and not smoking end points to the process of change from smoking to nonsmoking, questions have been raised about the need to elucidate more clearly other variables that may be implicit in the stages of change (intention to change, past quit attempts, current behavior, and the duration of the current behavior) but that are not explicitly assessed in research studies of stages of change and quitting (Etter and Sutton 2002). Recently, West (2005) has questioned the stages of change paradigm as a description of the cessation process. He found that the majority of smokers stop smoking impulsively, without going through stages of precontemplation and contemplation. Of course, this does not mean that concerns about health and the other harmful effects of smoking have not played an important role in the attempt to quit.

Quitting Attempts

Understanding which smokers will eventually take steps to quit, who will be successful at quitting, and how long smoking abstinence will endure can be difficult to discern from the literature. Difficulties arise because periods of cessation vary, as do definitions of "abstinence." Definitions of smoking cessation in the literature typically range from a 24-hour point-prevalence abstinence rate to a 6-month prolonged period of abstinence (Velicer and Prochaska 2004). Some researchers account for whether the smoker has had smoking lapses or was totally abstinent during the period of cessation reviewed (Hughes et al. 2004). Cessation outcomes can also vary depending on whether quitting was unaided or assisted with behavioral or pharmacological therapies. What is clear is that smoking careers can be long in duration. Birth cohort data from NHIS indicate that half of 15- to 17-year-olds who reported smoking at least 100 cigarettes in their lifetime will likely continue to smoke for 16 to 20 years (Pierce and Gilpin 1996). The literature also reinforces the view that nicotine addiction and tobacco dependence show some similarities with chronic diseases that are characterized by periods of relapse and remission (Fiore et al. 2000); thus the path to smoking cessation will include cycles of abstinence, lapses, relapse, and abstinence.

Smokers who move from contemplating quitting to action typically fail. A study of self-quitters (Garvey et al. 1992) found that the majority of relapses occurred in the first few days and weeks post-cessation. Although most self-quitters (87.2 percent) relapsed within 1 year of their quit date, the majority of relapses occurred in the first few days and weeks after stopping: 13 percent relapsed by 1 day after quitting, 32 percent by 3 days, 49 percent by 1 week, and 62 percent by 2 weeks.

The results of another study of motivated self-quitters support the findings of an early relapse to smoking (Hughes et al. 1992). That study reported smoking cessation results by the use of two measures: one measure that reflected complete abstinence and another measure that reflected some smoking (smoking an average of one cigarette per day or less since the last follow-up and observer verification of no smoking of more than 10 cigarettes on any 2 days). The study findings, which used biochemical verification, indicated that 33 percent of self-quitters were abstinent at 2 days, 24 percent at 7 days, 22 percent at 14 days, 19 percent at 1 month, 11 percent at 3 months, 8 percent at 6 months, and 3 percent at 6 months. By using the more relaxed criteria, 47 percent were abstinent at 2 days, 38 percent at 7 days, 32 percent at 14 days, 27 percent at 1 month, 20 percent at 3 months, and 11 percent at 6 months.

Under a worst case scenario of unsuccessful quitting attempts, Piasecki and colleagues described cessation attempt "fatigue," or a decrease in motivation and ability to stay abstinent (Piasecki et al. 2002). Cessation attempt fatigue is noted to be associated with lower expectations for cessation success, a reduced ability to cope or to believe in having the capacity to quit or stay abstinent, and fewer resources to exert control over behaviors or actions related to tobacco use. Smoking lapses and relapses to smoking, however, do not necessarily represent total quit failures but, rather, represent learning experiences along the pathway to cessation.

Early on in a cessation attempt, smokers may face a number of circumstances that encourage a smoking lapse, including symptoms associated with nicotine addiction (withdrawal, negative affect, urges, and cravings), the presence of social environmental factors such as smokers in the environment, or easy access to tobacco products (Brauer et al. 1996; Piasecki 2006). Although any smoking behavior after quitting has been identified as a very strong predictor of an eventual relapse (Kenford et al. 1994; Shiffman et al. 2006; Westman et al. 1997), it may not necessarily be a final outcome. Hyland and colleagues (2006) found that quit attempts in the previous year and a longer duration of past quit attempts were important predictors of new quit attempts, suggesting that some smokers will continue to attempt to abstain from smoking, despite past lapses or relapses (Hyland et al. 2006).

Other researchers note that smokers with failed quit attempts may reduce the intensity of smoking and the level of addiction for several months after a relapse (Knoke et al. 2006). The ability to reduce smoking levels may prime relapsed smokers to be more successful in latter quit attempts. Results from the Community Intervention Trial for Smoking Cessation (surveys from 1988, 1993, and 2001) found a significant increase in quitting among participants who were able to reduce their daily cigarette consumption by 50 percent. Those who reduced their cigarette consumption by more than 50 percent were 1.7 times more likely to quit smoking by 2001 than those who did not reduce their cigarette consumption (Hyland et al. 2005).

Smokers who attempt to quit smoking with the use of some assistance tend to fare better than self-quitters; however, many smokers may not be informed about effective cessation methods (Hammond et al. 2004). Although it is not the intention of the committee to provide an exhaustive review of cessation therapies, it is important to highlight current guidelines for assisting smokers with quitting. The U.S. Department of Health and Human Services' Clinical Practice Guideline for Treating Tobacco Use and Dependence identifies three counseling and behavioral therapies that are effective in helping smokers quit. These include providing smokers with practical counseling that focuses on (1) problem-solving skills and skills training for relapse prevention and stress management, (2) providing social support as part of treatment, and (3) helping smokers obtain social support outside of treatment.

Current guidelines also recommend eight effective pharmacotherapies that can assist smokers in their attempts to quit. Five therapies are nicotine-based (nicotine gums, patches, nasal sprays, inhalers, lozenges/tablets), two are antidepression medications (bupropion and nortriptyline), and one is a medication (clonidine) that is used for the treatment of hypertension (Fiore et al. 2000; Foulds 2006; Henningfield et al. 2005). Recently, varenicline, a nicotinic cholinergic receptor partial agonist, has been marketed for smoking cessation. Bupropion, nicotine inhalers, nasal sprays, and nicotine patches are considered first-line medication treatments that double long-term abstinence rates compared with those achieved with placebo. Nicotine gum, also a first-line treatment, improves the long-term abstinence rate by about 30 to 80 percent. There is emerging evidence from a few studies that selected use of combinations of nicotine replacement therapies (a nicotine patch with either a nicotine gum or a nicotine nasal spray) may have greater efficacy than a single form of nicotine replacement, but this has not been proven (Fiore et al. 2000).

Summary

The previous sections can be summarized succinctly: nicotine in cigarettes and other forms of tobacco is highly addictive. Once addiction takes hold, it is difficult to stop using nicotine-containing products, although a number of therapies can improve the chances of quitting. Tobacco use is also harmful to one's health and to the health of others. Since 1964 (see Box 2-1 for a list of Surgeon General reports published from 1964 to 2006) the evidence has been building that, "smoking harms nearly every organ of the body, causing many diseases and reducing the health of smokers in general" (CDC 2004). More recently, the Surgeon General reported that, "secondhand smoke causes premature death and disease in children and in adults who do not smoke" (DHHS 2006). As a result, 90 percent of smokers regret having started to smoke, 70 percent want to quit and have made at least one quit attempt, and, at any given time, 40 percent are actively trying to quit or are thinking of quitting within the next six months.

SMOKING INITIATION

Given the clear and consistent evidence that smoking is addictive, quitting is difficult, and smoking is harmful to the health of everyone exposed to tobacco smoke, why do new smokers emerge each year? Because about 90 percent of adult smokers initiated smoking before the age of 18 years (DHHS 1994), addressing this question requires an understanding of why youths begin to smoke. Explanations of adolescent risk taking, including tobacco use, often point to adolescents' underestimation of the chance that a negative outcome will occur to them (Elkind 1967; Reyna and Farley 2006; Slovic 2001), a sense of personal invulnerability to harm (Elkind 1967, 1978), a failure to appreciate the personal applicability of known risks (Arnett 2000; Romer and Jamieson 2001b), and a general immaturity that impairs judgment (Steinberg and Cauffman 1996). Theories of health behavior have incorporated this notion, theorizing that perceptions of low risk are related to engagement in health-compromising behaviors (see, for example, the Health Belief Model (Rosenstock 1974), the Theory of Planned Behavior (Ajzen 1985), Self-Regulation Theory (Kanfer 1970), and theories of decision making [e.g., (Janis and Mann 1977)]; see also Transtheoretical Model of Change (Pallonen et al. 1998; Prochaska 1994; Prochaska and DiClemente 1983; Prochaska et al. 1992). This section provides a review of the literature on adolescents' and young adults' tobacco-related perceptions.

Perceptions of Risks of Using Tobacco

The literature on perceptions about tobacco use among adolescents and young adults is reviewed elsewhere in this report. A number of studies have assessed the extent to which adolescents and young adults recognize and appreciate the risks of smoking. Although some studies show that smokers either overestimate (Borland 1997; Kristiansen et al. 1983; Viscusi 1990; 1991; Viscusi et al. 2000) or underestimate (Schoenbrun 1997; Sutton 1997) the particular risks of smoking compared with the actual risk from epidemiological data, most studies agree that adolescents and young adults are aware of many of the risks involved with tobacco use. In particular, they are aware that smoking involves a significant risk of lung cancer and other health outcomes (Jamieson and Romer 2001a). However, the literature also indicates that adolescents are not aware of the full extent to which smoking is harmful (Arnett 2000; Covington and Omelich 1992; Eiser and Harding 1983; Halpern-Felsher et al. 2004; Hansen and Malotte 1986; Leventhal et al. 1987; Virgili et al. 1991), nor do they fully understand the extent to which tobacco use can shorten the life span (Romer and Jamieson 2001a). More importantly, adolescents are less likely to believe that the risk of addiction and the related health consequences apply to them. To complicate matters, adolescents show an incomplete understanding of the addictive nature of tobacco use that is related, in part, to their inaccurate assessment of smoking risks and their belief that they can quit at any time and therefore avoid addiction (Arnett 2000; Slovic 1998). Furthermore, they believe that smoking risks can be counteracted by altering the amount that they smoke, when they smoke, or what they smoke (e.g., "light" versus regular cigarettes) (Kropp and Halpern-Felsher 2004).

Whether such perceptions, or misperceptions, actually motivate or predict tobacco use is a complicated question. For example, although the concept of adolescent invulnerability is widely used to explain why adolescents smoke, the few studies that have examined the relationship between personal risk perceptions and tobacco use have yielded mixed results. Although some studies find that adolescents who have smoked perceive greater personal risks (Gerrard et al. 1996; Johnson et al. 2002; Resnicow et al. 1999), others show that smokers perceive less personal risk (Arnett 2000; Covington and Omelich 1992; Eiser and Harding 1983; Goldberg et al. 2002; Urberg and Robbins 1981; 1984; Virgili et al. 1991). The following sections details smokers' (particularly adolescent smokers') risk-related beliefs regarding several such aspects of tobacco use.

Beliefs Regarding the Effects of Smoking

Adolescent smokers tend to overestimate some smoking risks and underestimate others. In general, they understand that smoking causes lung cancer, but they also overestimate the degree to which it does. Jamieson and Romer reported that among 14- to 22-year olds surveyed in the Annenberg Tobacco Survey, 70 percent of smokers and 79 percent of nonsmokers overestimated the risk of lung cancer attributed to smoking (Jamieson and Romer 2001b). The survey respondents also underestimated the degree to which smoking can shorten a smoker's life. Although the majority of smokers (68 percent) and nonsmokers (79 percent) recognize that smoking shortens one's life, close to 26 percent of smokers and 18 percent of nonsmokers responded that they did not know whether this was actually the case. When asked more specifically about the number of years that smoking can shorten a life span, 44 percent of smokers and 48 percent of nonsmokers correctly identified that smoking can shorten one's life by 5 to 10 years; however, 28 percent of smokers and 19 percent of nonsmokers reported that they did not know. A high proportion of respondents also reported inaccurate assessments of the lethality of smoking compared with those of other behaviors. Many of those surveyed failed to recognize that smoking causes more deaths than gunshots and car accidents (42 percent) or alcohol and the use of other drugs (62 percent).

Another important finding from the Annenberg Tobacco Study concerns "optimism bias," that is, smokers' belief that the smoking risk is lower for themselves than for others engaging in similar behaviors (Weinstein 1989). In other words, an abstract understanding of the nature and the magnitude of smoking risks does not necessarily translate into a personalized appreciation of the hazards to oneself. In their analysis of the survey data, Romer and Jamieson found that, among smokers who correctly estimated that half of lifetime smokers die from smoking-related causes, 40 percent viewed their own smoking as less than "very risky" (the scale ranged from "very risky" to "not at all risky"). Among respondents who estimated that 60 percent or more of lifetime smokers die from smoking-related causes, 25 percent did not view their own smoking as very risky (Romer and Jamieson 2001a). Arnett reported similar results from a survey of both adolescents and adults (Arnett 2000). Arnett found that in both of these groups, smokers were more than twice as likely as nonsmokers to doubt that they would die from smoking, even if they were to smoke for 30 to 40 years. Moreover, a nontrivial proportion of adolescent smokers (29 percent) doubted slightly or strongly that they would die from smoking if they smoked for 30 to 40 years. Other studies have also shown that participants who reported that they smoked rated the chance that a negative health outcome as well as a negative social outcome (e.g., getting into trouble) would occur lower than did participants who did not smoke (Arnett 2000; Halpern-Felsher et al. 2004; Virgili et al. 1991). Furthermore, risk perceptions vary by level of smoking (Chassin et al. 2000; Halpern-Felsher et al. 2004; Soldz and Cui 2002) or stage of smoking (Pallonen et al. 1998; Prokhorov et al. 2002), with individuals who have smoked longer and more often perceiving fewer risks than those who have smoked for shorter periods and less often. Similarly, studies have found that perceived health and social risks are related to behavioral intentions and that these intentions are the most important and immediate determinants of behavior (Ajzen 1985; Distefan et al. 1998; Fishbein and Ajzen 1975; Pallonen et al. 1998; Parsons et al. 1997; Prokhorov et al. 2002).

Beliefs Regarding Addiction and Cessation

Researchers have also examined the extent to which adolescents understand the grip of addiction and the implications of addiction on quitting. The results of these studies indicate that, although adolescents might be aware of the health and long-term risks of smoking in general, they are much less aware of the addictive nature of smoking. There are also indications that adolescent smokers might be less worried about the long-term risks of smoking, in part because they believe that they can quit smoking easily and at any time.

Weinstein and colleagues examined youth and adult smokers' beliefs about the difficulty of quitting smoking and the nature of addiction (Weinstein et al. 2004). On the basis of data from two nationwide surveys, they found that most (96 percent) smokers, both youth and adults, agreed that the longer you smoke, the harder it is to quit. A high proportion of both groups also agreed that signs of addiction appear very quickly if a teenager starts smoking half a pack of cigarettes a day: 80 percent of youth and 79 percent of adults said signs of addiction appeared in a few months or less. The youths examined in that study also tended to claim that they were less addicted than the average smoker.

Similarly, Jamieson and Romer found that a substantial proportion of smokers understood that the properties of tobacco are addictive, but they did not fully appreciate the implications for quitting (Jamieson and Romer 2001b). Their survey results showed that, whereas 82 percent of smokers agreed that cigarettes have addictive chemical properties, nearly 60 percent of those smokers believed that quitting is either very easy or possible for most people if they really try. These findings are consistent with those reported by Arnett who showed that nearly 60 percent of adolescents believed that they could smoke for a few years and then quit (Arnett 2000). However, most of them do not quit. Smoking continues beyond the high school years, with 63 percent of 12th grade daily smokers still smoking daily 7 to 9 years later, even though only 3 percent of them estimated in high school that they would still be smoking in 5 years (Johnston et al. 2004).

Beliefs Regarding So-Called "Light" Cigarettes

Another area where smokers, including adolescents, have a distorted understanding of the risks of smoking is in the comparative effects of so-called "light" cigarettes and regular cigarettes. Adolescents often smoke "light" cigarettes to counteract the risks of smoking. In a study conducted by Kropp and Halpern-Felsher, the participants were found to believe—incorrectly—that they would be significantly less likely to get lung cancer (and other adverse health outcomes) if they smoked "light" cigarettes rather than regular cigarettes (Kropp and Halpern-Felsher 2004). Adolescents also mistakenly thought that it would take significantly longer to become addicted to "light" cigarettes and that their chances of quitting smoking were higher with "light" cigarettes than with regular cigarettes, even though it is now well established that most smokers achieve the same level of exposure to nicotine and tobacco-related toxins when they smoke so-called "light" cigarettes (IOM 2001). They also "agreed" or "strongly agreed" that regular cigarettes deliver more tar than "light" cigarettes and that "light" cigarettes deliver less nicotine than regular cigarettes. Although some of the adolescents in that study were aware of the health risks and addictive properties associated with "light" cigarettes, the data showed that some 22 percent of the adolescents were uncertain about the differences between regular and "light" cigarettes and that between 25 percent and 35 percent of the adolescents mistakenly thought that health risks were more likely to be associated with regular cigarettes than with "light" cigarettes.

Adolescent Weighing of Risks and Benefits in Smoking Initiation

Halpern-Felsher and colleagues (Appendix E) also discuss other personal and behavioral factors that influence smoking behavior in adolescents, including the reasons adolescents smoke and how they weigh smoking pros and cons. According to Halpern-Felsher and colleagues, the motivation for adolescents to start smoking can result from a variety of factors: curiosity about a means to relieve stress and boredom, peer and social influence, parental influence, and as a means to decrease appetite or increase the intoxicating effects of alcohol and drugs (Conrad et al. 1992; Turner et al. 2006; Vuckovic et al. 2003).

Although adolescents tend to minimize the risks of smoking, they also have a tendency to exaggerate the benefits of smoking, especially given the influences of a variety of factors such as those mentioned above. One tool used to understand how perceived benefits motivate individuals to smoke, compared with how perceived risks deter smoking, is the Decisional Balance Inventory which incorporates a weighing of both the benefits (pros) and the risks (cons) in predicting behavior and behavioral change. The tool assesses three factors: social pros (e.g., kids who smoke have more friends), coping pros (e.g., smoking relieves tension), and cons (e.g., smoking stinks). Using this Inventory, Prokhorov and colleagues found that scores on the smoking pros scale increased and that those on the cons scale decreased, as adolescents were more susceptible to smoking (Prokhorov et al. 2002). Pallonen also found a positive relationship between perceived smoking benefits and nonsmokers' likelihood of smoking, whereas the cons of smoking were less predictive of smoking (Pallonen et al. 1998). Researchers have also noted that adolescent smokers tend to perceive that benefits are more likely to occur and that risks are less likely to occur compared with adolescents who have not smoked (Goldberg et al. 2002; Halpern-Felsher et al. 2004).

Summary

In summary, research suggests that adolescents misperceive the magnitude of smoking harms and the addictive properties of tobacco and fail to appreciate the long-term dangers of smoking, especially when they apply the dangers to their own behavior. When taken together with the general tendencies of adolescents to take a short-term perspective and to given substantial weight to peer influences, they tend to unduly discount the risks and overstate the benefits of smoking. These distorted risk perceptions are associated with adolescents' decisions to initiate tobacco use, a decision that they will later regret.

ATYPICAL PATTERNS OF TOBACCO USE

The discussion has thus far focused on what may be regarded as the "standard" pattern of tobacco use. The typical case of tobacco addiction involves a person who began smoking as a teenager; rapidly escalated to daily use and to nicotine addiction; and eventually has a "smoking career" of 15 to 20 years of frequent daily use, characterized by heavy regret and punctuated by unsuccessful efforts to quit. In this section, the committee calls attention to patterns of smoking that deviate from this typical pattern (e.g., an increase in occasional, and perhaps non-addictive or less addictive, smoking to highlight the challenges that they pose for tobacco use prevention and control efforts).

One pattern of occasional smoking is nondaily smoking. Most smokers smoke cigarettes every day. Nondaily smoking was once thought to occur only in the first few years of initiation, before the development of nicotine dependence. However, research conducted since 1990 suggests that occasional smoking is becoming more frequent among U.S. smokers, whereas daily smoking is declining. A survey of 32 Minnesota work sites conducted from 1987 to 1990 found that 18.3 percent of smokers were nondaily smokers (Hennrikus et al. 1996). At follow-up two years later, 21.5 percent were nondaily smokers, suggesting that the rate of occasional smoking was increasing. Results from the Behavior Risk Factor Surveillance Survey (BRFSS) showed that the median proportion of "some-day" smokers among adults aged 18 years and older increased from 17.2 percent in 1996 to 24.0 percent in 2001 (CDC 2003). However, whether such an increase in nondaily smoking is occurring remains uncertain. Data from NHIS of individuals 18 years and older do not support this finding; the mean rate of some-day smoking remained fairly constant between 1993 (18.4 percent) and 2004 (18.7 percent) (CDC 2005a; Hyland et al. 2005).

Nondaily smokers among adults are younger, are highly educated, have higher income levels, are more likely to be racial and ethnic minorities (African American, Hispanic, and Asian) and male, and are more likely to have begun smoking after age 19 years (CDC 2003; Hassmiller et al. 2003; Husten et al. 1998; Hyland et al. 2005). About half of nondaily smokers had been regular smokers of 10 or more cigarettes per day in the past. Many more nondaily smokers than daily smokers reported a strong intent to quit smoking.

The rate of nondaily smoking varies widely by state. An analysis of nondaily smokers based on NHIS longitudinal data from 1996 through 2002 revealed wide state-by-state variations in the rate of nondaily smoking (as a proportion of all current smokers), ranging from 15.2 percent in Kentucky to 41.2 percent in Washington, D.C. (CDC 2003). From 1996 to 2001, the prevalence of nondaily smoking increased in 38 states. Nondaily smokers were more likely to be young and were slightly more likely to be men than women. The nondaily smoking prevalence was, in general, the highest in states or territories with the lowest overall smoking prevalence (such as California, Utah, and Puerto Rico) and the lowest in states with the highest smoking prevalence (for example, Kentucky and West Virginia).

Nondaily smoking may represent a transitional stage toward quitting for some smokers. In the 1990 California Tobacco Survey of smokers 18 years of age or older, 15.4 percent of smokers were classified as occasional smokers (smoking on some days but not every day and smoking on 25 days or less in the past month) (Evans et al. 1992). Two-thirds of these smokers were considered not to be in the process of taking up smoking based on their age (25 years or older). Twenty percent of occasional smokers had been daily smokers in the previous year, indicating that it is possible to switch from daily to occasional smoking. Furthermore, many of the occasional smokers were planning to quit within the next 6 months, suggesting that occasional smoking may be a transition to quitting (Evans et al. 1992).

Several explanations for an increasing prevalence of nondaily smoking have been proposed (CDC 2003). These include some tobacco control interventions that make it more difficult to smoke, such as smoking bans in public places and the increased price of cigarettes in recent years. Another explanation is that some nondaily smokers are still in the uptake phase of smoking or have previously been daily smokers who are in the process of trying to quit. The recent increase in initiation of smoking among individuals over 19 years of age may also contribute to the increased prevalence of nondaily smokers. Individuals who start smoking at a later age perhaps become less dependent in general than those who start at a younger age.

Another atypical pattern of smoking that poses a quandary for tobacco prevention and control efforts is daily light smoking (i.e., smoking less than five cigarettes per day). Since 1993, data from NHIS show that the proportion of light smokers has increased from 2.9 percent in 1993 to 4.8 percent in 2004 (CDC 2005a). Although these light smokers (or "chippers") may smoke daily, they do not develop nicotine dependence. They are, however, similar to dependent smokers on a number of parameters, including puff number and duration, as well as blood nicotine absorption and elimination levels. They also show cardiovascular responses similar to those of dependent smokers (Brauer et al. 1996; Shiffman 1989; Shiffman et al. 1990, 1992). These findings challenge classical theories of nicotine dependence (Shiffman 1989).

Studies that have examined the smoking attitudes and behaviors of smokers have also found perplexing similarities and differences between those of light smokers and those of dependent smokers. Presson and colleagues found that future chippers closely resembled future heavy smokers in viewing smoking as not very harmful to their health (Presson et al. 2002). Future chippers differed from heavy smokers, however, in that they had social environments with low levels of risk (i.e., low levels of smoking among peers and family members). Other studies have found that light smokers and heavy smokers tend to differ in their motives and attitudes toward smoking. Smoking behavior among light smokers tends to be influenced by social and sensory motives (the pleasure of handling cigarettes and smoking itself) rather than pharmacological or addiction-related reasons, such as cravings and habit (Shiffman et al. 1994). Notwithstanding the lack of classical nicotine dependence among low-level smokers, the scientific evidence on the harmful effects of exposure to low levels of nicotine (DHHS 2006) and the potential transitional nature of individuals in this subpopulation of smokers argue for focusing special attention on helping these individuals stop smoking.

POPULATIONS AT GREATER RISK OF CONTINUING SMOKING

A variety of individual and group characteristics and behaviors have been associated with higher rates of tobacco product use. Wallace (Appendix P) provides a review of some of these populations: adult smokers with mental illness, children and adolescents with mental illness and conduct disorders, inmates in correctional institutions, military recruits, homeless individuals, gamblers, and some individuals with disabling conditions.

Wallace notes that there have been a few recent national surveys suggesting that the majority of cigarettes in the United States are sold to persons with a lifetime history of some type of psychiatric morbidity, but this needs additional confirmation (Breslau 1995; Breslau et al. 1991, 1993, 1994; Grant et al. 2004; Hughes et al. 1986; Lasser et al. 2000).

Children with psychiatric and behavioral comorbidities and adverse experiences are at risk for smoking initiation. Children with attention-deficit/ hyperactivity disorder (ADHD) were found to have a higher risk of cigarette use initiation and smoking maintenance, as well as abuse of other substances, than those in non-ADHD comparison groups (Daley 2004; Lambert and Hartsough 1998; Wilens et al. 1997). Wallace also notes that a body of literature has associated a host of adverse experiences—including direct physical or sexual abuse, the presence of depressive effect, suicide attempts, sexually transmitted diseases, and an impoverished, dysfunctional household environment—with substantially increased risks of smoking initiation (De Von Figueroa-Moseley et al. 2004; Dube et al. 2003; Mcnutt et al. 2002; Nichols and Harlow 2004).

Furthermore, Wallace notes that, although the research literature is not extensive, higher rates of smoking have been documented among incarcerated individuals, homeless individuals, and other populations. Among these populations, the highest rates of smoking have been reported among inmates. Hughes and Boland (1992) and Lightfoot and Hodgins (1988) reported a 77 percent smoking rate in the past 6 months among inmates in a penitentiary for men. High rates (71 percent) of current smoking have also been reported among women arrested in New York City (Durrah and Rosenberg 2004). The higher rates of smoking among prisoners may be influenced by the intersection of a number of other factors associated with higher rates of smoking, such as substance abuse, lower socioeconomic status, and high rates of psychiatric comorbidities among incarcerated individuals (Andersen 2004).

The literature describes a group of "hardcore" smokers who have never attempted to quit smoking. This subgroup of smokers is often described as a small but intractable public health problem. Using data from the 1998-99 Tobacco Use Supplement of the Current Population Survey, Augustson and Marcus (2004) defined "hardcore" smokers as established daily smokers (smoking for at least 5 years) who smoke more than 15 cigarettes per day with no reported history of quit attempts and who are over 25 years of age (Emery et al. 2000). They found that "hardcore" smokers represent 24.7 percent of heavy chronic smokers, 17.6 percent of all established smokers, and 13.7 percent of all current smokers. They are also more likely to be male, unmarried, not working, and to have lower education levels. Warner and Burns (2003) suggest that "hardcore" smokers represent members of a group of smokers whose behavior may be especially resistant to change (Warner and Burns 2003).

Genetic vulnerability may be one reason some "hardcore" smokers find it difficult to stop smoking. Emerging genetic and pharmacogenetic studies have identified a potential role for gene variances in frustrated cessation attempts. One study, for example, found that smokers with a variant CYP2B6 gene have increased cravings for cigarettes following cessation and are about one and one half times more likely to relapse during treatment (Lerman et al. 2002). Information on genetic variants related to dopamine, serotonin, and nicotine metabolism, as well as other mechanisms that play important roles in nicotine addiction and maintenance, will be important to understand and better assist "hardcore" smokers and other smokers who have difficulty quitting.

There seems to be little doubt that a subset of the population of long term smokers is more heavily addicted and less amenable to cessation inteventions. It is likely that these smokers are particularly vulnerable to nicotine addiction on the basis of predisposing personal characteristics and environmental stresses. These observations have two important implications: first, it is clear that specialized cessation interventions will be needed to assist them with quitting. Second, a realistic assessment of the prospects of achieving a substantial reduction in the prevalence of tobacco use must take the size of the "hardcore" target populations into account.

CONCLUSION

Smoking prevalence reflects the combined effects in any given period of the changes in the number of new smokers and in the number of smokers who have quit (Niaura and Abrams 2002). This chapter has provided an abridged overview of an extensive body of literature on the factors that affect the trends in smoking prevalence, with particular attention given to how the unique nature of nicotine addiction poses significant challenges to the success of tobacco control efforts.

At the center of the story emerging from this literature is the fact that nicotine addiction stimulates and sustains long-term tobacco use, with all of its serious health hazards and social costs. The literature also indicates that, although an overwhelming majority of smokers (90 percent) regret having begun to smoke, overcoming the grip of addiction and the associated withdrawal symptoms is difficult; most smokers must try quitting several times before they are successful. Progress in helping smokers who want to quit and achieve successful and permanent cessation requires that a variety of cessation technologies, both clinical and population-based, be readily available to the smoking population, that they be used, and that they be effective. This task is discussed further in Chapter 5 of this report.

While tackling the difficult challenge of helping addicted smokers quit, the fact that thousands of individuals begin smoking each day must also be addressed. Most of these new smokers are youth and adolescents who, in part because of their developmental stage, do not clearly understand the full range of risks and consequences of smoking or who discount these long-term health risks because of a belief that they do not apply to them personally.

These distortions of judgment include a failure of youth and adolescents to appreciate the risk and grip of addiction when they begin smoking. Tolerance and dependence to nicotine can occur early on after initiation (Bottorff et al. 2004; DHHS 1994; DiFranza et al. 2000; IOM 1994), and the early initiation of smoking is related to the number of years that a person will smoke and the quantity of cigarettes smoked per day in childhood. Less is known about initiation and subsequent intensity after adolescence (Escobedo et al. 1993; Taioli and Wynder 1991). Unfortunately, many youths view themselves as invulnerable to addiction and its associated harm. They are also sensitive to the social factors and norms that promote smoking, such as the influences exerted by peers, family members, and the exposure to smoking in the media. These influences tend to override the information about the risks of smoking. Therefore, to substantially reduce the rate of smoking initiation, it will be necessary to do a better job of counteracting the perceived benefits of smoking and to develop new tools that make the personal risks of starting to smoke more salient.

All new smokers are not young, however. Some initiate smoking during their college years, which helps to explain why some new smokers have characteristics that differ from those of usual smokers: they tend to have higher levels of education and income than other smokers. It is also noteworthy that some new smokers smoke at lower levels, and some never reach a level of dependence. It will be important for tobacco control experts to pay close attention to these emerging trends and to design appropriate interventions to respond to them.

On the other side of the ledger are smokers who have a more difficult time quitting. "Hardcore" smokers with a long career of smoking and individuals with psychiatric comorbidities or special circumstances, including incarceration and homelessness, have not been the primary targets of traditional cessation treatments or research studies. Achieving success in substantially reducing tobacco use will require taking stock of the progress made with current tobacco prevention and control strategies, identifying where they fall short in responding to emerging smoking trends, and identifying the characteristics and behaviors of subpopulations of smokers. Success will also require the rigorous implementation of known, effective strategies and pushing the envelope to develop new and innovative approaches that can build on the existing tools and strategies used to help people quit smoking.

REFERENCES

Ajzen I. 1985. *From Intentions to Actions. Action Control from Cognition to Behavior.* New York: Springer-Verlag.

Andersen HS. 2004. Mental health in prison populations. A review—with special emphasis on a study of Danish prisoners on remand. Acta Psychiatrica Scandinavica. *Supplementum* (424):5-59.

Arnett JJ. 2000. Optimistic bias in adolescent and adult smokers and nonsmokers. *Addictive Behaviors* 25(4):625-632.

Augustson E, Marcus S. 2004. Use of the current population survey to characterize subpopulations of continued smokers: a national perspective on the "hardcore" smoker phenomenon. *Nicotine and Tobacco Research* 6(4):621-629.

Borland R. 1997. What do people's estimates of smoking-related risk mean? *Psychology and Health* 12:513-521.

Bottorff JL, Johnson JL, Moffat B, Grewal J, Ratner PA, Kalaw C. 2004. Adolescent constructions of nicotine addiction. *Canadian Journal of Nursing Research* 36(1):22-39.

Brauer LH, Behm FM, Lane JD, Westman EC, Perkins C, Rose JE. 2001. Individual differences in smoking reward from de-nicotinized cigarettes. *Nicotine and Tobacco Research* 3(2):101-109.

Brauer LH, Hatsukami D, Hanson K, Shiffman S. 1996. Smoking topography in tobacco chippers and dependent smokers. *Addictive Behaviors* 21(2):233-238.

Breslau N. 1995. Psychiatric comorbidity of smoking and nicotine dependence. *Behavior Genetics* 25(2):95-101.

Breslau N, Andreski P, Kilbey MM. 1991. Nicotine dependence in an urban population of young adults: prevalence and co-morbidity with depression, anxiety and other substance dependencies. *NIDA Research Monograph* 105:458-459.

Breslau N, Kilbey MM, Andreski P. 1993. Nicotine dependence and major depression. New evidence from a prospective investigation. *Archives of General Psychiatry* 50(1):31-35.

Breslau N, Kilbey MM, Andreski P. 1994. DSM-III-R nicotine dependence in young adults: prevalence, correlates and associated psychiatric disorders. *Addiction* 89(6):743-754.

CDC (Centers for Disease Control and Prevention). 2003. Prevalence of current cigarette smoking among adults and changes in prevalence of current and some day smoking—United States, 1996 2001. *MMWR (Morbidity and Mortality Weekly Report)* 52(14):303-304, 306-307.

CDC. 2004. *The Health Consequences of Smoking: A Report of the Surgeon General.* Web Page. Available at: http://www.cdc.gov/tobacco/data_statistics/sgr/sgr_2004/index.htm; accessed May 25, 2007.

CDC. 2005a. Cigarette smoking among adults—United States, 2004. *MMWR (Morbidity and Mortality Weekly Report)* 54(44):1121-1124.

CDC. 2005b. State-specific prevalence of cigarette smoking and quitting among adults—United States, 2004. *MMWR (Morbidity and Mortality Weekly Report)* 54(44):1124-1127.

CDC. 2006. *Surgeon General's Reports.* Web Page. Available at: http://www.cdc.gov/Tobacco/sgr/index.htm; accessed August 17, 2006.

Chassin L, Presson CC, Pitts SC, Sherman SJ. 2000. The natural history of cigarette smoking from adolescence to adulthood in a midwestern community sample: multiple trajectories and their psychosocial correlates. *Health Psychology* 19(3):223-231.

Conrad KM, Flay BR, Hill D. 1992. Why children start smoking cigarettes: predictors of onset. *British Journal of Addiction* 87(12):1711-1724.

Covington MV, Omelich CL. 1992. *Perceived Costs and Benefits of Cigarette Smoking Among Adolescents: Need Instruments, Self-Anger and Anxiety Factors. Anxiety: Recent Developments in Cognitive, Psychophysiological and Health Research.* Washington, DC: Hemisphere Publishing Corporation. Pp. 245-261.

Daley KC. 2004. Update on attention-deficit/hyperactivity disorder. *Current Opinion in Pediatrics* 16(2):217-226.

Dani JA, De Biasi M. 2001. Cellular mechanisms of nicotine addiction. *Pharmacology, Biochemistry and Behavior* 70(4):439-446.

De Von Figueroa-Moseley C, Landrine H, Klonoff EA. 2004. Sexual abuse and smoking among college student women. *Addictive Behaviors* 29(2):245-251.

DHHS (U.S. Department of Health and Human Services). 1988. *The Health Consequences of Smoking: Nicotine Addiction (A Report of the Surgeon General).* Rockville, MD: U.S. Department of Health and Human Services, Centers for Disease Control and Prevention, Center for Health Promotion and Education, Office on Smoking and Health.

DHHS. 1994. *Preventing Tobacco Use Among Young People (A Report of the Surgeon General).* Rockville, MD: U.S. Department of Health and Human Services, Centers for Disease Control and Prevention, Center for Health Promotion and Education, Office on Smoking and Health.

DHHS. 2006. *The Health Consequences of Involuntary Exposure to Tobacco Smoke: A Report of the Surgeon General.* Atlanta, GA: U.S. Department of Health and Human Services, Centers for Disease Control and Prevention, Coordinating Center for Health Promotion, National Center for Chronic Disease Prevention and Health Promotion, Office on Smoking and Health.

DiClemente CC, Prochaska JO, Fairhurst SK, Velicer WF, Velasquez MM, Rossi JS. 1991. The process of smoking cessation: an analysis of precontemplation, contemplation, and preparation stages of change. *Journal of Consulting and Clinical Psychology* 59(2):295-304.

DiFranza JR, Rigotti NA, McNeill AD, Ockene JK, Savageau JA, St Cyr D, Coleman M. 2000. Initial symptoms of nicotine dependence in adolescents. *Tobacco Control* 9(3):313-319.

Distefan JM, Gilpin EA, Choi WS, Pierce JP. 1998. Parental influences predict adolescent smoking in the United States, 1989-1993. *Journal of Adolescent Health* 22(6):466-474.

Dube SR, Felitti VJ, Dong M, Giles WH, Anda RF. 2003. The impact of adverse childhood experiences on health problems: evidence from four birth cohorts dating back to 1900. *Preventive Medicine* 37(3):268-277.

Durrah TL, Rosenberg TJ. 2004. Smoking among female arrestees: prevalence of daily smoking and smoking cessation efforts. *Addictive Behaviors* 29(5):1015-1019.

Eiser JR, Harding CM. 1983. Smoking, seat-belt use and perception of health risks. Addictive Behaviors 8(1):75-78.

Elkind D. 1967. Egocentrism in adolescence. *Child Development* 38(4):1025-1034.

Elkind D. 1978. Understanding the Young Adolescent. *Adolescence* 13:127-134.

Emery S, Gilpin EA, Ake C, Farkas AJ, Pierce JP. 2000. Characterizing and identifying "hardcore" smokers: implications for further reducing smoking prevalence. *American Journal of Public Health* 90(3):387-394.

Escobedo LG, Marcus SE, Holtzman D, Giovino GA. 1993. Sports participation, age at smoking initiation, and the risk of smoking among US high school students. *Journal of the American Medical Association* 269(11):1391-1395.

Etter JF. 2004. Associations between smoking prevalence, stages of change, cigarette consumption, and quit attempts across the United States. *Preventive Medicine* 38(3):369-373.

Etter JF, Perneger TV, Ronchi A. 1997. Distributions of smokers by stage: international comparison and association with smoking prevalence. *Preventive Medicine* 26(4):580-585.

Etter JF, Sutton S. 2002. Assessing "stage of change" in current and former smokers. *Addiction* 97(9):1171-1182.

Evans N, Gilpin E, Pierce J, Burns D, Borland R, Johnson M, Bal D. 1992. Occasional smoking among adults: evidence from the California Tobacco Survey. *Tobacco Control* 1:169-175.

Fiore MC, Bailey WC, and Cohen SJ. 2000. *Treating Tobacco Use and Dependence (Clinical Practice Guideline)*. Rockville, MD. U.S. Department of Health Human Services. Public Health Service.

Fishbein M and Ajzen I. 1975. *Belief, Attitude, Intention, and Behavior: An Introduction to Theory and Research*. Reading, MA: Addison-Wesley.

Fong GT, Hammond D, Laux FL, Zanna MP, Cummings KM, Borland R, Ross H. 2004. The near-universal experience of regret among smokers in four countries: findings from the International Tobacco Control Policy Evaluation Survey. *Nicotine and Tobacco Research* 6(Suppl 3):S341-S351.

Foulds J. 2006. The neurobiological basis for partial agonist treatment of nicotine dependence: varenicline. *International Journal of Clinical Practice* 60(5):571-576.

Garvey AJ, Bliss RE, Hitchcock JL, Heinold JW, Rosner B. 1992. Predictors of smoking relapse among self-quitters: a report from the Normative Aging Study. *Addictive Behaviors* 17(4):367-377.

Gerrard M, Gibbons FX, Benthin AC, Hessling RM. 1996. A longitudinal study of the reciprocal nature of risk behaviors and cognitions in adolescents: what you do shapes what you think, and vice versa. *Health Psychology* 15(5):344-354.

Goldberg JH, Halpern-Felsher BL, Millstein SG. 2002. Beyond invulnerability: the importance of benefits in adolescents' decision to drink alcohol. *Health Psychology* 21(5):477-484.

Goldstein M, Niaura R, Willey-Lessne C, Depue J, Eaton C, Rakowski W, Dube` C. 1997. Physicians counseling smokers: A population based survey of patients' perceptions of health care provider-delivered smoking cessation interventions. *Archives of Internal Medicine* 157(12):1313-1319.

Grant BF, Hasin DS, Chou SP, Stinson FS, Dawson DA. 2004. Nicotine dependence and psychiatric disorders in the United States: results from the national epidemiologic survey on alcohol and related conditions. *Archives of General Psychiatry* 61(11):1107 1115.

Hall W, Madden P, Lynskey M. 2002. The genetics of tobacco use: methods, findings and policy implications. *Tobacco Control* 11(2):119-124.

Halpern-Felsher B, Biehl M, Kropp RY, Rubinstein ML. 2004. Perceived risks and benefits of smoking: differences among adolescents with different smoking experiences and intentions. *Preventive Medicine* 39(3):559-567.

Hammond D, McDonald PW, Fong GT, Borland R. 2004. Do smokers know how to quit? Knowledge and perceived effectiveness of cessation assistance as predictors of cessation behaviour. *Addiction* 99(8):1042-1048.

Hansen WB, Malotte CK. 1986. Perceived personal immunity: the development of beliefs about susceptibility to the consequences of smoking. *Preventive Medicine* 15(4):363-372.

Hassmiller KM, Warner KE, Mendez D, Levy DT, Romano E. 2003. Nondaily smokers: who are they? *American Journal of Public Health* 93(8):1321-1327.

Heath AC, Kirk KM, Meyer JM, Martin NG. 1999. Genetic and social determinants of initiation and age at onset of smoking in Australian twins. *Behavior Genetics* 29(6):395-407.

Henningfield JE, Fant RV, Buchhalter AR, Stitzer ML. 2005. Pharmacotherapy for nicotine dependence. *A Cancer Journal for Clinicians* 55(5):281-299; quiz 322-323, 325.

Hennrikus DJ, Jeffery RW, Lando HA. 1996. Occasional smoking in a Minnesota working population. *American Journal of Public Health* 86(9):1260-1266.

Hughes GV, Boland FJ. 1992. The effects of caffeine and nicotine consumption on mood and somatic variables in a penitentiary inmate population. *Addictive Behaviors* 17(5):447-457.

Hughes JR. 1999. Four beliefs that may impede progress in the treatment of smoking. *Tobacco Control* 8(3):323-326.

Hughes JR. 2003. Motivating and helping smokers to stop smoking. *Journal of General Internal Medicine* 18(12):1053-1057.

Hughes JR, Gulliver SB, Fenwick JW, Valliere WA, Cruser K, Pepper S, Shea P, Solomon LJ, Flynn BS. 1992. Smoking cessation among self-quitters. *Health Psychology* 11(5):331-334.

Hughes JR, Hatsukami DK, Mitchell JE, Dahlgren LA. 1986. Prevalence of smoking among psychiatric outpatients. *American Journal of Psychiatry* 143(8):993-997.

Hughes JR, Keely J, Naud S. 2004. Shape of the relapse curve and long-term abstinence among untreated smokers. *Addiction* 99(1):29-38.

Husten CG, McCarty MC, Giovino GA, Chrismon JH, Zhu B. 1998. Intermittent smokers: a descriptive analysis of persons who have never smoked daily. *American Journal of Public Health* 88(1):86-89.

Hyland A, Borland R, Li Q, Yong HH, McNeill A, Fong GT, O'Connor RJ, Cummings KM. 2006. Individual-level predictors of cessation behaviours among participants in the International Tobacco Control (ITC) Four Country Survey. *Tobacco Control* 15(Suppl 3):iii83-iii94.

Hyland A, Levy DT, Rezaishiraz H, Hughes JR, Bauer JE, Giovino GA, Cummings KM. 2005. Reduction in amount smoked predicts future cessation. *Psychology of Addictive Behaviors* 19(2):221-225.

Hyland A, Li Q, Bauer JE, Giovino GA, Steger C, Cummings KM. 2004. Predictors of cessation in a cohort of current and former smokers followed over 13 years. *Nicotine and Tobacco Research* 6(Suppl 3):S363-S369.

Hyland A, Rezaishiraz H, Bauer J, Giovino GA, Cummings KM. 2005. Characteristics of low-level smokers. *Nicotine and Tobacco Research* 7(3):461-468.

Hymowitz N, Cummings KM, Hyland A, Lynn WR, Pechacek TF, Hartwell TD. 1997. Predictors of smoking cessation in a cohort of adult smokers followed for five years. *Tobacco Control* 6(Suppl 2):S57-S62.

IOM (Institute of Medicine). 1994. *Growing Up Tobacco Free: Preventing Nicotine Addiction in Children and Youth.* Washington, DC: National Academy Press.

IOM. 2001. *Clearing the Smoke: Assessing the Science Base for Tobacco Harm Reduction.* Washington, DC: National Academy Press.

Jamieson P, Romer D. 2001a. A Profile of Smokers and Smoking. In Slovic P, Editor. *Smoking: Risk, Perception, and Policy.* Thousand Oaks, CA: Sage Publications. Pp. 29-47.

Jamieson P, Romer D. 2001b. What Do Young People Think They Know About the Risks of Smoking? In Slovic P, Editor. *Smoking: Risk, Perception, and Policy.* Thousand Oaks, CA: Sage Publications. Pp. 51-63.

Janis IL, Mann L. 1977. *Decision Making: A Psychological Analysis of Conflict, Choice, and Commitment.* New York: Free Press.

Johnson RJ, McCaul KD, Klein WM. 2002. Risk involvement and risk perception among adolescents and young adults. *Journal of Behavioral Medicine* 25(1):67-82.

Johnston L, O'Malley P, Bachman J, Schulenberg J. 2004. *Cigarette Smoking Among American Teens Continues to Decline, but More Slowly Than in the Past.* Web Page. Available at: http://www.monitoringthefuture.org/pressreleases/04cigpr_complete.pdf; accessed April 6, 1905.

Kanfer FH. 1970. *Self Regulation: Research, Issues and Speculations.* New York, Appleton Century-Crofts.

Kendler KS, Neale MC, Sullivan P, Corey LA, Gardner CO, Prescott CA. 1999. A population-based twin study in women of smoking initiation and nicotine dependence. *Psychological Medicine* 29(2):299-308.

Kenford SL, Fiore MC, Jorenby DE, Smith SS, Wetter D, Baker TB. 1994. Predicting smoking cessation. Who will quit with and without the nicotine patch. *Journal of the American Medical Association* 271(8):589-594.

Knoke JD, Anderson CM, Burns DM. 2006. Does a failed quit attempt reduce cigarette consumption following resumption of smoking? The effects of time and quit attempts on the longitudinal analysis of self-reported cigarette smoking intensity. *Nicotine and Tobacco Research* 8(3):415-423.

Koopmans JR, Slutske WS, Heath AC, Neale MC, Boomsma DI. 1999. The genetics of smoking initiation and quantity smoked in Dutch adolescent and young adult twins. *Behavior Genetics* 29(6):383-393.

Kristiansen CM, Harding CM, Elser JR. 1983. Beliefs About the Relationship Between Smoking and Death. *Basic and Applied Social Psychology* 4:253-261.

Kropp RY, Halpern-Felsher B. 2004. Adolescents' beliefs about the risks involved in smoking "light" cigarettes. *Pediatrics* 114(4):e445-e451.

Lambert NM, Hartsough CS. 1998. Prospective study of tobacco smoking and substance dependencies among samples of ADHD and non-ADHD participants. *Journal of Learning Disabilities* 31(6):533-544.

Larabie LC. 2005. To what extent do smokers plan quit attempts? *Tobacco Control* 14(6):425-428.

Lasser K, Boyd JW, Woolhandler S, Himmelstein DU, McCormick D, Bor DH. 2000. Smoking and mental illness: A population-based prevalence study. *Journal of the American Medical Association* 284(20):2606-2610.

Lee AM, Tyndale RF. 2006. Drugs and genotypes: how pharmacogenetic information could improve smoking cessation treatment. *Journal of Psychopharmacology* 20(Suppl 4):7-14.

Lerman C, Berrettini W. 2003. Elucidating the role of genetic factors in smoking behavior and nicotine dependence. *American Journal of Medical Genetics*. Part B, Neuropsychiatric Genetics 118(1):48-54.

Lerman C, Shields PG, Wileyto EP, Audrain J, Pinto A, Hawk L, Krishnan S, Niaura R, Epstein L. 2002. Pharmacogenetic investigation of smoking cessation treatment. *Pharmacogenetics* 12(8):627-634.

Lerman C, Wileyto EP, Patterson F, Rukstalis M, Audrain-McGovern J, Restine S, Shields PG, Kaufmann V, Redden D, Benowitz N, Berrettini WH. 2004. The functional mu opioid receptor (OPRM1) Asn40Asp variant predicts short-term response to nicotine replacement therapy in a clinical trial. *Pharmacogenomics* 4(3):184-192.

Leventhal H, Glynn K, Fleming R. 1987. Is the smoking decision an "informed choice"? Effect of smoking risk factors on smoking beliefs. *Journal of the American Medical Association* 257(24):3373-3376.

Li MD. 2003. The genetics of smoking related behavior: a brief review. *American Journal of the Medical Sciences* 326(4):168-173.

Li MD. 2006. The genetics of nicotine dependence. *Current Psychiatry Reports* 8(2):158-164.

Lightfoot LO, Hodgins D. 1988. A survey of alcohol and drug problems in incarcerated offenders. *International Journal of the Addictions* 23(7):687-706.

Madden PA, Heath AC, Pedersen NL, Kaprio J, Koskenvuo MJ, Martin NG. 1999. The genetics of smoking persistence in men and women: a multicultural study. *Behavior Genetics* 29(6):423-431.

Malaiyandi V, Sellers EM, Tyndale RF. 2005. Implications of CYP2A6 genetic variation for smoking behaviors and nicotine dependence. *Clinical Pharmacology and Therapeutics* 77(3):145-158.

McCaul KD, Hockemeyer JR, Johnson RJ, Zetocha K, Quinlan K, Glasgow RE. 2006. Motivation to quit using cigarettes: a review. *Addictive Behaviors* 31(1):42-56.

Mcnutt LA, Carlson BE, Persaud M, Postmus J. 2002. Cumulative abuse experiences, physical health and health behaviors. *Annals of Epidemiology* 12(2):123-130.

Naqvi NH, Bechara A. 2005. The airway sensory impact of nicotine contributes to the conditioned reinforcing effects of individual puffs from cigarettes. *Pharmacology, Biochemistry and Behavior* 81(4):821-829.

Niaura R, Abrams DB. 2002. Smoking cessation: progress, priorities, and prospectus. *Journal of Consulting and Clinical Psychology* 70(3):494-509.

Nichols HB, Harlow BL. 2004. Childhood abuse and risk of smoking onset. *Journal of Epidemiology and Community Health* 58(5):402-406.

O'Brien CP. 2001. Drug addiction and abuse. In : Hardman JG and Limbird LE, eds. *The Pharmacological Basis of Therapeutics* . 10 ed. New York: Goodman and Gilman. Pp. 621-642

Pallonen UE, Prochaska JO, Velicer WF, Prokhorov AV, Smith NF. 1998. Stages of acquisition and cessation for adolescent smoking: an empirical integration. *Addictive Behaviors* 23(3):303-324.

Parsons JT, Siegel AW, Cousins JH. 1997. Late adolescent risk-taking: effects of perceived benefits and perceived risks on behavioral intentions and behavioral change. *Journal of Adolescence* 20:381-392.

Piasecki TM. 2006. Relapse to smoking. *Clinical Psychology Review* 26(2):196-215.

Piasecki TM, Fiore MC, McCarthy DE, Baker TB. 2002. Have we lost our way? The need for dynamic formulations of smoking relapse proneness. *Addiction* 97(9):1093-1108.

Pierce JP, Gilpin E. 1996. How long will today's new adolescent smoker be addicted to cigarettes? *American Journal of Public Health* 86(2):253-256.

Presson CC, Chassin L, Sherman SJ. 2002. Psychosocial antecedents of tobacco chipping. *Health Psychology* 21(4):384-392.

Prochaska JO. 1994. Strong and weak principles for progressing from precontemplation to action on the basis of twelve problem behaviors. *Health Psychology* 13(1):47-51.

Prochaska JO, DiClemente CC. 1983. Stages and processes of self-change of smoking: toward an integrative model of change. *Journal of Consulting and Clinical Psychology* 51(3):390-395.

Prochaska JO, DiClemente CC, Norcross JC. 1992. In search of how people change. Applications to addictive behaviors. *American Psychologist* 47(9):1102-1114.

Prokhorov AV, de Moor CA, Hudmon KS, Hu S, Kelder SH, Gritz ER. 2002. Predicting initiation of smoking in adolescents: evidence for integrating the stages of change and susceptibility to smoking constructs. *Addictive Behaviors* 27(5):697-712.

Resnicow K, Smith M, Harrison L, Drucker E. 1999. Correlates of occasional cigarette and marijuana use: are teens harm reducing? *Addictive Behaviors* 24(2):251-266.

Reyna VF, Farley F. 2006. Risk and rationality in adolescent decision-making. *Psychological Science in the Public Interest* 7(1):1-44.

Romer D, Jamieson P. 2001a. Do adolescents appreciate the risks of smoking? Evidence from a national survey. *Journal of Adolescent Health* 29(1):12-21.

Romer D, Jamieson P. 2001b. The Role of Perceived Risk in Starting and Stopping Smoking. In Slovic P, Editor. *Smoking: Risk, Perception, and Policy.* Thousand Oaks, CA: Sage Publications. Pp. 64-80.

Rose JE. 1988. The role of upper airway stimulation in smoking. *Progress in Clinical and Biological Research* 261:95-106.

Rose JE. 2006. Nicotine and nonnicotine factors in cigarette addiction. *Psychopharmacology* 184(3-4):274-285.

Rose JE, Behm FM, Westman EC, Bates JE, Salley A. 2003. Pharmacologic and sensorimotor components of satiation in cigarette smoking. *Pharmacology, Biochemistry and Behavior* 76(2):243-250.

Rose JE, Behm FM, Westman EC, Johnson M. 2000. Dissociating nicotine and nonnicotine components of cigarette smoking. *Pharmacology, Biochemistry and Behavior* 67(1):71-81.

Rose JE, Westman EC, Behm FM, Johnson MP, Goldberg JS. 1999. Blockade of smoking satisfaction using the peripheral nicotinic antagonist trimethaphan. *Pharmacology, Biochemistry and Behavior* 62(1):165-712.

Rosenstock IM. 1974. *Historical Origins of the Health Benefit Model.* The Health Belief Model and Personal Health Behavior. Thorofare, NJ: Charles B. Sclack. Pp. 1-8.

Royal College of Physicians. 2000. *Nicotine Addiction in Britain.* London, England: Royal College of Physicians.

Russell MAII, Wilson C, Taylor C, Baker CD. 1979. Effect of general practitioners' advice against smoking. *British Medical Journal* 2(231).

Schoenbrun M. 1997. Do smokers understand the mortality effect of smoking? *American Journal of Public Health* 87:755-759.

Schroeder SA. 2005. What to do with a patient who smokes. *Journal of the American Medical Association* 294(4):482-487.

Shiffman S. 1989. Tobacco "chippers"—individual differences in tobacco dependence. *Psychopharmacology* 97(4):539-547.

Shiffman S. 2004. *Smoking Cessation.* Presentation at the October 14, 2004, Meeting of the IOM Committee on Reducing Tobacco Use: Strategies, Barriers, and Opportunities, Chicago, IL.

Shiffman S, Ferguson SG, Gwaltney CJ. 2006. Immediate hedonic response to smoking lapses: relationship to smoking relapse, and effects of nicotine replacement therapy. *Psychopharmacology* 184(3-4):608-618.

Shiffman S, Fischer LB, Zettler-Segal M, Benowitz NL. 1990. Nicotine exposure among non-dependent smokers. *Archives of General Psychiatry* 47(4):333-336.

Shiffman S, Kassel JD, Paty J, Gnys M, Zettler-Segal M. 1994. Smoking typology profiles of chippers and regular smokers. *Journal of Substance Abuse* 6(1):21-35.

Shiffman S, Zettler-Segal M, Kassel J, Paty J, Benowitz NL, O'Brien G. 1992. Nicotine elimination and tolerance in non-dependent cigarette smokers. *Psychopharmacology* 109(4):449-456.

Slovic P. 1998. Do adolescent smokers know the risks? *Duke Law Journal* 47(6):1133-1141.

Slovic P. 2001. *Smoking: Risk, Perception, and Policy.* Thousand Oaks, CA: Sage Publications.

Soldz S, Cui X. 2002. Pathways through adolescent smoking: a 7-year longitudinal grouping analysis. *Health Psychology* 21(5):495-504.

Steinberg L, Cauffman E. 1996. Maturity of judgment in adolescence: Psychosocial factors in adolescent decision making. *Law and Human Behavior* 20:249-272.

Sullivan PF, Kendler KS. 1999. The genetic epidemiology of smoking. *Nicotine and Tobacco Research* 1(Suppl 2):S51-S57; discussion S69-S70.

Sutton SR. 1997. Are smokers unrealistically optimistic about the health risks? *Risk and Human Behaviour Newsletter* 1:3-5.

Swan GE, Valdes AM, Ring IIZ, Khroyan TV, Jack LM, Ton CC, Curry SJ, McAfee T. 2005. Dopamine receptor DRD2 genotype and smoking cessation outcome following treatment with bupropion SR. *Pharmacogenomics* 5(1):21-29.

Taioli E, Wynder EL. 1991. Effect of the age at which smoking begins on frequency of smoking in adulthood. *New England Journal of Medicine* 325(13):968-969.

Tapper AR, McKinney SL, Nashmi R, Schwarz J, Deshpande P, Labarca C, Whiteaker P, Marks MJ, Collins AC, Lester HA. 2004. Nicotine Activation of 4* Receptors: Sufficient for Reward, Tolerance, and Sensitization. *Science* 306(5698):1029-1032.

Tremblay M, Gervais A, Lacroix C, O'Loughlin J, Makni H, Paradis G. 2001. Physicians taking action against smoking: an intervention program to optimize smoking cessation counselling by Montreal general practitioners. *Canadian Medical Association Journal* 165(5):601-607.

Turner K, West P, Gordon J, Young R, Sweeting H. 2006. Could the peer group explain school differences in pupil smoking rates? An exploratory study. *Social Science and Medicine* 62(10):2513-2525.

Tyndale RF. 2003. Genetics of alcohol and tobacco use in humans. *Annals of Medicine* 35(2):94-121.

Urberg K, Robbins R. 1981. Adolescent perception of the costs and benefits associated with cigarette smoking: sex differences and peer influence. *Journal of Youth and Adolescence* 10(5):353-361.

Urberg K, Robbins R. 1984. Perceived vulnerability in adolescents to the health consequences of cigarette smoking. *Preventive Medicine* 13(4):367-376.

Velicer WF, Norman GJ, Fava JL, Prochaska JO. 1999. Testing 40 predictions from the transtheoretical model. *Addictive Behaviors* 24(4):455-469.

Velicer WF, Prochaska JO. 2004. A comparison of four self-report smoking cessation outcome measures. *Addictive Behaviors* 29(1):51-60.

Virgili M, Owen N, Sverson HH. 1991. Adolescents' smoking behavior and risk perceptions. *Journal of Substance Abuse* 3(3):315-324.

Viscusi WK. 1990. Do smokers underestimate risks? *Journal of Economy* 98(6):1254-1270.

Viscusi WK. 1991. Age variations in risk perceptions and smoking decisions. *Review of Economics and Statistics* 73:577-588.

Viscusi WK, Carvalho I, Antonanzas F, Rovira J, Brana FJ, Portillo F. 2000. Smoking risks in Spain: part III—determinants of smoking behavior. *Journal of Risk and Uncertainty* 21(2-3):213-234.

Vuckovic N, Polen MR, Hollis JF. 2003. The problem is getting us to stop. What teens say about smoking cessation. *Preventive Medicine* 37(3):209-218.

Warner KE, Burns DM. 2003. Hardening and the hard-core smoker: concepts, evidence, and implications. *Nicotine and Tobacco Research* 5(1):37-48.

Weinstein N, Slovic P, Waters E, Gibson G. 2004. Public understanding of the illnesses caused by cigarette smoking. *Nicotine and Tobacco Research* 6(2):349-355.

Weinstein ND. 1989. Optimistic biases about personal risks. *Science* 246(4935):1232-1233.

West R. 2005. Time for a change: putting the Transtheoretical (Stages of Change) Model to rest. *Addiction* 100(8):1036-1039.

Westman EC, Behm FM, Rose JE. 1995. Airway sensory replacement combined with nicotine replacement for smoking cessation. A randomized, placebo-controlled trial using a citric acid inhaler. *Chest* 107(5):1358-1364.

Westman EC, Behm FM, Simel DL, Rose JE. 1997. Smoking behavior on the first day of a quit attempt predicts long-term abstinence. *Archives of Internal Medicine* 157(3):335-340.

Wewers ME, Stillman FA, Hartman AM, Shopland DR. 2003. Distribution of daily smokers by stage of change: Current Population Survey results. *Preventive Medicine* 36(6):710-720.

WHO (World Health Organization). 2003. *Policy Recommendations for Smoking Cessation and Treatment of Tobacco*. Web Page. Available at: http://www.who.int/tobacco/resources/publications/tobacco_dependence/en/index.html; accessed June 6, 2007.

Wilens TE, Biederman J, Mick E, Faraone SV, Spencer T. 1997. Attention deficit hyperactivity disorder (ADHD) is associated with early onset substance use disorders. *Journal of Nervous and Mental Disease* 185(8):475-482.

3

Containing the Tobacco Problem

The trends in cigarette smoking charted in Chapter 1 reflect the push and pull of social forces that tend to promote tobacco use and those that tend to reduce it. Tobacco use in the United States dates back to before colonization, and it has probably had its detractors almost as long. This chapter reviews public health efforts to contain tobacco use over the past four decades. It is not meant to present a nuanced account of the economic, political, and social forces that have shaped the nation's response to tobacco use over this period. Fortunately, interested readers can find the full story in recent books by Richard Kluger and Allan Brandt (Brandt 2007; Kluger 1997). The brief review presented below is designed to highlight key features of the story as seen through the lens of public health.

The introduction of mass-produced, finished cigarettes in the 1880s was followed by mass marketing campaigns that have made cigarettes one of the most highly promoted products in the nation's history. As the appeal of cigarette smoking grew, however, so did the strength and vehemence of the antitobacco activists. Some opponents had moral or religious objections to smoking, and they and others decried its presumed health dangers in the context of a contemporary populist health and hygiene movement. Cigarettes were called a "poison" and even "coffin nails" during those antitobacco campaigns (Burnham 1989; DHHS 2000; Tate 1999).

The antitobacco activists claimed some victories in the early 20th century, including the passage of laws in several states that prohibited tobacco use by both adults and minors (DHHS 2000; Outlook 1901). Their gains, however, were short-lived. Smoking was becoming embedded in the American culture. Cigarette use among soldiers in the Civil War—as in wars to follow—helped promote its popularity and respectability (DHHS 2000). There was no medical consensus regarding health dangers; in fact, many physicians openly smoked and sometimes even promoted the product (DHHS 2000; Walsh 1937). The anti-tobacco forces were unable to stem the growing popularity of cigarettes over the first half of the next century (DHHS 2000; Schudson 1984).

By the middle of the 20th century, researchers were studying the health effects of smoking. In 1952, an article in Reader's Digest reporting on the emerging evidence linking smoking and cancer aroused public concern (Norr 1952). More than 10 years later, publication of the 1964 Surgeon General's report (HEW 1964) was widely regarded as a turning point in the history of smoking in the United States and the point of departure for the modern tobacco control movement (DHHS 2000).

The 1964 report consolidated the growing body of research that linked smoking to lung cancer, chronic bronchitis, and emphysema, disseminating the emerging data on tobacco's adverse effects to a wide audience (HEW 1964). The report's authoritative voice—the Surgeon General is the country's top health officer—and compelling documentation were impossible to ignore. The steady growth in smoking prevalence that had begun in 1920s came to a halt.

After publication of the report, public debate over smoking could never again be divorced from its documented adverse health effects. Smoking could no longer be viewed exclusively as a matter of consumer choice based on the idea that tobacco is an ordinary consumer good. Smoking had officially become a medical problem and a public health challenge. As the 1964 report stated, "cigarette smoking is a health hazard of sufficient importance in the United States to warrant appropriate remedial action" (HEW 1964).

The Surgeon General's report stimulated a significant change in public attitudes about smoking and new public health and public policy responses. The story of the past four decades, however, is not one of unmitigated public health success. The decades following the report's release can be divided into two periods. The first phase, which lasted through the late 1980s, was characterized by largely unsuccessful efforts by those involved in the antismoking movement to gain political footing against the tobacco industry, a commercial giant with many tools at its disposal. Beginning in the mid-1980s, however, the understanding of the tobacco problem and the tools used to combat it underwent dramatic transformations. Smoking came to be recognized as a form of drug addiction, one that typically begins by the age of 18 years and that is fostered by the marketing and other actions of cigarette companies. In addition, the harms that smoking causes to nonsmokers, as well as smokers, also changed the political landscape of tobacco control efforts.

PUBLIC HEALTH TAKES ON THE TOBACCO INDUSTRY: 1964–1988

The initial declines in smoking following the release of the 1964 Surgeon General's report came largely from motivated smokers quitting in response to the highly publicized and frightening findings about tobacco's dangers. With some 70 million tobacco users in the country and with so many Americans—from farmers, factory workers, and cigarette manufacturers to retailers, advertising agencies, and the media—tied economically to smoking, however, dramatic political change did not occur overnight. Moreover, in the turbulent 1960s, the country's attention was focused on such pressing political issues as civil rights, Vietnam, and the War on Poverty (Kluger 1996).

Educational Initiatives

Public education was the first line "remedial action" taken in response to the Surgeon General's call. The American Cancer Society was an early leader. Other voluntary health groups, such as the American Lung Association and the American Heart Association, with their core missions of public education, were also well positioned to take early leadership roles. The three groups worked independently of one another until 1981, when they formed the Coalition on Smoking OR Health. State and local leaders of these organizations began to form similar coalitions in their areas, extending the antismoking effort in states and local communities (DHHS 2000). The American Medical Association (AMA) did not become an advocate for tobacco control until the mid-1980s, when Board of Trustees member Ronald Davis urged the AMA to testify before Congress (Kluger 1996).

New programs to aid in smoking cessation and prevention were developed and implemented. The 1960s saw a rapid introduction of new behavioral approaches to smoking cessation, with novel ideas appearing almost every year. By the 1980s, pharmacological approaches were attracting attention. The National Cancer Institute's Smoking and Tobacco Control Program was a major source of research funding (Shiffman 1993).

School-based prevention programs were also developed and introduced in the 1970s and 1980s, sometimes as a part of alcohol or other substance abuse programs. These programs used a variety of approaches, which varied on the basis of local preferences. Later, the Centers for Disease Control and Prevention issued its Guidelines for School Health Programs to Prevent Tobacco Use and Addiction to provide a national framework and impetus for these programs (CDC 1994).

It took time for antismoking coalitions to coalesce, but anti-tobacco advocacy and grassroots efforts came to play a key role in containing the tobacco problem. A notable early development came in 1966 when John F. Banzhaf successfully petitioned the Federal Communications Commission (FCC) to invoke the Fairness Doctrine and mandate reply time on television and radio for the cigarette commercials glamorizing smoking. This action ultimately led to an FCC requirement, beginning in 1967, that stations run one free counter advertisement from health groups for every three cigarette commercials that they aired. The American Cancer Society, working with top advertising agencies that donated their time, took the lead in producing graphic and compelling counter advertisements. Banzhaf went on to form Action on Smoking and Health, a national antismoking consumer organization that was reported to have 60,000 members by 1979 (Kluger 1996).

Congressional initiatives gave some support to the public education efforts, giving what seemed to be at least a symbolic win to the nascent tobacco control movement. Within a year of the publication of the Surgeon General's report, the U.S. Congress passed the Cigarette Labeling and Advertising Act of 1965, which required cigarettes packages to contain the message "Warning: Cigarette Smoking May Be Hazardous To Your Health" (CDC 2005).

As additional scientific evidence documenting the dangers of smoking continued to emerge, the 1969 Public Health Cigarette Smoking Act upgraded the warning to read "Warning: The Surgeon General Has Determined That Cigarette Smoking Is Dangerous To Your Health" (CDC 2005). The law also banned all cigarette advertising on television and radio, effective January 1, 1971 (Borio 1993).

By 1981 a Federal Trade Commission (FTC) staff report had concluded that the health warning on packages was "worn out" and was having little impact on public knowledge and attitudes about smoking. The warning was too abstract and difficult to remember, and it was not seen as personally relevant (Hinds 1982). Congress responded with the Comprehensive Smoking Education Act of 1984, which required the use of four, more specific, labels on cigarette packages and cigarette advertisements that would be rotated on a regular basis (CDC 2005).

The new warnings reflected the steady flow of research findings tying smoking to increasing numbers of serious conditions. By the time that the 1989 Surgeon General's report was released, the list of conditions that scientific studies had linked to smoking included various cancers—including lung, laryngeal, oral, and esophageal cancers—as well as pulmonary disease, heart disease, and fetal growth retardation. This growing body of research helped power the tobacco control movement.

The Tobacco Industry's Response

Even as public health forces were coalescing and making policy inroads, the tobacco industry was fully engaged as a formidable opponent. Tobacco has been entrenched in American society for so long that it is extremely difficult to sort out the precise roles of various commercial, medical, social, and cultural forces in sustaining the tobacco problem. The tobacco industry's forceful strategies, however, have provided a powerful counterforce to the public health effort. As the 2000 Surgeon General's report would later state, in admittedly simplified terms: "The history of tobacco use can be thought of as a conflict between tobacco as an agent of economic gain and tobacco as an agent of human harm" (DHHS 2000).

The medical establishment was initially slow to embrace the imperatives of the growing findings about smoking and heath. The tobacco industry, on the other hand, quickly sprung into action in the early 1950s to counter the studies connecting smoking to higher mortality rates. In the late 1950s, cigarette manufacturers created the Tobacco Institute, which claimed to represent not only cigarette producers and distributors but also hundreds of thousands of farmers and others with economic interests in tobacco (Kluger 1996). The Tobacco Institute was the driver of the industry's extensive public relations and lobbying campaigns for decades. It sought to underscore the economic importance of tobacco and, together with the industry's Council for Tobacco Research (initially called the Tobacco Industry Research Council), to undermine the scientific evidence identifying the risks of smoking and documenting its effects on health. By disputing the scientific findings about the dangers of smoking, the industry sought to reassure its customers and to obscure the public's understanding of the risks.

The industry also assertively sought to counter and displace the message about the dangers of smoking with a message tapping into the American spirit of individualism, freedom, and unease with government paternalism. The industry's message was simple: Smoking is an individual's free choice and no one else's business and certainly not the government's business.

Although the voluntary health organizations leading the early public education effort tended to avoid controversy and politics, tobacco interests built a powerful presence on Capitol Hill. They sustained their influence by lobbying, making campaign contributions, and building allegiances with members from tobacco growing states, many of whom held key leadership positions (Kluger 1996).

Through their efforts, tobacco industry advocates were able to influence key legislation. For example, Congress denied the Consumer Product Safety Commission jurisdiction over cigarettes, reversing the position taken by the agency's first chairman, who said that the commission had authority to regulate or even ban cigarettes. Tobacco was also expressly exempted from regulation under the Toxic Substances Control Act (1976), even though the law was intended to regulate chemical substances which present "unreasonable risk of injury to health of the environment." Although the nicotine in tobacco is highly addictive, tobacco is also explicitly exempted from regulation under the Controlled Substances Act (1970). Without these congressionally enacted exemptions, tobacco products would have been subject to strong regulation—indeed, they theoretically could have been removed from the market under these statutes if the applicable regulatory agency had been so inclined (Kluger 1996).

As they sought protection from potentially damaging legislation, tobacco companies also spent billions of dollars marketing cigarettes to ensure a steady stream of customers. Their products were killing some 400,000 people a year and causing widespread morbidity, while the public health community scrambled to stem the damage. The major companies, aggressively competing for market share and for new smokers, hired top public relations companies to reshape the image of old brands and draw in new populations of smokers (Kluger 1996).

With women accounting for an increasing proportion of smokers and with the women's liberation movement advocating for female freedom and independence, women became a ready target for tobacco industry marketing. In 1967, companies rapidly increased their advertising in women's magazines and Philip Morris launched its Virginia Slims cigarette featuring the memorable slogan "You've Come a Long Way Baby." The rate of smoking initiation among girls younger than age 18 years rose abruptly in 1967, the year that the Virginia Slims campaign began, peaking in 1973 at more than double the rate in 1967 (Pierce et al. 1994).

By the late 1980s, the R.J. Reynolds Company recast its Camel cigarette brand with a cartoon figure, Joe Camel, and initiated a marketing effort that would prove especially popular with young people. Following this image redesign, Camel's youth market share ballooned. Although the tobacco companies insisted for decades that they were not targeting underage smokers, industry papers that would later become public indicated otherwise (Kluger 1996).

The tobacco companies also competed for smokers who were concerned about the dangers of smoking by marketing a succession of new low-tar and "light" cigarettes that offered smokers an alternative to quitting. These products emit lower levels of tar, carbon monoxide, and nicotine than other cigarettes, as measured by the standard FTC machine testing method. The implication that low-tar cigarettes would therefore reduce the dangers of smoking made these products the choice of increasingly large numbers of customers. Research later showed, however, that the benefits of low-tar products are not what the FTC figures might suggest, because smokers alter their smoking patterns to compensate for the reduced nicotine delivery and because the standard smoking machine used by the FTC does not accurately simulate how smokers smoke. Therefore, people who switched to these brands did not significantly lower their health risks (Harris et al. 2004; IOM 2001; NCI 2001).

Companies also turned their attentions internationally, as free trade agreements and the collapse of communism in the late 1980s opened markets in Asia and Eastern Europe that previously were controlled by local monopolies. The big international tobacco companies introduced marketing campaigns in countries that until then had not seen extravagant cigarette advertisements, due to the state previously controlling all tobacco sales. The introduction of more varied and better-tasting American cigarettes, sometimes cheaper thanks to market competition, exported the tobacco problem to developing countries, even as rates were declining in the United States (Sugarman 2001). As a result, more than 95 percent of the world's smokers now live outside the United States. According to World Health Organization projections, by the year 2020, 10 million people will die annually from tobacco-related illnesses, and 70 percent of these individuals will be in developing countries (WHO 2005).

Even when Congress passed legislation that seemed to promote the tobacco control effort, the public health gains often turned out to be illusory. The 1965 health warning legislation, for example, actually represented an important success for tobacco interests. Without it, a much tougher FTC proposal would have taken effect, putting in place a stronger warning on packages and also on advertisements. Congress temporarily blocked a warning on advertisements, a requirement that the industry was eager to avoid. Preemption language in the bill also stripped states of the authority to impose tougher requirements on packages or advertisements. The legislation kept regulatory action centered in Congress, where tobacco interests were most powerful (DHHS 2000).

The industry also recognized—though it presented a contrary message to the public—that the mild warnings that Congress required in the 1965 and 1969 acts might prove helpful in suits by smokers who claimed that the companies had not informed them of the dangers of smoking. Indeed, in 1992, the U.S. Supreme Court ruled in a case brought on behalf of a smoker, Rose Cipollone, that the 1969 act preempts state tort suits based on negligent failure to warn of the dangers of smoking, to the extent that such suits were based on a claim that the manufacturers' and sellers' post-1969 advertising ought to have included additional or more clearly stated warnings about the health consequences of cigarette smoking (Rabin 2001a). The trade-offs involved in the labeling legislation, as well as doubts about the impact of the product warnings, have led some public health experts to question whether the legislation was a public health victory (IOM 1994). Surgeon General Luther Terry, who issued the 1964 report, would later go so far as to call the 1965 law, "a hoax on the American people" (DHHS 2000).

The broadcast ban on tobacco advertising was probably also a net benefit to the industry. Between 1967 and 1970, when public health advocates aired counter advertisements as part of the Fairness Doctrine, cigarette consumption dropped at a much faster rate than either before or after this period (DHHS 1989). Several studies have found that the ads were driving at least some of the downturn in smoking (Farrelly et al. 2003; Hamilton 1972; O'Keefe 1971; Warner 1989). When the congressional broadcast ban took effect (without much industry resistance), those advertisements disappeared from the nation's living rooms, and the tobacco control movement lost one of its more effective tools for reducing tobacco use. Whatever the public health benefits of banning broadcast tobacco advertising, it was to the industry's advantage to get the counter advertisements off the air.

After the television advertising ban, tobacco companies vastly increased their marketing budgets, shifting a large portion of advertising dollars into promotional activities aimed at (1) putting cigarettes in the hands of prospective users; (2) positioning cigarettes in prominent and accessible places at points of sale; and (3) creating good will for the companies with the public, community leaders, and politicians (IOM 1994). In 1975, the tobacco industry spent $491 million on all types of cigarette advertising and promotion in the United States. By 1985 that figure had nearly quintupled to $2.48 billon, and it continues to multiply (FTC 2005).

The industry prevailed in the courts as well. Of more than 200 tort claims filed on behalf of individual smokers between the mid-1950s and the early 1990s, not a single lawsuit succeeded. Tort litigation against the tobacco industry seemed to be dead. In a first wave of litigation, which began in the 1950s, the companies successfully argued that, absent a foreseeable risk of harm, consumers must bear the risks of using nondefective products. In the second wave, which began in the early 1980s, the industry successfully argued that smokers continued to smoke even with knowledge of the associated health risks (Rabin 1993).

The industry message that smoking was an individual choice—indeed, a right—and that others had no business depriving smokers of that pleasure resonated powerfully within American society. Even as antismoking forces were gathering steam and public knowledge of the dangers of smoking was high, smoking was widely seen as a personal decision, even if it was a self-destructive one. For those who were not smokers or tied to the tobacco industry, it could be a justification for steering clear of the controversy over smoking. As the remainder of this chapter reveals, however, new and increasing concerns about the health consequences of tobacco use would soon begin to reshape public opinion regarding smoking.

The Campaign Against Secondhand Smoke

Research about the harmful effects of secondhand smoke began to emerge in the 1970s. As nonsmokers sought to assert their right to a smoke-free environment, they introduced a new justification for tobacco control.

Eventually, this movement would weaken the claims of smokers' rights and transform public perceptions and the tobacco policy debate. In the end, this shift also played a major role in reducing smoking altogether by changing social norms and helping smokers quit or reduce smoking.

Early research on secondhand smoke left many uncertainties about the nature and scope of the risk that tobacco smoke posed to nonsmokers, and specific scientific findings supporting nonsmokers' rights claims did not emerge until the late 1980s. However, public health officials and grassroots antismoking groups—particularly the Group Against Smokers' Pollution, or GASP, founded in 1971—did not wait. They embraced the early indications that smoking could harm nonsmokers, while locating their campaign for smoke-free environments in the context of a broader environmental protection movement along with a growing consumer health consciousness (Bayer and Colgrove 2002).

The 1972 Surgeon General's report (HEW 1972) noted the potential hazards of secondhand smoke. By the mid-1970s, government at all levels and private companies were beginning to respond to calls for smoke-free areas. In 1973, domestic airlines were required to have a no-smoking section, and a year later smoking was restricted on interstate buses. Much of the action was taking place at the state and local levels. In 1973, Arizona became the first state to create smoke-free public places; in 1974, Connecticut became the first state with a law restricting smoking in restaurants; and in 1975, Minnesota became the first state to have a comprehensive workplace smoking ban (DHHS 2000).

The tobacco industry tried to focus attention on the lack of definitive data about the risks of secondhand smoke, but the threat to nonsmokers had caught the attention of the media and the public. By the late 1970s, a Roper poll commissioned by the Tobacco Institute found that almost 60 percent of respondents believed that smoking was probably harmful to nonsmokers, and even 40 percent of smokers agreed that their smoking probably endangered others (The Roper Organization Inc. 1978).

The campaign against secondhand smoke continued to gain momentum in the 1980s, with states and localities passing a variety of restrictions on smoking in public places. By 1986, 41 states and the District of Columbia had statutes restricting smoking (Bayer and Colgrove 2002). That year, reports from the National Academy of Sciences and the Surgeon General contributed to the sense of urgency about secondhand smoke. The report by the National Academy's National Research Council stated that secondhand tobacco smoke increases the risk of lung cancer in nonsmokers by 30 percent and is harmful to children (NRC 1986). Surgeon General C. Everett Koop's 1986 report (DHHS 1986), Health Consequences of Involuntary Smoking, acknowledged the limitations of the data but called for immediate measures to protect nonsmokers.

Congress banned smoking on all airline flights of 2 hours or less in 1987, and 3 years later effectively extended that prohibition to all domestic flights. Smoking was also banned in federal buildings and in child care facilities that received federal funds.

The 1992 release of the Environmental Protection Agency's landmark report, Respiratory Health Effects of Passive Smoking: Lung Cancer and Other Disorders, added to the momentum for smoke-free spaces (EPA 1992). The report concluded that secondhand smoke is a Class A carcinogen, meaning that it is a definite cause of human cancer. According to the Environmental Protection Agency report, secondhand smoke causes some 3,000 deaths from lung cancer a year among nonsmokers.

Secondhand smoke gave new momentum to the efforts of tobacco control advocates, setting the stage for a fundamental shift in the political dynamic of tobacco control and in the public discourse and understanding of tobacco control efforts during the last decade of the 20th century.

ADVANCES IN TOBACCO CONTROL: 1988–2005

The tobacco control movement coalesced around the secondhand smoke issue, which turned out to be only the first of several issues to pose unprecedented challenges to commercial tobacco interests. While the science on the adverse effects of secondhand smoke continued to emerge, a second scientific front opened to counter the industry focus on freedom of choice: advances in neuroscience demonstrated that nicotine is a highly addictive drug. This finding permanently transformed the debate about smoking and reshaped the public policy agenda. The emphasis on addiction also cast smoking among adolescents and youth in a new light and stimulated a third front in the tobacco wars.

Nicotine: An Addictive Drug

Historically, the term addiction has been associated with stereotypical images of compulsive drug use, deviance, and criminality; heroin has been viewed as the prototypical addictive drug in the United States (HEW 1964). Beginning in the mid-1960s, however, scientific criteria for addiction (often labeled "drug dependence") have emphasized the hallmark behavioral features of drug use, including a loss of control, and experts in the field have attempted to disassociate the clinical condition itself from the social and moral connotations and images traditionally linked with the term addiction. Equally important have been the major advances in neuroscience research that have identified the neurobiological substrates of addiction (IOM 1996) (see Chapter 2).

By the early 1980s, researchers reported that laboratory animals worked to acquire nicotine; this behavior is a hallmark of addiction to a substance.

Studies also demonstrated nicotine's psychoactive effects, another component of addiction. Brain mechanisms for behavioral reinforcement and
compulsive use were characterized (IOM 2001). Epidemiological studies
showing that large majorities of smokers had tried and failed to quit added
to the evidence of addiction.

The 1988 Surgeon General's report (DHHS 1988), Health Consequences of Smoking: Nicotine Addiction, detailed how nicotine meets the
criteria for an addictive drug, concluding that smokers smoke because they
are addicted and that nicotine is the addictive agent. A growing number
of scientific and medical organizations, including the World Health Organization, the American Medical Association, and the American Psychiatric
Association, declared nicotine addictive or dependence producing.

The medical consensus that nicotine is an addictive drug transformed
the concept of smoking from a bad habit of weak-willed people to a patho-
physiological process that produces compulsive behavior. Increasingly, scientific studies have documented the pharmacological and structural effects
of nicotine on the nervous system, which ultimately leads to specifiable
changes in the brain.

The highly addictive nature of nicotine undermines the tobacco industry's longstanding position that smoking is a "free choice" and, by drawing
attention to the similarities between tobacco addiction and addiction to
other psychoactive drugs, establishes the empirical and ethical foundation
for more aggressive regulation. Although the FDA regulates nicotine patches
and other nicotine-containing products used as aids for smoking cessation,
FDA commissioners had traditionally declined to assert any jurisdiction
over cigarettes. In the late 1980s, Scott Ballin, director of the Coalition on
Smoking OR Health, petitioned the FDA to regulate low-tar cigarettes and
the new smokeless brand Premier on the basis of their implied health claims
that these products are less harmful than ordinary cigarettes (Kessler 2000).
In response to the petition, FDA Commissioner David Kessler decided to explore a broader regulatory approach than one based on the "implied health
claims" associated with low-tar cigarettes. In 1991, he created a team of
FDA lawyers, scientists, and policy makers to study the policy implications
of the finding that nicotine is an addictive drug. In particular, they explored
whether the FDA could regulate nicotine under the Federal Food, Drug, and
Cosmetic Act (Kessler 2000).

The statutory definition of drugs under the FDA law refers to "articles
(other than food) intended to affect the structure or any function of the
body." Kessler's team would spend the next several years documenting
both that nicotine affects the structure or function of the body and that the
tobacco industry intends it to have that effect. The phrase "intended to"
required evidence that nicotine was not merely an unavoidable component
of tobacco but was also an ingredient that cigarette makers intended to

affect the structure or function of the body. Using internal industry documents that had become available in lawsuits and from industry insiders, FDA policy makers documented in the industry's own words how tobacco companies manipulate nicotine levels and rely on the addictive qualities of nicotine to hook users (Kessler 2000).

Most Smokers Become Addicted as Adolescents

In the early 1990s, as the FDA tobacco team was exploring policy options, national experts on tobacco use had begun to highlight the importance of smoking among youth. Studies showed that nearly 90 percent of adult smokers began smoking by the time they were 18 years old and that every day some 3,000 young people began to smoke (DHHS 1994; IOM 1994; Pierce et al. 1989). In 1992, Congress passed the so-called Synar Amendment to limit youth access to tobacco by requiring states to control access as a condition of receiving federal substance abuse block grants (IOM 1994).

In 1994, two major reports highlighted the problem of smoking among youth: the Surgeon General issued Preventing Tobacco Use Among Young People (DHHS 1994), and the Institute of Medicine (IOM) released Growing Up Tobacco Free: Preventing Nicotine Addiction in Children and Youth (IOM 1994). Those reports described the problem of initiation of smoking and nicotine addiction among youth and the factors promoting use of tobacco use among young people. The IOM report recommended specific actions that could be used to address the problem, including proposals to curtail youth access to tobacco products, restrict youth-oriented tobacco marketing, limit advertising to a text-only format, narrow the preemption provision of the 1969 federal cigarette labeling law, and enact comprehensive federal regulation of tobacco products.

The recognition that most smokers become addicted in their teens further undermined the industry arguments against regulation based on free choice. Secondhand smoke findings demonstrated that smoking endangers nonsmokers, evidence of nicotine addiction established that the decision to continue smoking is not always a free choice, and now studies showed that the overwhelming majority of smokers are already on the path toward addiction before they turn 18 years of age (IOM 1994). The public may respond negatively to paternalistic, "Nanny State" policies aimed at changing the behavior of competent adults, but protecting children is a powerful justification for regulating dangerous products. Moreover, industry marketing in the 1990s (epitomized by R.J. Reynolds' Joe Camel campaign) clearly had special appeal to children and teens and suggested that the industry was actually targeting young people, a suspicion subsequently borne out by internal industry documents.

The focus on youth and the revelations in industry documents caught on with the public. A 1993 Roper poll asked a sample of registered voters whether they mostly agreed or mostly disagreed with the following statement: "Even though tobacco companies say they don't want kids to smoke, they really do everything they can to get teenagers and young people to take up smoking" (Marttila and Kiley Inc. 1993a). Of those polled, 64 percent said they mostly agreed, while 73 percent of the respondents reported an unfavorable or very unfavorable overall impression of the tobacco industry (Marttila and Kiley Inc. 1993b).

FDA Commissioner Kessler decided to focus the FDA regulatory approach on tobacco use among youth. Kessler, a pediatrician, called nicotine addiction a "pediatric disease" (Hilts 1995). On August 23, 1996, he joined President Bill Clinton in the White House Rose Garden to announce historic regulations that, for the first time, would put cigarettes under FDA control. The regulations declared cigarettes "nicotine-delivery devices" (DHHS 2000). Relying on the scientific foundation laid in the 1994 reports by the Surgeon General and the IOM, the new FDA regulations limited youth access to tobacco and controlled tobacco advertising and promotion targeted at young people. Immediately, tobacco companies challenged the regulations in federal court, initiating litigation that would eventually find its way to the U.S. Supreme Court (DHHS 2000).

States Take the Lead

In the early 1990s, while the FDA was exploring a federal role in regulating tobacco, states and localities had already begun to take action to contain the tobacco problem. Grassroots antitobacco advocacy was a driving force behind the creation of smoke-free spaces, and increasingly activists began to initiate other antismoking programs at the state and local levels. New antitobacco coalitions in the states began to effect important policy changes.

The burst of state action began in 1988, when the people of California passed Proposition 99, a referendum that increased the excise tax on tobacco from 10 to 35 cents per pack and earmarked 20 percent of the new revenues for a statewide antismoking campaign. California designed and put in place a comprehensive program that included mass media counter marketing campaigns, school-based programs, community-based interventions, and a research component. Massachusetts, Arizona, and a succession of other states followed with citizen referenda or legislation increasing tobacco excise taxes to various degrees and designating some of the money for antitobacco activities.

Historically, federal, state, and local governments have taxed cigarettes primarily to generate revenues, especially in response to budget crises. In recent years, however, many states have viewed tobacco excise tax increases as a tool for reducing demand for tobacco while providing funding for public health measures (Rabin and Sugarman 2001). Many studies have found that the overall consumption of cigarettes declines with increases in the price of cigarettes (DHHS 2000) (see Chapter 5). Although figures on the "price elasticity" of demand for cigarettes vary somewhat, the general rule is that a 10 percent increase in the real price reduces overall consumption by about 4 percent and the rate of smoking among youth by 7 percent.

In addition to tax revenues, in the 1990s states received funds from philanthropic organizations and the federal government to create comprehensive tobacco control programs. The National Cancer Institute's American Stop Smoking Intervention Study (ASSIST) demonstration program, a partnership with the American Cancer Society, funded 17 state health departments from 1991 to 1999. The program's goal was to "alter states' social, cultural, economic, and environmental factors that promote smoking" (NCI 2005). The Centers for Disease Control and Prevention's Initiatives to Mobilize for the Prevention and Control of Tobacco program (IMPACT) funded tobacco control initiatives in the other states (except California).

Also in the early 1990s, the Robert Wood Johnson Foundation (RWJF), under President Steven Schroeder, became the first philanthropy in the United States to make a major commitment to tobacco control. Over the next decade, the RWJF invested more than $400 million dollars in research, policy, and communications programs aimed at reducing the harm caused by tobacco (Bornemeier 2005). In 1994, RWJF created the SmokeLess States program, administered by the AMA, to support nongovernmental coalitions to educate the public and policy makers about the risks of tobacco use. The program was meant to augment the federal funding that was going to state governments and expand upon the innovations under way in California.

By the mid-1990s, every state had funds from one or more of these sources to build tobacco control programs. In 1999, the CDC replaced ASSIST and IMPACT with a nationwide program that provided funds to all 50 states and the District of Columbia. The SmokeLess States program continued until 2004. Comprehensive state programs contained various initiatives, such as launching counter advertising and public education campaigns, establishing smoke-free workplaces and public spaces, increasing prices through taxation, supporting treatment programs for tobacco dependence, enforcing youth access restrictions, and monitoring performance and evaluating programs (IOM/NRC 2000). Some states, including California, Massachusetts, and Florida, pioneered innovative models that included edgy youth-oriented media campaigns that challenged youth not to let the tobacco industry manipulate them into smoking.

The state-based programs reflected a shift in tobacco control—from a reliance on efforts directed at individual behavioral change to community approaches designed to change social and environmental influences on smoking behavior. Research suggested that this new emphasis would be beneficial, as studies had shown that interventions directed solely at individuals were not likely to result in large-scale declines in smoking prevalence (NCI 1991).

The tobacco industry recognized the potential of this new approach for reducing tobacco use and sought to defeat local initiatives and limit the scope and impact of the increasing activities of the states. The industry charged that advocacy activities amounted to illegal lobbying by public agencies (Aguinaga-Bialous and Glantz 1999; Gerlach and Larkin 2005). An evaluation of the ASSIST program, based in part on internal industry documents, found that the industry's strategy was to burden the states with requests for documents under the federal Freedom of Information Act and accuse ASSIST staff and local coalition members with using funds for illegal lobbying, causing confusion over what actions the ASSIST program could legally take (NCI 2005). To stem the movement toward smoke-free spaces, the industry tried, often successfully, to convince state legislatures to enact lax statewide laws while precluding more stringent local ordinances (ANR 2004).

New Litigation Strategies

Commercial tobacco interests were also becoming increasingly engaged on another battleground. From the 1950s until the early 1990s, tobacco companies were consistently victorious against tobacco control efforts in the courts. Litigation had thus shown little promise as a tool for tobacco control (Rabin 1993). However, the findings about nicotine addiction, the revelations that companies had concealed and misrepresented health information, and new opportunities to aggregate cases in so-called class actions transformed the litigation landscape in the 1990s (Rabin 2001a).

Attorneys who had previously not been involved in tobacco litigation began suing tobacco companies on behalf of large groups of smokers (Rabin 2001b). The first tobacco class action was Broin v. Philip Morris, filed in 1991 on behalf of flight attendants who claimed that they were injured by secondhand smoke prior to the airline smoking ban. A $349 million settlement was reached before the trial concluded.

The nationwide class action suit Castano v. American Tobacco, filed in 1994, brought together some of the country's leading plaintiff attorneys. Nicotine addiction was the centerpiece of the case, which drew on emerging evidence that companies tried to conceal and misrepresent the addictive properties of nicotine and that they knowingly addicted their customers. Although a federal appellate court eventually decertified the class in the Castano case, subsequent individual tort suits and class actions suits continued to develop the addiction argument. Some suits were successful, although not all rulings were upheld on appeal. Other pending cases accuse tobacco companies of fraud over use of words like "light" and "low-tar" to imply that cigarettes with these characteristics are less hazardous to a person's health. Potentially the most significant case of this kind, Schwab v. Philip Morris, was certified as a class action in a federal district court in New York in 2006. The "third wave" of tobacco litigation, beginning in 1994, has been summarized by Douglas et al. (2006) and Janofsky (2005). In what proved to be a pivotal legal milestone in the history of tobacco control, in 1994 Mississippi Attorney General Michael Moore filed a suit against the tobacco companies to recover the state's Medicaid expenditures on residents with tobacco-related illnesses. Because the state was the injured party under Moore's legal theory, he bypassed the industry's customary defense in suits filed by smokers that the smokers were responsible for their own injuries (Fisher 2001). Soon every state filed similar suits.

Moore and several other state attorneys general negotiated a so-called global settlement with the major tobacco companies in 1997. The proposed agreement would have bound the industry to various tobacco control efforts, including restrictions on advertising and promotion, and would have accepted FDA jurisdiction over cigarettes. The agreement would also have settled all pending state suits and would have immunized the companies from all class action litigation. According to Stanford law professor (and committee member) Robert Rabin: "Beyond doubt, [the agreement] was a testament to the awesome threat posed by the [states'] litigation strategy" (Rabin 2001b).

Congressional approval was required for the agreement to be binding. Legislation sponsored by Senator John McCain to implement the settlement and put in place other measures favored by tobacco control advocates became a target for aggressive lobbying by both those for and those against the bill. The legislation divided the tobacco control advocates, with some leaders—including David Kessler and former Surgeon General C. Everett Koop—opposing it on the ground that it was too favorable to the tobacco companies. The proposed legislation was caught up in a filibuster and never received a floor vote (Pertschuk 2001).

However, a short time later—on November 23, 1998—the attorneys general of 46 states, the District of Columbia (and American territories such as Guam and Puerto Rico) signed the Master Settlement Agreement (MSA) with the major tobacco companies (National Association of Attorneys General 1998).

The MSA required companies to pay an estimated $206 billion to the 46 states between 2000 and 2025. (Four states—Florida, Minnesota, Mississippi, and Texas—had previously reached a settlement that obligated the companies to pay those states more than $40 billion.) Because the MSA did not envision FDA jurisdiction or other federal action, it did not require congressional approval; the required approval came from state legislatures and the courts.

The MSA also required the companies to support a new charitable foundation—which came to be the American Legacy Foundation—to reduce teenage smoking and substance abuse and to prevent tobacco-related diseases. The MSA placed numerous restrictions on industry marketing and promotion, including the elimination of cartoon characters and billboard advertising and restrictions on tobacco company sponsorships of various events. The MSA also constrained the industry's political activity, disbanding the Tobacco Institute and the Council for Tobacco Research, and included a number of other provisions (National Association of Attorneys General 1998).

In return for these concessions, the tobacco companies that signed the agreement received protection from lawsuits by state Medicaid programs. The agreement also contained provisions to protect manufacturers from new competitors by providing for reductions in their required payments if the participating companies lost market share to other companies as a result of the agreement.

The MSA did not prohibit suits by or on behalf of smokers or by the federal government. In 1999, the Clinton Administration filed a landmark lawsuit against the major cigarette companies under the Racketeer Influenced and Corrupt Organizations Act (RICO) and the Bush Administration continued to prosecute the litigation. On the basis of the evidence introduced at the trial, which began in 2004 in the U.S. District Court for the District of Columbia, the federal government argued that the companies "engaged in and executed—and continue to engage in and execute—a massive 50-year scheme to defraud the public, including consumers of cigarettes, in violation of RICO," and that the companies' "past and ongoing conduct indicates a reasonable likelihood of future violations." Although the government originally sought "disgorgement of Defendants' ill-gotten gains," the U.S. Court of Appeals for the District of Columbia Circuit ruled out disgorgement and limited the scope of the remedy to "forward-looking" actions designed to prevent continued RICO violations. District Judge Gladys Kessler subsequently found that the defendants were liable under RICO and imposed a remedial order aimed at preventing future violations including bans on the use of misleading terms such as "light" and requiring corrective statements in a variety of channels to overcome the defendants' past efforts to deny the addictive character and adverse health effects of smoking. (For further discussion of the RICO remedy, see Chapter 6.)

Momentum Builds

Major advances in tobacco control occurred both in the courts and in legislatures during a short period of time, thereby reversing the political momentum that long seemed to favor the tobacco industry in Congress and state legislatures. Thus, by end of the 1990s, tobacco control advocates were energized and optimistic about further gains in the 50-year effort to end the tobacco problem. At about this time, the architects of Healthy People 2010 (DHHS 2002) set an ambitious goal of reducing the prevalence of smoking among adults (defined as smoking at least 100 cigarettes in their lifetimes and who now report smoking cigarettes every day or on some days) in half—from the 1998 baseline of 24 percent, to 12 percent in 2010. For high school students the target was a 54 percent drop from the 1999 smoking prevalence rate of 35 percent to a rate of 16 percent in 2010 (smokers in high school were defined as those having smoked one or more cigarettes in the previous 30 days).

Despite setbacks and persistent opposition, important milestones in tobacco control were attained in the 1990s and early 2000s. The MSA and the four-state settlement placed some controls on the industry and provided for large payments to the states. The American Legacy Foundation, established and funded pursuant to the MSA, sponsored a nationwide counter advertising campaign, the first in 30 years. The campaign, modeled on the "truth" campaign in Florida, was linked to 22 percent of the decline in the rate of smoking among youth between 1999 and 2002. The overall rate of smoking among students in grades 8, 10, and 12 dropped from 25.3 percent to 18 percent during that period. This translates into approximately 300,000 fewer young smokers (Farrelly et al. 2005) (see Chapter 5 and Slater, Appendix N).

Studies have also linked comprehensive tobacco control activities to decreases in smoking among youth. A recent study of state expenditures on tobacco control found, "clear evidence that tobacco control funding is inversely related to the percentage of youth who smoke and the average number of cigarettes smoked by young smokers" (DHHS 1994; Tauras et al. 2005). The smoking rates in states with the most aggressive programs declined more than the national average. Recently, in Maine, for example, the rates of smoking declined 59 percent among middle schools students and 48 percent among high school students between 1997, when the state began its campaign, and 2003 (Tobacco Free Kids 2004).

Aggressive state antismoking campaigns also contributed to the overall decrease in the prevalence of smoking among adults beginning in the late 1990s. Early evidence of the impact of these programs came from the California Tobacco Control Program, which was associated with nearly twice the rate of decline in smoking prevalence as that in the rest of the United

States between 1989 and 1993 (Gilpin et al. 2001). The National Cancer Policy Board (a joint program of the IOM and the National Research Council) examined the evidence on the effectiveness of state programs and concluded in a 2000 report that, "multi-faceted state tobacco control programs are effective in reducing tobacco use" (IOM/NRC 2000). The evidence on the effects of the state programs is reviewed in Chapter 5.

A growing number of states, localities, and workplaces have become smoke free. Nine states—California, Connecticut, Delaware, Maine, New York, Massachusetts, Rhode Island, Vermont, and Washington—have comprehensive, statewide smoke-free laws (ALA 2005, 2006). The laws in Florida, Idaho, and Utah exempt only stand-alone bars. Studies and economic data show that fears that restaurants and bars would suffer economically from smoking bans have not generally been borne out. Some of the strongest evidence of the impact of secondhand smoke policies comes from New York City, where a comprehensive smoking ban took effect on March 30, 2003. In the year after the law took effect, business receipts for restaurants and bars increased, the rate of employment rose, and the number of liquor licenses increased. Virtually all establishments are complying with the law, which has the support of most New Yorkers (Tobacco Free Kids 2006). According to a 2005 report, 18.4 percent of adults in New York City smoke, a decline from 19.2 percent a year earlier and a decline from 21.6 percent from 2 years earlier. These declines are significantly steeper than those for the nation overall (Perez-Pena 2005).

A substantial increase in cigarette prices has also occurred over the past decade. The federal excise taxes on cigarettes rose from 24 cents to 39 cents per pack between 1993 and 2002, many states raised their cigarette taxes, and the major manufacturers increased prices by about a dollar per pack, including 45 cents a pack to cover the cost of the MSA (Capehart 2001). In 1997, premium brands cost about $1.90 per pack, and by 2003 the cost had increased to about $3.60 a pack, with higher prices in states with higher taxes (Derthick 2004).

The exposure of the tobacco companies' deceptive marketing practices not only resulted in widespread criticism of the industry but also created a new justification for legal action and regulation. A dramatic measure of how much had changed was the new corporate stance of the country's largest cigarette company, Philip Morris USA. In the fall of 1999, Philip Morris acknowledged in a public statement that smoking causes cancer and that nicotine is addictive (Meier 1999). A few months later, Philip Morris officially took the position that cigarettes should be regulated (AP 2000). Only a few years earlier, the company's chief executive officer (who had since left the company), along with the chief executive officers of other major tobacco companies, testified before a congressional committee (under oath) that he did not believe that nicotine is addictive (Waxman 1994).

More effective smoking cessation techniques that use pharmacological and behavioral methods recently became available, although many smokers still lack access to quitting services. The federal government released clinical practice guidelines to provide health care professionals with the latest information available on effective treatment strategies to help smokers quit. A subcommittee of the federal government's Interagency Committee on Smoking and Health developed a National Action Plan for Tobacco Cessation aimed at preventing 3 million premature deaths and helping 5 million smokers quit. In February 2004, the day before the plan was released at a news conference, Secretary of Health and Human Services Tommy Thompson announced the establishment of the National Quitline Network with an allocation of $25 million per year. The subcommittee estimated to reach its goals; however, the cost of the quit line would be $3.2 billion a year. Ten months later, Thompson announced the toll-free number for this quit line (1-800-QUITNOW). In early 2005, the Centers for Medicare and Medicaid Services announced that smoking cessation counseling would become a covered Medicare benefit, the second of the subcommittee's six recommendations to be addressed (Michael Fiore, personal communication, June 30, 2005).

One important objective of many tobacco control advocates has not been realized, however. In 2000, the U.S. Supreme Court ruled 5-4 that the Federal Food, Drug, and Cosmetic Act does not give the FDA the authority to regulate tobacco (FDA v. Brown & Williamson Tobacco Corp. [98-1152] 529 U.S. 120, 2000). This left in place the incongruous situation in which the FDA and other agencies have authority over products that cause far less harm than cigarettes while cigarettes continue to evade meaningful federal regulation.

After the Supreme Court's decision, attention turned to Congress. In 2004, a Senate bill giving the FDA the authority to regulate tobacco was attached to a $10 billion buyout of tobacco growers. Although the bill passed by a large margin in the Senate, the provisions related to the FDA were eliminated in conference committee. Comprehensive and bipartisan bills were reintroduced in 2007. Like its predecessors, the Family Smoking Prevention and Tobacco Control Act (S.625 and HR 1008) would give the FDA wide-ranging authority over the manufacture, distribution, and promotion of tobacco products (Legal Resource Center for Tobacco Regulation 2005).

Among other important provisions, S.625 and HR 1008 would revive the 1996 FDA Tobacco Rule, strengthen cigarette package warnings and authorize the FDA to prescribe stronger warnings in the future, and give the FDA the authority to require cigarettes to meet health-based performance standards. The bill has widespread support among tobacco control advocates as well as the endorsement of Philip Morris USA. Notwithstanding the broad powers that it would give the FDA, some tobacco control advocates oppose it because it would legitimize tobacco products and might deter the development and marketing of reduced-risk products.

Since the 1980s, tobacco companies have experimented with novel tobacco- and cigarette-like products designed to reduce the toxicity of smoking and the level of secondhand smoke emissions. These products have taken various forms over the years, including cigarette-like devices that heat rather than burn tobacco and, more recently, cigarettes with reduced carcinogen emissions. Harm reduction products, also referred to as PREPs (potential reduced-exposure products), are potentially beneficial, but there is not yet enough scientific evidence to determine their effectiveness in reducing harm from smoking (IOM 2001).

Companies have test marketed PREPs in recent years, but few have been introduced and few are marketed nationally. In 2005, Vermont, joined by several other states, sued the R.J. Reynolds company over the company's claims that its Eclipse cigarette, which heats tobacco without actually burning it, might reduce the risk of cancer and other health problems (AP 2005).

Although congressional action on tobacco had been stalled since 2004 until recently, important litigation victories have continued to occur. In 2006, U.S. District Judge Gladys Kessler ruled in favor of the federal government in its massive RICO case against the tobacco companies alleging that they had engaged in misleading conduct for decades as part of a broad conspiracy (United States v. Philip Morris USA Inc., et al., 99-CV-2496, 2006). As noted above, Judge Kessler's remedial order was limited to actions designed to prevent future violations of RICO because earlier rulings had precluded "backward-looking" remedies such as disgorgement of the profits made by the defendant cigarette manufacturers:

[T]he Court is enjoining Defendants from further use of deceptive brand descriptors which implicitly or explicitly convey to the smoker and potential smoker that they are less hazardous to health than full flavor cigarettes, including the popular descriptors "low tar," "light," "ultra light," "mild," and "natural." The Court is also ordering Defendants to issue corrective statements in major newspapers, on the three leading television networks, on cigarette "onserts," and in retail displays, regarding: (1) the adverse health effects of smoking; (2) the addictiveness of smoking and nicotine; (3) the lack of any significant health benefit from smoking "low tar," "light," "ultra light," "mild," and "natural" cigarettes; (4) Defendants' manipulation of cigarette design and composition to ensure optimum nicotine delivery; and (5) the adverse health effects of exposure to secondhand smoke.

Judge Kessler's RICO rulings regarding liability and remedy are now on appeal. In addition, findings similar to those made by Judge Kessler have provided the factual foundation for substantial punitive damages awards in states courts. Although some of these awards have been reduced on appeal on the grounds that they were unconstitutionally excessive, the courts have rarely questioned the factual basis for the findings or the suitability of some award for punitive damages for the industry's "reprehensible conduct" (see generally, Guardino and Daynard 2005).

TOBACCO CONTROL IN THE YEARS AHEAD: WILL PROGRESS CONTINUE?

Has Momentum Slowed?

The public health community has made significant progress over the past decade, but there are also worrisome signs that progress may be stalling. It is difficult to sustain public attention on an endemic health problem over an extended period. Other pressing public health concerns, such as obesity and disparities in the provision of health care, have increasingly commanded the attention of both public and private leaders in the health care sector. Budgetary constraints in federal agencies, such as NIH and the CDC have affected tobacco control research. Moreover, in recent years many states have chosen to cut tobacco control funding and to divert MSA payments to needs other than tobacco control (GAO 2006).

Billions of dollars are flowing to the states from the MSA and the accompanying four-state settlement. By the end of 2003, the 46 MSA states had received more than $46 billion. Each state determines how much of that money will be allocated for tobacco control activities, however, and with states experiencing serious budget shortfalls in the early years of the new millenium, many chose to divert substantial portions of those funds to help balance budgets and meet other state needs. Additionally, some states used the stream of money to secure bonds, forfeiting future MSA funds to get money immediately. Even when the states were not experiencing such a deep financial crisis, less than 5 percent of MSA funds to the states were being spent on tobacco control (Gross et al. 2002; Schroeder 2002).

The CDC has recommended minimum levels that states need to spend to achieve successful tobacco prevention and cessation (CDC 1999). As of December 2004, only three states—Delaware, Maine, and Mississippi—met that minimum. The District of Columbia and 37 states fund tobacco control programs at less than half the CDC minimum or provide no funds at all. Some of the states with the most innovative programs, including Minnesota, Florida, and Massachusetts, have substantially reduced their tobacco control budgets. 2005 marked the third straight year that states overall cut their tobacco control expenditures (Campaign for Tobacco Free Kids 2004).

When support for tobacco control wanes, earlier progress in reducing tobacco use can quickly be reversed by the social forces that tend to promote smoking. Industry expenditures on traditional advertising have declined in the wake of the marketing restrictions imposed by the MSA. However, promotional activities remain very strong, as the companies concentrate on direct contact with potential consumers and retail promotions, particularly price discounts. As a result of a heavy emphasis on price promotions, tobacco companies spent a record $15.15 billion on cigarette advertising and promotion in the United States in 2003 (the year for which latest data are available), which represents an increase of 21.5 percent over that in 2002, 35.0 percent over that in 2001, and 58 percent over that in 2000. The amount for the 2003 is more than twice what companies were spending just 5 years earlier (FTC 2005). As marketing to underage smokers has been curtailed, companies have increasingly targeted the 18- to 21-year-old market (Tobacco Free Kids 2005).

Tobacco companies are spending $28 on marketing tobacco products for every dollar that the states spend on tobacco prevention efforts, according to a report by a coalition of public health agencies. Stated in another way, tobacco companies spend more money on marketing in a single day than 46 states and the District of Columbia spend on preventing smoking in a year (Tobacco Free Kids 2004).

The market share of nonparticipating discount cigarettes marketers has increased since the agreement was signed, even though MSA provisions were designed to avoid such an increase. As a result, most funding for the American Legacy Foundation ended after 5 years because continued funding was conditioned on maintenance of at least a 99.05 percent market share among the four companies that signed the agreement (American Legacy Foundation 2003).

Many smokers still lack access to effective cessation services; and physicians do not routinely address tobacco use with patients, despite the dissemination of national clinical guidelines. Several recommendations of the Interagency Committee on Smoking and Health, including investing in research into new tobacco dependence interventions, have not been addressed. Current treatments result in long-term success at quitting among only 10 to 30 percent of smokers (Fiore et al. 2004).

The Consequences of Unchanged or Weakened Tobacco Policies and Programs

In sum, over the last decade considerable progress in building a strong foundation for continued efforts to reduce tobacco use has been made, but the momentum appears to have slowed. Indeed, there are genuine reasons for concern that the infrastructure for tobacco control is eroding while the tobacco industry's efforts to promote and maintain demand are continuing to increase. It is these concerns that led the American Legacy Foundation to ask the IOM to evaluate strategies that can be used to continue to reduce tobacco use and to examine barriers to the implementation of those strategies. As a part of this undertaking, the committee believed that it was necessary to consider the likely consequences not only of intensified tobacco control activities but also of standing still or even a weakened investment in tobacco control efforts. Thus the committee decided to explore the available tools for projecting trends in tobacco use under different sets of assumptions. Scientists who do this type of work create mathematical models of the "system" of tobacco use, quantifying the factors that affect the outcomes of interest, such as the prevalence of use, tobacco-related mortality, and health expenditures.

No one can ever be certain what will happen in the future, and predictions in this domain are complicated by the fact that the system of tobacco use is complex in the technical, as well as the everyday, sense of the word. However, certain aspects of future patterns of use, morbidity, and mortality are relatively predictable because they display considerable inertia and lagged behavior. For example, even if, starting today, not one additional person were to begin smoking, the prevalence of tobacco use would still decline relatively slowly over time. Likewise, even if, starting today, every current smoker were to decide to quit and were able to do so permanently, there would still be substantial smoking-related morbidity and premature mortality for many years to come.

The committee's charge requires it to estimate the consequences of adopting or not adopting particular tobacco control policies and programs on future patterns of use. Making that sort of projection is inevitably somewhat speculative. Careful use of certain technical tools can lead to better-informed projections than mere human intuition can produce, however, particularly for systems with lags and inertia. Accordingly, the committee surveyed the macrolevel tobacco policy simulation literature thoroughly and commissioned analyses based on two macro- or population-level tobacco simulation models: the SimSmoke model (Levy, Appendix J) and the System Dynamic Model (Mendez, Appendix K). Although the committee is confident that these two models represent the state of the art in the domain of tobacco policy, it is important to emphasize that this body of knowledge is rather incomplete compared with the enormous knowledge base concerning the individual-level consequences of smoking and past and current patterns of smoking. The models may also appear to be incomplete compared with the completeness of the policy simulation tools available in other policy domains. (Particular limitations of the state of the art in tobacco policy modeling are outlined in Chapter 7.) The limitations of the models must be taken into account in deciding how much weight should be given to projections based on them.

Both of the models used in the committee's analyses are what might be called "compartmental" or "stocks-and-flows" models. They track over time the number of people in various "states," such as the number of female smokers in the past year between the ages of 25 and 34 years. Levels of these "stocks" change over time because of "flows" in and out because of smoking initiation, cessation, and relapse and underlying demographic changes (aging, death, etc.). For the present purposes, the most important difference between these two models concerns what each takes as inputs. The System Dynamic Model projects the consequences of particular initiation and cessation rates. It answers questions of the form, "Suppose that the rate of smoking initiation fell by 10 percent. What would that imply for smoking prevalence in 15 years?" The SimSmoke model backs up one step and uses policies as inputs. The SimSmoke model's policy modules translate evidence pertaining to historical policy actions into estimated effects on flow rates, which then, in turn, affect smoking prevalence over time.

The modeling commissioned by the committee is focused on smoking prevalence because the committee believes that prevalence can be projected more reliably than smoking-related morbidity and mortality. (As indicated above, however, that does not mean that model-based projections of future rates of smoking prevalence are necessarily accurate; the accuracy of these projections is limited by the inevitable uncertainty of the future and by the limitations of the models or the data used by the modelers.)

Projections Based on the Status Quo

The first question of interest to the committee in carrying out its charge is what trends can be expected in tobacco use prevalence if the level and intensity of tobacco control remain unchanged. Figures 3-1 and 3-2 give those projections by use of the SimSmoke model and System Dynamic Model, respectively. Specifically, the SimSmoke model projects what would happen if the tobacco control policies of 2005 were maintained with no additions or retrenchments. The System Dynamic Model shows what might occur if the smoking initiation and cessation rates of 2005 were maintained in the future. The models reveal that there is good news and bad news for public health with regard to reducing tobacco use in the future.

The good news is that both models show that, even if tobacco control activities remain at present levels, smoking prevalence will decline from 2006's estimated 20.9 percent to a little less than 16 percent in 2025. This continued decline will occur because of the system's inertia: there are currently more middle-aged and older smokers than there would have been

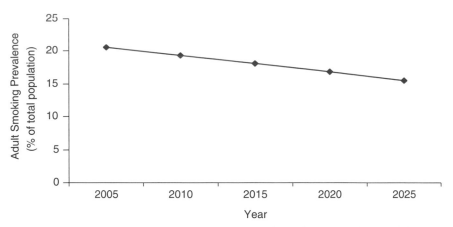

FIGURE 3-1 Estimated adult smoking prevalence from the SimSmoke Model (2005 to 2025) assuming no change in the tobacco control environment (status quo scenario).

had those birth cohorts passed through the ages of tobacco initiation under higher tobacco prices and stronger tobacco controls. Over time, as those birth cohorts are replaced by aging younger cohorts who had lower rates of smoking initiation, the prevalence of smoking will continue to decline.

The System Dynamic Model projects further into the future than SimSmoke, in this case, until the year 2050; and this projection gives the

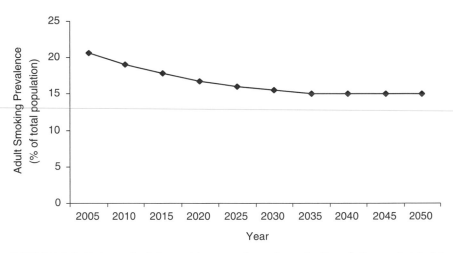

FIGURE 3-2 Estimated adult smoking prevalence from the System Dynamic Model (2005 to 2050) assuming no change in the tobacco control environment (status quo scenario).

had news. One must keep in mind that the further into the future that one projects, the greater the uncertainty of the projection is; however, the System Dynamic Model shows that shortly after 2025, the decline in prevalence will plateau well above the Healthy People 2010 target of 12 percent, halting at about 15 percent.

Projections Based on Weakened Tobacco Control

Both of these two, independent models give similar projections under base-case conditions, but future conditions could look quite different. As noted above, the risk of backsliding in tobacco control is considerable. With this in mind, the SimSmoke model was used to project a worst-case scenario based on a weakening of tobacco control policies and programs. Table 3-1 (Table 4 from Levy, Appendix J) shows the SimSmoke model projections of the consequences of various adverse changes in the baseline assumptions about the intensity of various tobacco control policies and programs. Specifically, the envisioned changes are reductions in tobacco prices of 40 and 80 cents per pack (whether these are due to reduced production costs, tax cuts, or price reductions in the face of competition from discount brands and Internet sales); the elimination of enforcement and publicity for clean air laws (but leaving the laws in place), elimination of media campaigns aimed at adults and youth, such as the American Legacy Foundation and Massachusetts state campaigns; elimination of quit lines; and, finally, the effects of all these changes together.

Any of these actions alone would increase the smoking prevalence in 2025 relative to the baseline or status quo projection of 15.5 percent prevalence. If all of these retrenchments occurred, the projected smoking prevalence in 2025 would be 17.1 percent, which would result in approximately 4 million more people smoking than would otherwise be the case (see also

TABLE 3-1 SimSmoke Model Prediction of Trends in Adult Smoking Prevalence (2005 to 2025) Assuming a Decline in Selected Tobacco Control Measures

Measure	Smoking Prevalence (%)				
	2005	2010	2015	2020	2025
40-cent-per-pack price reduction	20.6	19.6	18.6	17.6	16.3
80-cent-per-pack price reduction	20.6	19.9	18.9	18.0	16.7
Clean air law reduction	20.6	19.3	18.1	17.0	15.6
Adult media campaign reduction	20.6	19.4	18.2	17.0	15.7
Youth media campaign reduction	20.6	19.3	18.3	17.2	15.8
Cessation program reduction	20.6	19.3	18.1	17.0	15.6
All	20.6	20.0	19.2	18.4	17.1

Figure 3-3). Although the momentum generated by the last four decades of tobacco control is unlikely to be erased altogether, these projections do show that a weakened commitment to tobacco control will affect millions of lives; and the model does not take into account new smoking fads, other changes in demand, or industry innovations.

In Chapter 1, the committee observed that the patterns and trends of tobacco use differ substantially in different regions and states and that these differences arise to some extent from differences in the nature and the intensity of tobacco control activities. To depict the range of possible outcomes, the System Dynamic Model was used to project what would happen to smoking prevalence if, over the next 4 years (by 2010), the entire country's smoking initiation rates rose and smoking cessation rates fell to match those prevailing in Kentucky, the state with highest smoking prevalence, in 2005. If this were to occur, national smoking prevalence could rise—and could rise substantially, to 23.5 percent by 2025, an increase of approximately 11 million smokers. It is unlikely that tobacco control initiatives throughout the country would lose ground so quickly, but this calculation graphically makes the point that the inertial continuation of past trends should not be taken for granted. The committee also used the System Dynamic Model to estimate the changes in smoking prevalence that would occur if the country were to reach Kentucky's 2005 smoking initiation and smoking cessation levels in 2015 and 2020, scenarios that are more realistic. As shown in Figure 3-4, the results were equally disturbing: even imagining that it would take 15 years for smoking initiation and smoking cessation rates to reach Kentucky's levels, the model predicts that there would be more than 17 million more smokers by 2025 than under the status quo scenario displayed in Figure 3-5.

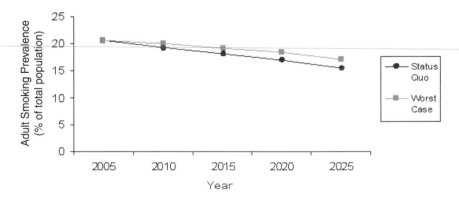

FIGURE 3-3 Comparison of SimSmoke Model estimates of adult smoking prevalence (2005 to 2025) under the status quo and worst-case scenarios.

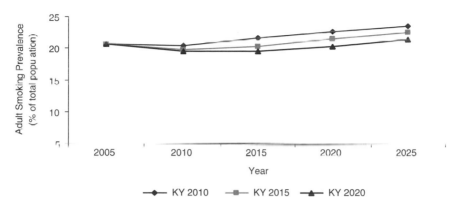

FIGURE 3-4 System Dynamic Model estimated adult smoking prevalence assuming the U.S. matched the 2004 initiation and cessation rates of Kentucky by 2010, 2015, and 2020.

Conversely, the committee wondered what would happen to overall national tobacco use prevalence if, over the next few years, tobacco control efforts intensified to the point that the entire country had initiation and cessation rates by 2010 that matched those of California in 2004. California was selected for this purpose because it is, to some extent, a model state with respect to both tobacco control policies and tobacco use. The projected trajectory is parallel to the national projection, but it plateaus at substantially lower levels, eventually reaching the 10 percent target of Healthy People 2010—albeit in 2050, almost two generations later than the 2010 milestone (Figure 3-6). Accordingly, there would appear to be substantial room for advances in tobacco control efforts to make a positive

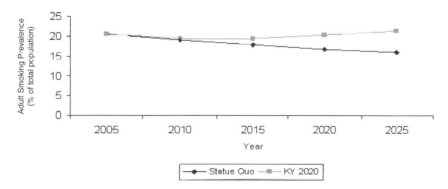

FIGURE 3-5 System Dynamic Model estimated adult smoking prevalence comparing Kentucky 2020 scenario with the status quo scenario.

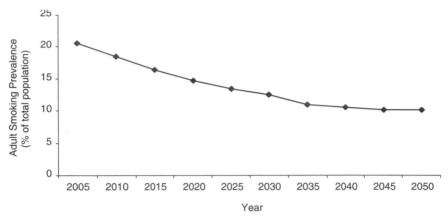

FIGURE 3-6 System Dynamic Model estimated adult smoking prevalence assuming the U.S. reaches California's 2004 initiation and cessation rates by 2010.

difference. The effects of intensified tobacco control activities are explored in Chapter 5.

SUMMARY

This chapter has documented the progress in building a strong foundation for state tobacco control activities that has been made over the last decade. However, there are genuine reasons for concern that the infrastructure for tobacco control is eroding while the tobacco industry's efforts to promote and maintain demand are continuing to increase.

The committee has tried to project the likely public health consequences of intensified or weakened investments in tobacco control compared with those of standing still. The good news is that even if tobacco control activities remain at present levels, smoking prevalence is likely to decline from 2006's estimated 20.9 percent to a little less than 16 percent in 2025. As noted above, this continued decline will occur because of the system's inertia: There are currently more middle-aged and older smokers than there would have been had their birth cohorts passed through the ages of tobacco initiation under higher tobacco prices and stronger tobacco controls. Over time, as those birth cohorts are replaced by aging younger cohorts who had lower rates of initiation, the prevalence of tobacco use will continue to decline. Shortly after 2025, however, the decline in prevalence appears likely to plateau at about 15 percent, well above the Healthy People 2010 target of 12 percent.

This steady-state scenario should be compared with a worst-case scenario, based on a weakening of tobacco control policies and programs.

If a significant retrenchment occurred, the projected smoking prevalence in 2025 would be about 17 percent, resulting in approximately 4 million more people smoking than would otherwise occur. Although the momentum generated by the last four decades of tobacco control is unlikely to be erased altogether, these projections do show that a weakened commitment to tobacco control will affect millions of lives; and the model does not take into account new smoking fads, other changes in demand, or industry innovations.

Finally, the committee projected the likely effect on overall national tobacco use prevalence if, over the next few years, tobacco control efforts intensified to the point that the initiation and cessation rates for the entire country were equivalent to those for California in 2004. The projected trajectory is parallel to the national projection, but it plateaus at substantially lower levels, eventually reaching 10 percent—albeit in 2050, almost two generations from now.

With these projections in mind, the committee considered what steps should be taken, not only to solidify progress already achieved and prevent backsliding, but also to set the country on a sure course for reducing tobacco use substantially by 2025. Part Two of the report presents the committee's "Blueprint for the Nation."

REFERENCES

Aguinaga-Bialous S, Glantz SA. 1999. Arizona's tobacco control initiative illustrates the need for continuing oversight by tobacco control advocates. *Tobacco Control* 8(2):141-151.

ALA (American Lung Association). 2005. *State of Tobacco Control: 2005*. New York: American Lung Association.

ALA. 2006. *American Lung Association Says More State Taking Strong Action to Protect Citizens From Tobacco Use*. Web Page. Available at: http://www.lungusa.org/site/apps/nl/content3.asp?c=dvLUK9OO0E&b=40408&ct=2059325; accessed July 24, 2006.

American Legacy Foundation. 2003. *American Legacy Foundation Calls Lorillard Plan to Tie Up Funding Unwarranted And Harmful*. Web Page. Available at: http://www.americanlegacy.org/americanlegacy/skins/alf/display.aspx?CategoryID=160386b2-d43a-4f67-890a-98e135a8ee6c&ObjectID=ab6fa256-833a-4d26-9f57-a3d8019874a8&Action=display_user_object&Mode=user&ModuleID=ad3a024a b2d6-4593-874f-9b66136bc614; accessed July 21, 2006.

ANR (Americans for Nonsmokers' Rights). 2004. *Preemption: Tobacco Control's #1 Enemy*. Berkeley, CA: Americans for Nonsmokers' Rights Foundation.

AP (Associated Press). 2000, February 29. Phillip Morris open to tobacco regulation. *USA Today*.

AP. 2005, July 27. Vermont: State Files Suit Against Tobacco Company. *The New York Times*.

Bayer R, Colgrove J. 2002. Science, politics, and ideology in the campaign against environmental tobacco smoke. *American Journal of Public Health* 92(6):949-954.

Borio G. 1993. *Tobacco Timeline*. Web Page. Available at: http://www.tobacco.org/resources/history/Tobacco_Historynotes.html; accessed August 4, 2006.

Bornemeier J. 2005. Taking on Tobacco: The Robert Wood Johnson Foundation's Assault on Smoking. Issacs S, Knickman J, Eds. *To Improve Health and Health Care, Vol. VIII.* San Francisco, CA: Jossey-Bass. Pp. 3-28.

Brandt AM. 2007. *The Cigarette Century: The Rise, Fall, and Deadly Persistence of the Product That Defined America.* New York: Basic Books.

Burnham JC. 1989. American physicians and tobacco use: two Surgeons General, 1929 and 1964. *Bulletin of the History of Medicine* 63(1):1-31.

Capehart TC. 2001. *Trends in the Cigarette Industry After the Master Settlement Agreement.* Washington, DC: Economic Research Service, U.S. Department of Agriculture.

CDC (Centers for Disease Control and Prevention). 1994. Guidelines for school health programs to prevent tobacco use and addiction. *MMWR (Morbidity and Mortality Weekly Report)* 43(RR-2):1-18.

CDC. 1999. *Best Practices for Comprehensive Tobacco Control Programs—August 1999.* Atlanta, GA: U.S. Department of Health and Human Services, Centers for Disease Control and Prevention, National Center for Chronic Disease Prevention and Health Promotion, Office on Smoking and Health.

CDC. 2005. *Selected Actions of the U.S. Government Regarding the Regulation of Tobacco Sales, Marketing, and Use.* Web Page. Available at: http://www.cdc.gov/tobacco/overview/regulate.htm; accessed July 24, 2006.

Derthick MA. 2004. *Up In Smoke: From Legislation to Litigation in Tobacco Politics.* Washington, DC: CQ Press.

DHHS (U.S. Department of Health and Human Services). 1986. *The Health Consequences of Involuntary Smoking: A Report of the Surgeon General.* Rockville, MD: U.S. Department of Health and Human Services, Centers for Disease Control and Prevention, Center for Health Promotion and Education, Office on Smoking and Health.

DHHS. 1988. *The Health Consequences of Smoking: Nicotine Addiction (A Report of the Surgeon General).* Rockville, MD: U.S. Department of Health and Human Services, Centers for Disease Control and Prevention, Center for Health Promotion and Education, Office on Smoking and Health.

DHHS. 1989. *Reducing the Health Consequences of Smoking: 25 Years of Progress (A Report of the Surgeon General).* Rockville, MD: U.S. Department of Health and Human Services, Centers for Disease Control and Prevention, Center for Chronic Disease Prevention and Health Promotion, Office on Smoking and Health.

DHHS. 1994. *Preventing Tobacco Use Among Young People (A Report of the Surgeon General).* Rockville, MD: U.S. Department of Health and Human Services, Centers for Disease Control and Prevention, Center for Health Promotion and Education, Office on Smoking and Health.

DHHS. 2000. *Reducing Tobacco Use: A Report of the Surgeon General.* Atlanta, GA: U.S. Department of Health and Human Services, Centers for Disease Control and Prevention, National Center for Chronic Disease Prevention and Health Promotion, Office on Smoking and Health.

DHHS. 2002. *Healthy People 2010: Understanding and Improving Health.* Washington, DC: U.S. Government Printing Office.

Douglas CE, Davis RM, Beasley JK. 2006. Epidemiology of the third wave of tobacco litigation in the United States, 1994-2005. *Tobacco Control* 15(Suppl 4):iv9-iv16.

EPA (Environmental Protection Agency). 1992. *Respiratory Health Effects of Passive Smoking: Lung Cancer and Other Disorders.* Washington DC: Office of Health and Environmental Assessment, Office of Research and Development, U.S. Environmental Protection Agency.

Farrelly MC, Davis KC, Haviland ML, Messeri P, Healton CG. 2005. Evidence of a dose—response relationship between "truth" antismoking ads and youth smoking prevalence. *American Journal of Public Health* 95(3):425-431.

Farrelly MC, Niederdeppe J, Yarsevich J. 2003. Youth tobacco prevention mass media campaigns: past, present, and future directions. *Tobacco Control* 12(Suppl 1):i35-i47.

Fiore MC, Croyle RT, Curry SJ, Cutler CM, Davis RM, Gordon C, Healton C, Koh HK, Orleans CT, Richling D, Satcher D, Seffrin J, Williams C, Williams LN, Keller PA, Baker TB. 2004. Preventing 3 million premature deaths and helping 5 million smokers quit: a national action plan for tobacco cessation. *American Journal of Public Health* 94(2):205-310.

Fisher L. 2001. Mississippi: the unsung hero of tobacco control, USA. *Cancer Causes and Control* 12:965-967.

FTC (Federal Trade Commission). 2005. *Cigarette Report for 2003*. Washington, DC: Federal Trade Commission.

GAO (General Accounting Office). 2006. *Tobacco Settlement: States' Allocations of Fiscal Year 2005 and Expected Fiscal Year 2006 Payments*. Washington, DC: GAO.

Gerlach KK, Larkin MA. 2005. *To Improve Health and Health Care, Vol. VIII*. San Francisco, CA: Jossey-Bass.

Gilpin EA, Emery SL, Farkas AJ, Distefan JM, White MM, Pierce JP. 2001. *The California Tobacco Control Program: A Decade of Progress, Results from the California Tobacco Surveys, 1990–1998 (Final Report)*. La Jolla, CA: University of California, San Diego.

Gross CP, Soffer B, Bach PB, Rajkumar R, Forman HP. 2002. State expenditures for tobacco-control programs and the tobacco settlement. *New England Journal of Medicine* 347(14):1080-1086.

Guardino SD, Daynard RA. 2005 (unpublished). *Punishing Tobacco Industry Misconduct: The Case for Exceeding a Single Digit Ratio Between Punitive and Compulsory Charges*. Web Page. Available at: http://law.bepress.com/cgi/viewcontent.cgi?article=2236&context=expresso; accessed July 26, 2007.

Hamilton JL. 1972. The demand for cigarettes: advertising, health scare, and the cigarette advertising ban. *Review of Economics and Statistics* 54:401-411.

Harris JE, Thun MJ, Mondul AM, Calle EE. 2004. Cigarette tar yields in relation to mortality from lung cancer in the cancer prevention study II prospective cohort, 1982-8. *BMJ* 328(7431):72.

HEW (Department of Health, Education, and Welfare). 1964. *Smoking and Health: Report of the Advisory Committee to the Surgeon General of the Public Health Service*. Washington, DC: U.S. Department of Health, Education, and Welfare; Public Health Service.

HEW. 1972. *The Health Consequences of Smoking: A Report of the Surgeon General 1972*. Washington, DC: Health Services and Mental Health Administration, Public Health Service, U.S. Department of Health, Education, and Welfare.

Hilts PJ. 1995, March 9. FDA head calls smoking a pediatric disease. *The New York Times*.

Hinds MD. 1982, January 30. Tougher cigarette warnings gain support. *The New York Times*.

IOM (Institute of Medicine). 1994. *Growing Up Tobacco Free: Preventing Nicotine Addiction in Children and Youth*. Washington, DC: National Academy Press.

IOM. 1996. *Pathways of Addiction: Opportunities in Drug Abuse Research*. Washington, DC: National Academy Press.

IOM. 2001. *Clearing the Smoke: Assessing the Science Base for Tobacco Harm Reduction*. Washington, DC: National Academy Press.

IOM/NRC (National Research Council). 2000. *State Programs Can Reduce Tobacco Use*. Washington, DC: National Academy Press.

Janofsky M. 2005, August 11. Big Tobacco, in Court Again. But the Stock Is Still Up. *The New York Times*. P. 21.

Kessler D. 2000. *A Question of Intent: A Great American Battle with a Deadly Industry*. New York: PublicAffairs.

Kluger R. 1996. *Ashes to Ashes: America's Hundred-Year Cigarette War, the Public Health, and the Unabashed Triumph of Philip Morris.* New York: Alfred A. Knopf.

Kluger R. 1997. *Ashes to Ashes, American's Hundred-Year Cigarette War, the Public Health, and the Unabashed Triumph of Philip Morris.* New York: Vintage Books.

Legal Resource Center for Tobacco Regulation Litigation and Advocacy, University of Maryland School of Law. 2005. Congress Considers FDA Regulation of Tobacco Products. *Tobacco Regulation Review* 4(1):1,3.

Marttila and Kiley Inc. 1993a. Even though tobacco companies say they don't want kids to smoke, they really do everything they can to get teenagers and young people to take up smoking. *Public Opinion Online (for Roper Center at University of Connecticut).*

Marttila and Kiley Inc. 1993b. Overall impression of the tobacco industry is very favorable, somewhat favorable, somewhat unfavorable, or very unfavorable. *Public Opinion Online (for Roper Center at University of Connecticut).*

Meier B. 1999, October 13. Phillip Morris admits evidence shows smoking causes cancer. *The New York Times.*

National Association of Attorneys General. 1998. *Master Settlement Agreement.* Web Page. Available at: http://www.naag.org/upload/1109185724_1032468605_cigmsa.pdf; accessed August 2, 2005.

NCI (National Cancer Institute). 1991. *Strategies to Control Tobacco Use in the Unites States: A Blueprint for Public Health Action in the 1990s (Monograph 1).* Bethesda, MD: National Institutes of Health.

NCI. 2001. *Risks Associated with Smoking Cigarettes with Low Machine-Measured Yields of Tar and Nicotine (Monograph 13).* Bethesda, MD: National Institutes of Health.

NCI. 2005. ASSIST: Shaping the Future of Tobacco Prevention and Control. *Tobacco Control Monograph Series.* Vol. 8, NIH Publication Number 05-5645. Bethesda, MD: National Institutes of Health.

Norr R. 1952. Cancer by the Carton. *The Reader's Digest*:7-8.

NRC (National Research Council). 1986. *Environmental Tobacco Smoke: Measuring Exposures and Assessing Health Effects.* Washington, DC: National Academy Press.

O'Keefe M. 1971. The anti-smoking commercials: a study of television's impact on behavior. *Public Opinion Quarterly* 35:242-248.

Outlook. 1901. The anti-cigarette crusade. *Outlook* 67(11):607-608.

Perez-Pena R. 2005, June 11. Smoking in State and City Is at New Low, Surveys Say. *The New York Times.*

Pertschuk M. 2001. *Smoke in Their Eyes: Lessons in Movement Leadership From the Tobacco Wars.* Nashville, TN: Vanderbilt University Press.

Pierce JP, Fiore MC, Novotny TE, Hatziandreu EJ, Davis RM. 1989. Trends in cigarette smoking in the United States. Projections to the year 2000. *Journal of the American Medical Association* 261(1):61-65.

Pierce JP, Lee L, Gilpin EA. 1994. Smoking initiation by adolescent girls, 1944 through 1988. An association with targeted advertising. *Journal of the American Medical Assocation* 271(8):608-611.

Rabin R. 1993. Institutional and Historical Perspectives on Tobacco Tort Litigation. Rabin R, Sugarman S, Editors. *Smoking Policy: Law, Politics, and Culture.* Pp. 110-130.

Rabin RL, Sugarman SD. 2001. *Regulating Tobacco: Premises and Policy Actions.* New York: Oxford University Press.

Rabin R. 2001a. The Third Wave of Tobacco Tort Litigation. Rabin RL, Sugarman SD, Eds. *Regulating Tobacco: Premises and Policy Options.* New York: Oxford University Press. Pp. 176-206.

Rabin R. 2001b. The tobacco litigation: a tentative assessment. *DePaul L. Rev.* 51:331-358.

Schroeder SA. 2002. Conflicting dispatches from the tobacco wars. *New England Journal of Medicine* 347(14):1106-1109.

Schudson M. 1984. *Advertising, the Uneasy Persuasion: Its Dubious Impact on American Society.* New York: Basic Books.

Shiffman S. 1993. Smoking cessation treatment: any progress? *Journal of Consulting and Clinical Psychology* 61(5):718-722.

Sugarman S. 2001. Rabin RL, Sugarman SD, Eds. International Aspects of Tobacco Control and the Proposed WHO Treaty. *Regulating Tobacco: Premises and Policy Options.* New York: Oxford University Press. Pp. 245-284.

Tate C. 1999. *Cigarette Wars: The Triumph of "The Littel White Slaver."* New York: Oxford University Press.

Tauras JA, Chaloupka FJ, Farrelly MC, Giovino GA, Wakefield M, Johnston LD, O'Malley PM, Kloska DD, Pechacek TF. 2005. State tobacco control spending and youth smoking. *American Journal of Public Health* 95(2):338-344.

The Roper Organization Inc. 1978. *A Study of Public Attitudes Toward Cigarette Smoking and the Tobacco Industry in 1978—Volume 1.*

Tobacco Free Kids. 2004. *A Broken Promise to Our Children: The 1998 State Tobacco Settlement Six Years Later.* Web Page. Available at: http://www.rwjf.org/files/research/TOBACCO%20FREE%20KIDS%20-%20fullreport%2012-04.pdf; accessed June 23, 2007.

Tobacco Free Kids. 2005. *Tobacco Company Marketing to College Students Since the Multistate Settlement Agreement Was Signed.* Web Page. Available at: http://www.tobaccofreekids.org/research/factsheets/pdf/0135.pdf; accessed April 5, 2006.

Tobacco Free Kids. 2006. *Smoke-Free Laws: Protecting Our Rights to Breathe Clean Air.* Web Page. Available at: http://tobaccofreekids.org/reports/shs/; accessed April 5, 2006.

Walsh JJ. 1937. Cigarettes and pathology. *Commonwealth* 25(24):665.

Warner KE. 1989. Effects of the antismoking campaign: an update. *American Journal of Public Health* 79(2):144-151.

Waxman H. 1994. *Hearing on the Regulation of Tobacco Products—House Committee on Energy and Commerce—Subcommittee on Health and the Environment.* Web Page. Available at: http://www.henrywaxman.house.gov/issues/health/tobacco_leg_highlights.htm; accessed August 7, 2006.

WHO (World Health Organization). August 2, 2005. *Tobacco.* Web Page. Available at: http://www.who.int/substance_abuse/facts/tobacco/en/ http://www.who.int/tobacco/ en/; accessed August 2, 2005.

PART II

A BLUEPRINT FOR REDUCING TOBACCO USE

4

Reducing Tobacco Use: A Policy Framework

T he committee was charged with developing a blueprint for reducing
tobacco use in the United States. As shown in Part I, a continued
gradual decline in the prevalence of tobacco use can probably be
expected over the next 20 years as a result of the social, economic, and
demographic forces already at work. However, reductions in tobacco use
substantial enough to eliminate tobacco use as a public health problem are
not likely to occur if the nation simply waits for past successes to continue.
Ending the tobacco problem will require the persistence and nimbleness
needed to counteract industry innovations in marketing and product design,
as well as the larger cultural and economic forces that tend to promote
and sustain tobacco use, especially among young people. The challenge is
heightened by the fact that heavy tobacco users may increasingly be harder
to reach effectively with the customary tools of tobacco control. Any slackening of the public health response not only will reduce forward progress
but also may lead to backsliding. Chapters 5 to 7 offer a detailed blueprint
for strong remedial actions to reduce tobacco use and aiming, eventually,
to erase tobacco as a significant public health problem. This chapter aims
to establish the normative context for the blueprint that follows.

PRODUCT SAFETY AND CONSUMER SOVEREIGNTY

At bottom, the tobacco problem is a product safety problem. In an
economic and social system that values freedom of choice, consumers are
generally permitted to select products and activities as they see fit. If they
want to assume risks, they are permitted to do exactly that. Government

does not guarantee absolute safety, nor should it. Of course, some dangers
are too high to be acceptable. So long as consumers are properly informed,
however, the presumption has traditionally been in favor of consumer
sovereignty and freedom of choice. Yet, even most libertarians will admit
that the tobacco market has been characterized by severe market failures,
including information asymmetry between producers and users, distorted
consumer choice due to information deficits, and product pricing that has
not reflected the full social costs of the product's use (especially the effects
on nonsmokers). They acknowledge the legitimacy of interventions aiming
to prevent youth smoking, to disseminate accurate information and correct
misinformation, and to assure that nonsmokers are protected from involuntary exposure to tobacco smoke if the market does not function properly.
The residual issue concerns the legitimacy of interventions that burden
smokers' choices for the purpose of getting them to quit. The overarching task for the nation is to consider thoughtfully how consumer freedom
can be respected while also taking into account the unique properties of
tobacco and tobacco products. The committee's major goal here is to set
forth a framework for reducing tobacco use, and its associated morbidity
and mortality, while being duly respectful of the interests of consumers and
the companies that satisfy consumer needs.

THE POLICY CONTEXT

During the first six decades of the 20th century, tobacco use became
deeply embedded in the economic and cultural life of the United States and
in many parts of the world, sowing the seeds of a massive public health
problem. The prevalence of smoking among adults in the United States was
42 percent in 1965. The tide turned in the 1960s as the adverse health effects
became known, but the prevalence of smoking among adults was still 21
percent in 2005. Absent a major initiative, the prevalence of smoking among
adults is likely to level off in 2025 at about 15 percent (see Chapter 3).

Aggressive policy initiatives were impeded for four decades by the tobacco industry's political and legal strategy of denying and obscuring the
addictive properties of nicotine and the real health effects of tobacco use.
All this also was reinforced by widespread popular acceptance of consumer
freedom to smoke (characterized by its defenders, somewhat ironically, as
the "right to be foolish"). In retrospect, it is surprising and puzzling that
strong measures to discourage smoking were regarded as unduly paternalistic even by people who otherwise might have been expected to favor strong
consumer protection measures. Laissez-faire more or less prevailed despite
the seriousness of the problem.

Until the late 1980s, the operating assumptions of tobacco policy in the
United States were rooted in the society's general preference for individual

liberty and freedom of choice, especially in matters that affect individual health. Thus, although it has been widely understood for many years that smoking poses serious health risks, the prevailing assumption was that the weighing of the benefits and the health risks of consumer products, including tobacco products, is up to the consumer and that government efforts to force people to make healthy choices would amount to an unacceptable form of paternalism. The underlying intuition is that people are and ought to be free to make their own choices and are responsible for the consequences of their choices. This perspective was also reflected in the unbroken line of jury verdicts and judicial decisions refusing to hold tobacco companies liable for smoking-induced disease and death among informed consumers.

The first major change in tobacco policy was consistent with the antipaternalism principle and with traditional economic theory. The nonsmokers' rights movement, which took root in California in the late 1970s, called attention to the fact that some of the costs of smoking are borne by third parties and urged lawmakers to adopt bans on smoking in public buildings and workplaces. The antismoking movement received a major boost when the U.S. Environmental Protection Agency classified environmental tobacco smoke as a carcinogen in 1992 (EPA 1992). Although the tobacco industry disputed the nature and the extent of the risks associated with exposure to sidestream smoke and continues to do so, the evidence documented suggesting the considerable health dangers of environmental tobacco smoke has been definitively summarized by the Surgeon General (DHHS 2006), and the moral legitimacy of smoking restrictions in enclosed public places is now taken for granted.

In the late 1990s, the weaknesses in the libertarian point of view began to seep into public understanding and to transform the policy debate about tobacco. This profound change in the political dynamic occurred as a result of three intertwined developments.

The first important development was a profound change in public understanding as the addictive nature of nicotine became scientifically established (DHHS 1989). The simultaneous proliferation of nicotine replacement treatments (NRTs) and other cessation tools, along with evidence of their effectiveness, helped to reinforce public understanding of the grip of nicotine addiction and the need for stronger measures to help people quit. This development also began to erode the anti-paternalism objection against efforts to reduce consumption directly on the grounds that many people who have become hooked would like to quit.

The second convergent development was a concerted focus on the problem of smoking initiation. It became clear that almost all adult smokers began smoking as teenagers and that prevention of the initiation of smoking needed to be a core aim of tobacco policy. (Although it is not the only aim, prevention of smoking initiation is essential if the nation is to achieve a long-term permanent reduction in prevalence.) Understanding of nicotine addiction as a "pediatric disease" (Kessler 1995) also strengthened the ethical case for aggressive efforts to reduce smoking initiation by teenagers, even if the measures also had spillover effects on adult smokers. Reports by the Surgeon General and the Institute of Medicine in 1994 established the scientific foundation for a youth-oriented policy initiative (eventually spearheaded by Food and Drug Administration [FDA] Commissioner David Kessler in 1995) and also galvanized public opinion against the tobacco industry for targeting young people (DHHS 1994; IOM 1994).

Third, the state Medicaid lawsuits and other tobacco litigation led to revelations of industry deception and duplicity and confirmed the industry's role in fostering and perpetuating tobacco use. These disclosures weakened the force of the antipaternalism principle as a constraint on tobacco policy and eroded the supposition that smokers have freely assumed the risks of smoking and are responsible for the often fatal consequences. Instead of being a champion of individual freedom and consumer sovereignty, the tobacco industry is now more often seen as a vector of disease and death, bringing public understanding into alignment with the premises of the public health community.

In sum, over the past 15 years, the operating assumptions of tobacco policy in the United States and elsewhere in the world have changed dramatically in part because of the fundamental realization that tobacco use is grounded in addiction to nicotine and that nicotine addiction typically begins before smokers become adults. Most smokers actually start smoking and become addicted while they are adolescents; and most addicted adult smokers want to quit, try to quit, and would rather be nonsmokers. The deeper public understanding of tobacco addiction has, over a short time, transformed the ethical and political context of tobacco policy-making. A widespread popular consensus in favor of aggressive policy initiatives is now emerging, and this shift in popular sentiment has also been accompanied by support across most of the political spectrum (see material in Chapter 5 on the proliferation of state laws and local ordinances prohibiting indoor smoking and on increases in state tobacco excise taxes).

THE ETHICAL CONTEXT

The committee believes that this shift in popular sentiment rests on a solid ethical footing, and that the blueprint is securely grounded in either of two ethical frameworks.

From a traditional public health perspective, the legitimacy and importance of reducing tobacco use is grounded in the enormous social costs attributable to tobacco-related disease: reducing tobacco use increases overall population health. Implementing the blueprint would reduce tobacco use and the attendant social costs to a degree that exceeds the costs of the proposed interventions. Moreover, studies of cost-effectiveness show that the tobacco control interventions are less costly per year of life saved and per quality-adjusted life year than many other standard public health interventions (see, for example, Cromwell et al. 1997; Tengs et al. 2001; Warner 1997). Admittedly, these traditional public health calculations do not include the "savings" to society in health care costs or social security payments attributable to premature death, but the committee does not regard these "savings" as a social benefit.

Once the question of "savings" due to premature mortality is set aside, the "public health" case for aggressive, cost-effective measures is generally acknowledged to be a powerful one. The main ethical objection raised to tobacco control policies has been raised by people who eschew the public health paradigm in favor of a non-consequentialist ethical paradigm grounded in an analysis of individual rights. In the context of tobacco use, the rights-based framework most often invoked is libertarian. The committee recognizes that strict adherents to this perspective may resist any regulation of consumer products, including tobacco, that is not designed to promote informed choice or to reduce external harms. However, product regulation is common in many domains, dating at least to the Pure Food and Drug Act of 1906, and certain characteristics of tobacco products might make tighter control acceptable even to those who tend to embrace a libertarian approach toward regulation of most consumer products. We outline those characteristics next.

The first point to be noted is that, even within a libertarian framework, each of the subsidiary goals of tobacco policy has some justification: reducing exposure to ETS prevents harm to people other than the smokers themselves, preventing initiation of tobacco use by youth is arguably justified by the recognized shortcomings of adolescent judgment, and promoting cessation helps to restore the liberty of smokers who do succeed in quitting (rather than contracting their liberty). In this respect, it is important to recall that 90 percent of adult smokers eventually regret having become smokers, about 70 percent have tried to quit, and—at any given moment—40 percent are either actively trying to quit or thinking about making a quit attempt within the next six months (see Chapter 2).

The most ethically controversial policies aiming to reduce tobacco use are those aimed exclusively at reducing use by the minority of adult smokers who do not want to quit. This is the nub of the so-called paternalism problem. However, since every intervention aimed at current smokers serves the interests and the express wishes of the subset of smokers who do want to quit, interventions designed to protect the health of adult smokers do not necessarily rest on a paternalistic foundation. Instead, they entail both liberty-enhancing effects (achieved by assisting addicted smokers to quit) and liberty-restricting effects (insofar as they also "burden" the choices of smokers who do not want to quit or who object to the restrictions or costs imposed on them). Thus ethical analysis of tobacco control interventions within the libertarian paradigm requires a weighing of the liberty-reducing effects of particular intervention against the liberty-enhancing effects of these interventions for nonsmokers whose freedom to avoid ETS exposure is protected, for youths whose long-run autonomy is preserved, and for adult smokers whose ability to quit is enhanced (and who therefore regard the intervention as a benefit rather than a cost).

Even within these boundaries, however, burdens on individual smokers that are intrusive or coercive do require heightened justification. The more restrictive the intervention (and, consequently, the greater the burden on smokers' freedom) the stronger the case must be that the intervention protects youths or nonsmokers or helps smokers quit. That important principle is embraced by the committee in its evaluation of each of the tobacco control interventions considered in the following chapters.

AN ASIDE ON THE PATERNALISM PROBLEM

It can also be argued that paternalism in this context is a justified response to irremediable deficiencies in smokers' capacity to successfully exercise self-interested decision-making about whether they should continue to smoke. Although the committee's blueprint need not rest on this argument, many committee members do find elements of it convincing, and that is why we summarize it here.

The argument runs as follows: (1) virtually all addicted adults begin smoking (and probably become addicted) while they are adolescents before they have developed the capacity to exercise mature judgment about whether or not to become a smoker; (2) the preferences expressed when people begin to smoke, which tend to ignore long-term health risks, are inconsistent with the health-oriented preferences they later come to have, and they soon regret the decision to have become a smoker; and (3) once smokers begin to be concerned about the health dangers of smoking, their judgment is often distorted by optimism bias ("the harms will happen to other people, not to me"), thereby weakening their motivation to quit.

Adolescent Initiation

As shown in Chapter 2, between 80–90 percent of smokers start smoking before they turn 18 years of age. When they begin to smoke, they typically lack a full and vivid appreciation of the consequences of smoking and the grip of addiction, even if they have a roughly accurate understanding of the statistical evidence. When young people begin to smoke, they typically fail to appreciate the serious possibility that they will continue smoking for many years (see Chapter 2).

Inconsistent Preferences and Regret

Many people neglect long-term risks to their health, simply because they tend to have a short-term perspective when they consider the risks and the benefits of a particular behavior. In the language of economists, they apply a high "discount rate" to future harms. This neglect of the long-term danger is especially serious for young people. Because the most serious health risks of smoking do not come to fruition for many years, young smokers often treat those risks as if they were trivial. Even adult smokers often fail to take adequate account of the associated risks, simply because those risks are not likely to materialize for decades. Smokers themselves will typically change their minds later on, reflecting a difference between their preferences when they start smoking and the preferences that they have later in life, when they want to quit. (Economists call this problem "inter-temporal inconsistency.") In short, when people begin to smoke, at whatever age, they tend to give more weight to the pleasures of smoking and too little weight to the possible impact of smoking on their long-term well-being. Once people have become addicted, they give more weight to the health concerns and regret having become smokers. Most of them want to stop.

Optimism Bias

In some domains, people are unrealistically optimistic about risks, believing that they are immune from the dangers that others who are similarly situated face. For smokers, the problem of unrealistic optimism takes three distinct forms. First, many smokers, even those who have an adequate sense of the statistical realities, falsely believe that they are unlikely to face the risks that most smokers face. Second, many smokers, both young and old, are unrealistically optimistic about their future health and their longevity if they quit at some later point. Third, many smokers believe, falsely, that they will quit in the near future. Taken together, these forms of unrealistic optimism can be deadly.

More than four decades after the Surgeon General's initial report (HEW 1964) on the health risks of smoking, policymakers have not addressed these three problems with anything like the seriousness that they deserve. To be sure, the problem of addiction plays a large role in current thinking; and both states and localities, along with the private sector, have adopted commendable steps to protect and to inform young people. However, the whole notion of consumer sovereignty—of unambivalent respect for private choices—runs into serious difficulty when the underlying product creates serious long-term individual and societal harms, has addictive properties, and is usually chosen by young people who fail to appreciate the associated risks.

TOBACCO PRODUCTS ARE INHERENTLY DANGEROUS

As they are now designed, tobacco cigarettes are inherently dangerous products that would not be allowed to enter the marketplace if their effects were known and if they were being introduced for the first time. For example, the nicotine in tobacco products would meet the criteria for classification of a Schedule 1 drug under the Controlled Substances Act, tobacco smoke could be classified as a "toxic substance" posing an "unreasonable risk" under the Toxic Substances Control Act, and tobacco cigarettes (and perhaps other tobacco products) could be characterized as "unreasonably dangerous product[s]" under the Consumer Product Safety Act, if tobacco products were not exempted from regulation by the specific exclusionary language in each of these statutes. If tobacco products were within FDA jurisdiction under the Federal Food, Drug, and Cosmetics Act, pre-market approval from the FDA would be required, and it could safely be predicted that such approval would not be forthcoming in light of the addictive properties of nicotine and the multitude of dangerous constituents in tobacco smoke.

However, tobacco products were introduced into the marketplace not only before their adverse effects were understood but also before any modern consumer protection or environmental health legislation had been enacted. The early efforts to suppress the sale of cigarettes, largely on moral and hygienic grounds, occurred at the state level, but most of the early bans had been repealed by 1925. The advent of mass production capabilities in the late 19th century, waning opposition from temperance groups during the first third of the 20th century, and the explosion of smoking during and after World War II catapulted the cigarette to the status of one of the most successfully marketed consumer products in the nation's history. Given such a deep entrenchment in the cultural, social, and commercial life of the country, it is hardly surprising that the burden of demonstrating the need for any substantial regulatory restriction has rested on the proponents of regulation. As indicated in Chapter 3, however, this burden has now been convincingly met. The harmfulness of cigarettes is no longer disputed, even by the manufacturers; and the rhetoric of personal freedom has been softened by a general recognition of the powerful grip of nicotine addiction, the purposeful manipulation of that addictive potential by the manufacturers, and the hazardous effects of secondhand smoke on nonsmokers. Hence the burden has been shifting to the tobacco companies to explain why they should be permitted to continue to promote and market this admittedly dangerous product.

The central point is that cigarettes and other tobacco products are not ordinary consumer products. For no other lawful consumer product can it be said that the acknowledged aim of national policy is to suppress consumption. For alcohol, the generally accepted aim of national policy is to suppress underage drinking and excessive or otherwise irresponsible use by adults; reducing adult consumption per se is not the nation's goal. Indeed, in many respects, state and federal governments aim to facilitate alcohol consumption, such as by liberalizing access (IOM/NRC 2004). Similarly, although firearms are indisputably dangerous products, and their unlawful sale, possession, and use is suppressed, their lawful use is widely regarded as a valued constitutional right, and many aspects of recent changes in state law have been designed to facilitate access to weapons by lawful purchasers and owners. In terms of its goal, tobacco policy has more in common with the nation's policy toward marijuana and other illegal drugs than it does with policies pertaining to alcohol or firearms.

It has become commonplace for critics of aggressive tobacco control measures to invoke the classic slippery slope argument, claiming that restrictions on tobacco will lead down the slope to measures taking away food and drinks that people like on the ground that they are not healthy enough. After all, it is said, if the "nanny state" is empowered to suppress tobacco use, it will go after the Big Mac® next. This argument underappreciates the extent to which tobacco products are unlike ordinary consumer products. Tobacco is a highly addictive, carcinogenic, and deadly product. Foods rich in fats or carbohydrates may lead to overweight and increase disease risks if consumed in excess, but they are not addictive or inherently dangerous. It therefore bears repeating that tobacco is the only lawful consumer product for which the nation's unequivocal aim is to suppress consumption altogether—rather than promoting informed, healthy choices and moderation.

That being the case, governments at all levels must play a central role in the effort to overcome and reverse the forces that create and sustain tobacco use. Governments have both the authority and the obligation to establish and sustain conditions under which people can be healthy while respecting the constitutional liberties and other important values (IOM 1988, 2003). People trust and expect the government to protect children from hazards such as poisons, lead, and tobacco; to prevent the tobacco industry from misleading people and drawing them into or sustaining an addictive behavior that they will regret; to counteract industry efforts to stimulate and sustain demand for its dangerous products; and to help people quit if they want to do so.

BLUEPRINT OUTLINE

The committee's blueprint for reducing tobacco use in the United States reflects a two-pronged strategy. The first prong envisions strengthening traditional tobacco control measures; the second envisions changing the regulatory landscape to permit new policy innovations. Chapter 5 reviews the current legal structure and framework of tobacco policy and focuses on intensifying and strengthening the tools of tobacco control known to be effective. The emphasis in that chapter is largely, although not exclusively, on state and local initiatives. This is because almost all of the energy and innovation in tobacco control are currently generated at the state and local levels and are undergirded by public health partnerships and supported by community-based advocacy efforts. Policy changes are typically enacted and implemented through state laws and local ordinances, although the federal government plays a secondary role—often supporting state and local efforts, but sometimes impeding them.

Chapter 6 envisions a much more substantial federal presence characterized by a fundamentally transformed legal structure under which a federal regulatory agency, most likely the FDA, is given plenary regulatory authority while the states are liberated to take aggressive actions now forbidden by federal law. Federal power would be exercised to bolster and support state efforts in the traditional domains of tobacco control while the agency takes bold steps in under-regulated areas, including the use of more effective health warnings and constraints on industry advertising and promotional activity, with particular attention given to claims regarding so-called reduced-risk products. The federal government would also play a more substantial role in funding and coordinating state tobacco control activities.

Chapter 7 presents opportunities for policy innovations that can open new frontiers of tobacco control. One such possibility is gradually reducing the nicotine content of cigarettes. Implementation of a nicotine-reduction strategy or any other bold initiative aiming to end the tobacco problem will require sophisticated policy research, and the committee urges the federal government to create a robust capacity for tobacco policy research and development.

REFERENCES

Cromwell J, Bartosch WJ, Fiore MC, Hasselblad V, Baker T. 1997. Cost-effectiveness of the clinical practice recommendations in the AHCPR guideline for smoking cessation. *Journal of the American Medical Association* 278(21).
DHHS (U.S. Department of Health and Human Services). 1989. *Reducing the Health Consequences of Smoking: 25 Years of Progress (A Report of the Surgeon General)*. Rockville, MD: U.S. Department of Health and Human Services, Centers for Disease Control and Prevention, Center for Chronic Disease Prevention and Health Promotion, Office on Smoking and Health.

DHHS. 1994. *Preventing Tobacco Use Among Young People (A Report of the Surgeon General)*. Rockville, MD: U.S. Department of Health and Human Services, Centers for Disease Control and Prevention, Center for Health Promotion and Education, Office on Smoking and Health.

DHHS. 2006. *The Health Consequences of Involuntary Exposure to Tobacco Smoke: A Report of the Surgeon General*. Atlanta, GA: U.S. Department of Health and Human Services, Centers for Disease Control and Prevention, Coordinating Center for Health Promotion, National Center for Chronic Disease Prevention and Health Promotion, Office on Smoking and Health.

EPA (Environmental Protection Agency). 1992. *Respiratory Health Effects of Passive Smoking: Lung Cancer and Other Disorders*. Washington, DC: Office of Health and Environmental Assessment, Office of Research and Development, U.S. Environmental Protection Agency.

HEW (Department of Health, Education, and Welfare). 1964. *Smoking and Health: Report of the Advisory Committee to the Surgeon General of the Public Health Service*. Washington, DC: U.S. Department of Health, Education, and Welfare; Public Health Service.

IOM (Institute of Medicine). 1988. *The Future of Public Health*. Washington, DC: National Academy Press.

IOM. 1994. *Growing Up Tobacco Free: Preventing Nicotine Addiction in Children and Youth*. Washington, DC: National Academy Press.

IOM. 2003. *The Future of the Public's Health in the 21st Century*. Washington, DC: The National Academies Press.

IOM/NRC (National Research Council). 2004. *Reducing Underage Drinking: A Collective Responsibility*. Washington, DC: The National Academies Press.

Kessler D. 1995. Nicotine addiction in young people. *New England Journal of Medicine* 333:186-189.

Tengs TO, Osgood ND, Chen LL. 2001. The cost-effectiveness of intensive national school-based anti-tobacco education: Results from the Tobacco Policy Model. *Preventive Medicine* 33(6):558-570.

Warner KE. 1997. Cost effectiveness of smoking-cessation therapies. *PharmacoEconomics* 11:538-549.

5

Strengthening Traditional Tobacco Control Measures

D uring the 1990s, substantial progress was made in laying the foundation for an effective tobacco control policy, but that progress has stalled for at least three reasons. First, it is difficult to sustain public attention on endemic problems; in particular, on the challenges of prevention and cessation. Public attention (including the priority-setting driven by public opinion) is easily diverted to the crisis of the moment, and in times of austerity, expenditures on prevention and cessation efforts always seem to be the most dispensable. These tendencies explain in part why the political commitment needed for a sustained effort is lacking. Second, the political and commercial power of the tobacco industry remains substantial, even following the disclosures of past misconduct arising out of recent state reimbursement litigation, the Master Settlement Agreement (MSA), and the U.S. Justice Department's suit under the Racketeering Influenced and Corrupt Organization Act. Third, all the tobacco control measures described in Chapter 3 have had to be implemented in the context of a largely unregulated market in which tobacco products continue to be aggressively promoted. These promotion efforts are still at work, and it is difficult for public health programs to keep up, especially when the economy falters and public revenues fall short. The behavioral potential of aggressive prevention and cessation efforts is amply illustrated by the successes achieved in California, Massachusetts, and other states. So, too, however, is the fragility of these efforts—when the money disappeared, so did the programs.

The nation needs to muster the political will to intensify the efforts implemented so successfully during the 1990s and to build on them. These comprehensive state programs, as well as their individual components, have been shown to be effective. Failure to sustain these efforts will cost lives. This chapter of the committee's report outlines the core components of tobacco control as they have been implemented within the existing legal structure. It should be emphasized, however, that one of the constraints on the current legal structure is that no federal agency has regulatory jurisdiction over tobacco products. Another constraint is that the federal statute regulating the labeling and advertising of cigarettes forecloses state regulation of advertising and marketing of cigarettes "based on smoking and health." This unfortunate circumstance, addressed in Chapter 6, preempts most state efforts to regulate the appearance, display, promotion, and placement of cigarettes in retail outlets.

Chapter 5 begins with a discussion of the effectiveness of comprehensive state programs, as well as the states' current approaches toward funding these programs. The states' expenditures for tobacco control are placed in the context of the revenue streams generated by tobacco excise taxes and payments received under the MSA.

The remainder of the chapter focuses on seven key substantive elements of comprehensive state programs:

- Tobacco excise taxes
- Smoking restrictions with broad coverage
- Youth-access restrictions with adequate enforcement
- Prevention programs based in schools, families, and health care systems
- Media campaigns
- Cessation programs
- Grassroots community advocacy

The recommendations made throughout the chapter are meant to set forth a blueprint for strengthening and intensifying current tobacco control policies and programs, assuming that the current legal structure of tobacco control remains unchanged. The chapter closes with a projection of the likely impact of following (or not following) this blueprint on the national prevalence of tobacco use over the next 20 years.

COMPREHENSIVE STATE PROGRAMS

During the early days of tobacco use prevention, after the publication of the 1964 Surgeon General's report (HEW 1964), many state health departments relied on the funds in their state budgets for tobacco control and treatment. Interventions tended to be targeted toward smoking cessation for individuals. By the late 1980s, however, funding for comprehensive state tobacco control programs increased, beginning with California and then expanding to all states.

California launched the first statewide comprehensive tobacco control program in 1990, one and a half years after the passage of Proposition 99. This landmark referendum mandated an increase in state tobacco taxes and directed 20 percent of the revenues to tobacco control programs (Bal 1998; Glantz and Balbach 2000; Najera 1998). At that time, the National Cancer Institute (NCI) was already preparing to launch the seven-year national American Stop Smoking Intervention Study (ASSIST) program. In 1991, the ASSIST program funded community-level interventions to prevent tobacco use in 17 states (NCI 2005; Stillman et al. 2003).

By the mid-1990s, every state in the United States had some funding for comprehensive tobacco control, either from the ASSIST program or from the Initiatives to Mobilize for the Prevention and Control of Tobacco Use (IMPACT) program, funded by the Centers for Disease Control and Prevention (CDC). In addition, from 1994 through 2000, some states[1] also received funding for tobacco control efforts from the Robert Wood Johnson Foundation's (RWJF) SmokeLess States program (Gerlach and Larkin 2005; Tauras et al. 2005). In addition to educational and cessation programs, the funding supported statewide coalitions of individuals and organizations that pursued action strategies to strengthen tobacco control policies.

The ASSIST program promoted three types of interventions: program services, policy changes, and mass media. However, the ASSIST program guidelines stated that "efforts to achieve priority public policy objectives should take precedence over efforts to support service delivery" (NCI 2005, p.23). Mass media initiatives were intended to support those policy changes. The four ASSIST program priority policy areas were eliminating environmental tobacco smoke (ETS), increasing tobacco excise taxes, limiting tobacco advertising and promotion, and reducing youth access (NCI 2005).

Evaluation of Comprehensive State Programs

In 2005, the CDC's Office on Smoking and Health (OSH) released a summary of the literature on evidence of the effectiveness of state tobacco control programs (Kuiper et al. 2005). Organized by major reviews and five outcome indicators (tobacco-related mortality, prevalence, consumption, cessation, and smoke-free legislation and policy), the results are generally organized by state. The evidence provided can be considered a guide to state health departments for measuring the success of their comprehensive

---

[1]Smokeless States funded all states and the District of Columbia in its final round of grants in 2000.

tobacco control programs. Of the five indicators of success, one is a health outcome—tobacco-related mortality—and three are markers that lead to improved health outcomes: decreases in smoking prevalence, decreases in consumption of tobacco products, and smoking cessation. The fifth indicator, smoke-free legislation and policy, is an intermediate outcome that alters the environment that supports tobacco use.

This review appeared six years after the publication of the CDC's Best Practices for Comprehensive Tobacco Control Programs. Published in 1999, Best Practices had concluded that the evidence was sufficiently compelling to encourage all states to pursue comprehensive programs. This conclusion was drawn on the basis of analyses of the excise tax-funded state programs in California, Massachusetts, Oregon, and Maine, as well as the agency's experience in providing assistance to four other states: Florida, Minnesota, Mississippi, and Texas. The 2005 review reiterates the effectiveness of these programs, while also documenting the successes of other state programs that have appeared since 1999.

Over the past decade and a half, a number of investigators have tried to assess the contribution of comprehensive state programs to policy changes and reductions in smoking (DHHS 2000; Elder et al. 1996; Siegel 2002; Stillman et al. 2003; Tauras et al. 2005; Wakefield and Chaloupka 2000; Warner 2000). By design, a comprehensive tobacco control program consists of several elements (e.g., antismoking media campaigns, counseling services, and school-based prevention initiatives), and some authors have focused on evaluating the effectiveness of individual program components. Later in this chapter, the committee refers, for instance, to several studies that have assessed the impacts of state-sponsored antismoking media campaigns on smoking prevalence and changes in smoking-related beliefs. This section reviews studies that have looked at the effects of comprehensive programs as a whole.

One study that evaluated state programs throughout the country found that a program's intensity had a very large negative correlation with the prevalence of current smoking ($r = -0.81$, $p < .0001$) and a large positive correlation with the quit rate ($r = 0.82$, $p < .0001$) among adults 30 to 39 years of age (Jemal et al. 2003). Another study determined that states with better-funded programs have lower prevalence and consumption rates (Tauras et al. 2005). However, many states have substantially cut their tobacco control programs' budgets in recent years.

Description of Programs

Over the course of the 1990s, several other states—including Arizona, Florida, Massachusetts, and Oregon—followed California's lead and developed their own comprehensive tobacco control programs (Wakefield and Chaloupka 2000). Studies reviewing the effects of each of these states' efforts have been published, and many of these are listed in CDC's 2005 literature summary (Kuiper et al. 2005). As the first two states in the country to implement comprehensive programs, California and Massachusetts have received a particularly large amount of attention. A specific examination of these two states' pioneering efforts reveals that comprehensive state programs can be effective in reducing tobacco use and tobacco-related disease, especially when they are fully funded and operational.

California

In November 1988, California voters passed Proposition 99, which increased the state tobacco tax by 25 cents per pack of cigarettes. One year later, the California Assembly passed legislation that distributed the revenue earned from the tobacco tax increase as follows: 35 percent for hospital services, 20 percent for a health education account, 10 percent for physician services, 5 percent for research, and 5 percent for environmental conservation concerns (25 percent of the funds remained unallocated). Funds from the health education and research accounts were used for the creation of a statewide tobacco control program. The California Tobacco Control Program (CTCP), the first of its kind in the country, debuted in the spring of 1990 (Bal 1998; Najera 1998; TEROC 2000).

Together, the California Department of Health Services (CDHS) and the California Department of Education (CDE), along with the University of California, support a decentralized network of local health departments (LHDs), schools, researchers, and competitive grantees that forms the core of the CTCP. The CDE's Healthy Kids Program Office oversees the program's school-based components, whereas the University of California administers various research activities through its Tobacco Related Disease Research Program. The Tobacco Control Section of CDHS, which receives approximately two-thirds of the available funds from the Health Education Account, coordinates the public health elements of the program. These elements include programs conducted at the local level by LHDs and community organizations; a statewide media campaign; cessation counseling services (such as the California Smokers' Helpline); a materials clearinghouse; and four networks that seek to better integrate California's African American, American Indian, Asian and Pacific Islander, and Hispanic populations into the state's tobacco control efforts. California has also coordinated its efforts with other tobacco control initiatives, including the RWJF's SmokeLess States program (CDHS 1998; State of California 2004; TEROC 2000, 2003).

Throughout the 1990s, the CTCP's funding fluctuated dramatically. Between 1989–1990 and 1995–1996, for instance, the program experienced a 60 percent reduction in funding (from $131.3 million to $53.4 million). In addition, although the CTCP's budget more than doubled between 1995–1996 and 1997–1998 (from $53.4 million to $140.7 million), funding declined yet again in 1998–1999 as well as in 1999–2000 (Independent Evaluation Consortium 2002).

In its first few years, before these major budget fluctuations, the CTCP embraced a mix of policy, media, and program interventions to address a range of factors contributing to tobacco use (CDHS 1998). By 1993, however, looming budget cuts necessitated a more focused approach. Anticipating funding reductions, program administrators revised the CTCP's structure and priorities to streamline the state's tobacco control efforts. Administrators refocused the program's activities into four clearly defined areas: (1) reducing exposure to secondhand smoke, (2) countering the influence of the tobacco industry, (3) reducing youth access to tobacco products, and (4) providing cessation services (CDHS 1998). Since then, however, the CTCP has suffered additional reductions in funding, including a budget cut of 30 percent ($46 million) in FY 2002. Consequently, the gap between tobacco control funding and tobacco industry spending has widened considerably, especially in comparison to the more intensive and better-funded early years of the program. By 2002, California—once the trailblazer in comprehensive tobacco control programming—had fallen to 20th in state rankings for per-capita funding for tobacco control (TEROC 2003).

Massachusetts

Massachusetts modeled much of its tobacco control program after that of the CTCP. In November 1992, Massachusetts voters passed a ballot initiative (commonly known as Question 1) that—like Proposition 99 in California four years earlier—increased the state tobacco tax by 25 cents per pack of cigarettes. Although the Massachusetts Constitution prohibits the earmarking of tax revenue (as the California legislature had done with money earned from its tobacco tax increase), the drafters of Question 1 composed language that urged—but did not mandate—the state to allocate revenue collected from the tobacco tax to a statewide tobacco control program. Following passage of the initiative, Massachusetts legislators soon allocated revenue from the tobacco tax to a newly created Health Protection Fund for the financing of a tobacco-control program (Cady 1998; Connolly and Robbins 1998; Nicholl 1998).

Administered by the Massachusetts Department of Public Health, the Massachusetts Tobacco Control Program (MTCP) began operating in October 1993 with the launch of a mass media campaign, which used a wide spectrum of media, including television, radio, newspapers, and billboards, to disseminate its antismoking message throughout the state. In the following months, the MTCP started implementing additional tobacco control initiatives with an emphasis on three priority areas: (1) preventing youth from starting to smoke, (2) reducing smoking prevalence among adults, and (3) reducing nonsmokers' exposure to ETS. Massachusetts, like California, embraced a localized approach to achieve these goals. Although the MTCP first managed local programs by program type, it soon restructured its operations by organizing localities into six regional networks. Representatives from local tobacco control programs, along with MTCP representatives, began meeting monthly within their respective regional networks to ensure statewide cohesion and better facilitate exchanges of information. In addition, the MTCP has funded community coalitions to organize mobilization efforts, as well as boards of health and LHDs, to enact and enforce tobacco control regulations. Statewide programming, meanwhile, has included the media campaign and the Try to Stop Resource Center, which offers the Smoker's Quitline, a website (*www.trytostop.org*) for smokers seeking cessation support, and educational materials. The Center for Tobacco Prevention and Control at the University of Massachusetts Medical School performs research on tobacco use and nicotine dependence (Connolly and Robbins 1998; Hamilton et al. 2002; MDPH 2002a, 2002b).

Massachusetts has also mirrored California in coordinating its activities with other tobacco control initiatives. From 1991 through 1999, for instance, Massachusetts was 1 of 17 states in the country to participate in the NCI's ASSIST program. Massachusetts participated in various training programs and information exchanges with its fellow ASSIST states, as well as with California and other states with tobacco control programs (Celebucki et al. 1998).

As with the CTCP, the MTCP's early years represented its most intensive period of funding and activity. From 1994 to 1997, for example, the $7.09 per-capita spent on tobacco control in Massachusetts represented the highest investment of its kind in the country. Budgetary cuts have threatened the effectiveness of the MTCP throughout its history, however, and even in the first 3 years of its existence, the MTCP experienced a pattern of decreasing expenditures (Wakefield and Chaloupka 2000). These early reductions, however, pale in comparison with the cuts that occurred at the beginning of the 2000s. Although funds from the MSA helped increase the MTCP's budget in FY 2000, funding levels dropped again in FY 2001. In addition, between FY 2002 and FY 2003, as the state faced acute budget shortfalls, it decreased the MTCP's budget from $34 million to $5.5 million. These cuts resulted in a serious reduction of the MTCP's activities, including the elimination of almost all local programming and the discontinuation of the media campaign. Since these cuts occurred, surviving elements of the program have operated at a level far below that of the previous decade (Hamilton et al. 2003; MDPH 2002a, 2006).

Description of Evaluations

From the start, both California and Massachusetts incorporated evaluation mechanisms into their tobacco control programs. California developed a multidimensional evaluation structure that comprised local program assessments, in-house surveys, and an independent review. Through the "10 percent" clause, which requires local grantees to devote 10 percent of their program budgets to evaluation, the state can review the effects of programs carried out at the local level, where most CTCP activities take place. The CDHS's in-house data-gathering efforts, meanwhile, have included the Behavior Risk Factor Survey, the California Adult Tobacco Survey, and the California Youth Tobacco Survey. CDHS contracts with the University of California San Diego (UCSD) to operate the much larger California Tobacco Survey (CTS). UCSD conducts this survey every 3 years through interviews of individuals from randomly selected households, and reaches approximately 78,000 adults and 6,000 youth. The CTS provides CDHS with statewide smoking prevalence rate estimates (broken down into county and regional estimates) as well as data on attitudinal changes (Russell 1998).

The CTCP's enabling legislation mandated an independent evaluation of the program. The Gallup Organization has conducted this independent review, subcontracting various elements of its evaluation to Stanford University and the University of Southern California (USC). In their reviews, Gallup and its subcontractors have examined the overall impact of the program as well as the relative effectiveness of its various components (media campaigns, local initiatives, school-based programs, etc.). Other surveys used in the evaluation of the CTCP include the CDHS's annual survey of the rate of illegal sales of tobacco products to minors and occasional surveys targeting specific issues, such as the Field Institute poll on the number of smoke-free bars in the state. The Evaluation Task Force, with members from across the United States and Canada, advises the state on evaluation efforts (Independent Evaluation Consortium 2002; Russell 1998).

Massachusetts has used a similar multidimensional approach to evaluating the MTCP's success in reducing tobacco use. From October 1993 through March 1994, MTCP conducted the Massachusetts Tobacco Survey, a baseline survey that collected data on tobacco use among adults and youth through randomized telephone interviews. Beginning in March 1995, MTCP began conducting the Massachusetts Adult Tobacco Survey, a monthly follow-up cross-sectional survey, to monitor changes in tobacco use and related attitudes. In addition, along with the RWJF, the MTCP funded longitudinal surveys to evaluate the program's impact on adults and youth. Finally, like California, Massachusetts commissioned an independent assessment of its tobacco control program. In evaluating the success of the

MTCP, Abt Associates Inc. has reviewed data on smoking prevalence, quit attempts, smoking cessation, exposure to ETS, incidents of tobacco sales to minors, and changes in attitudes regarding tobacco use and tobacco-control policy (Hamilton et al. 2002). Frequent budget cuts, however, have impacted the regularity of the MTCP's surveillance efforts, restricting the extent and consistency of program evaluation (Hamilton et al. 2002).

Findings Regarding Effects

The results of the evaluations and surveys mentioned above, along with the findings from a number of peer-reviewed studies, indicate that California and Massachusetts have made progress in their tobacco control efforts; this progress is most notable when the respective programs have been well-funded and fully-implemented. On the basis of data from the CDC's Behavior Risk Factor Surveillance System, Figure 5-1 illustrates the successes that both states have had in reducing tobacco use in comparison with the rest of the country. Figure 5-1 shows that a 23.2 percent reduc tion in the prevalence of current smoking in California took place between 1990 (the first full year of the state's tobacco control program) and 2005, whereas the reduction in the U.S. median during the same period was

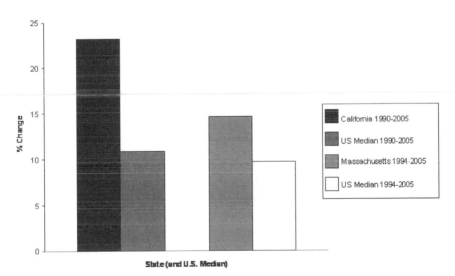

FIGURE 5-1 Percent reduction in current adult smokers in California and Massachusetts from the first year of their tobacco control programs (1990 and 1994, respectively) to 2005 (the year for which the most current data are available) compared with the percent reduction in the U.S. median for the same two time periods, based on data from the Behavior Risk Factor Surveillance System.
SOURCE: (CDC 2006a).

10.9 percent. In Massachusetts, meanwhile, a 14.6 percent reduction took place between 1994 (the first full year of the implementation of its tobacco control program) and 2005. During those same years, the U.S. median experienced a smaller reduction of 9.7 percent.

California

During the CTCP's early years, California experienced significant declines in the prevalence rate of smoking among adults. To determine whether the declines could be attributed to the program or to alternative factors (e.g., national trends or demographic changes) Siegel and colleagues (2000) compared data for California with data for the rest of the country. They found that California's rate of decline in adult smoking prevalence between 1990 and 1994 was 0.39 percent per year, whereas the rate of decline in the rest of the United States was only 0.05 percent per year. Restriction of the analysis to various demographic groups did not significantly affect the results. Consequently, Siegel and colleagues suggested that the greater reduction in adult smoking prevalence in California in comparison to that of the rest of the country in the early 1990s could be due to the implementation of the CTCP (Siegel et al. 2000).

It is important to note, however, that California's adult smoking prevalence rate has remained relatively level since the mid-1990s (CDHS 2002).[2] In an evaluation of the CTCP's activities from 1989 to 1996, Pierce and colleagues (1998) divided the program's first 7 years into two distinct periods. They found that during Period 1 (January 1989 to June 1993), adult smoking prevalence and per-capita cigarette consumption declined more than 50 percent faster than in previous years and more than 40 percent faster than in the rest of the United States. During Period 2 (July 1993 to December 1996), however, the rate of decline for both adult smoking prevalence and per-capita cigarette consumption slowed, with the prevalence declining at only 15 percent and consumption declining at only 34 percent of the Period 1 rate of decline. Furthermore, although the rate of decline in cigarette consumption remained substantially higher than the rate recorded in the rest of the United States during Period 2, California's rate of decline in adult smoking prevalence no longer exceeded that of the rest of the United States. This slowdown coincided with decreased financing of tobacco control programs by the state (Pierce et al. 1998).

Fichtenberg and Glantz (2000), meanwhile, analyzed the CTCP's effectiveness in relation to the rate of decline of deaths attributable to heart

---

[2]The increase in smoking prevalence in 1996 is generally considered to be a result of the fact that the CDC revised its definition of the term "current smoker," which resulted in the inclusion of more "occasional smokers."

disease in California. They found that between 1989 and 1992, both per-capita cigarette consumption rates and the annual rate of mortality from heart disease declined significantly more in California than in the rest of the country. Reflecting the trends noted above, however, the rates of decline slowed noticeably after 1992. Consequently, Fichtenberg and Glantz con-cluded that the CTCP was initially effective in reducing deaths from heart disease but that cutbacks in the scale and funding of the program weakened further progress (Fichtenberg and Glantz 2000).

The last independent evaluation of the CTCP to be released by the Gallup Organization and its partners (Stanford and USC) assessed the pro-gram's overall impact in relation to Californians' exposure to its various ele-ments and messages, as reported in surveys conducted in 1996–1997, 1998, and 2000. The evaluation concluded that the CTCP has had an impact on behavior, as counties with greater exposure to the program showed better outcomes than counties with less exposure, including a greater decline in adult smoking prevalence between 1996 and 2000, lower perceived access to cigarettes among 10th graders, and an increase from 1996 to 2000 in the proportion of adults with complete smoking bans in their homes (Inde-pendent Evaluation Consortium 2002).

The CTCP has also had success in reducing tobacco use among youth. A study released in 2005 associated the CTCP with reduced uptake and smoking rates among adolescents and young adults. The authors found that the rate of "ever puffing" declined by 70 percent among 12- to 13-year-olds from 1990 to 2002, by 53 percent among 14- to15-year-olds from 1992 to 2002, and by 34 percent among 16- to 17-year-olds from 1996 to 2002. The study identified similar patterns for smoking experimentation (smok-ing one or more cigarettes ever) and established smoking (smoking more than 100 cigarettes in a lifetime). Although the smoking prevalence among young adults (ages 18 to 24 years) remained constant in the rest of the country from 1992 to 2002, the prevalence among young adults in Califor-nia decreased significantly (by 18 percent) from 1998–1999 to 2001–2002 (Pierce et al. 2005). Gilpin and colleagues found a similar behavioral trend when they compared the results of two 3-year longitudinal studies (1993–1996 and 1996–1999) that measured smoking initiation rates at the baseline among California adolescents who had never smoked. The authors identified a lower rate of initiation at follow-up in the cohort of the second study than in that of the first study (Gilpin et al. 2005).

Data published by CDHS indicate that California has continued to make progress in reducing tobacco use among youth. According to CDHS, from 2000 to 2004, the 30-day smoking prevalence rate among high school students in California decreased from 21.6 percent to 13.2 percent (CDHS 2005). Figure 5-2 shows that although the rate of decline in smoking preva-lence among youth in California mirrored the rate of decline in the rest of

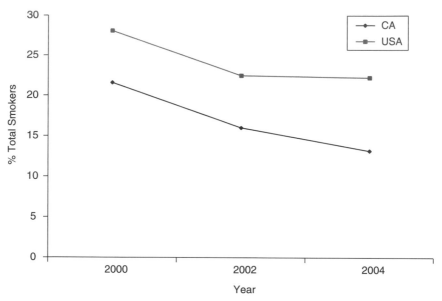

FIGURE 5-2 Thirty-day smoking prevalence among high school students (9th to 12th grades) in California and the United States between 2000 and 2004. Data for 2000 are from the National Youth Tobacco Survey, and data for 2002 and 2004 are from the California Student Tobacco Survey.
SOURCE: (CDHS 2005).

the country from 2000 to 2002, the smoking prevalence rate among youth declined at a greater rate in California than in the United States as a whole from 2002 to 2004. Figure 5-3 depicts the smoking rates among youth over the course of the 1990s in both California and the United States (excluding California). Although the rates rose in California as well as in the rest of the country in the early part of the decade, by the mid-1990s the smoking prevalence rate among youth in California began to decline, whereas the prevalence nationwide continued to increase for several more years.

Massachusetts

Like California, Massachusetts has made progress in reducing tobacco use, with both adult smoking prevalence and per-capita cigarette consumption trending downward since the implementation of the MTCP. Figure 5-1 illustrates Massachusetts's success in reducing the prevalence of smoking among adults, showing that from 1994 to 2005 Massachusetts experienced

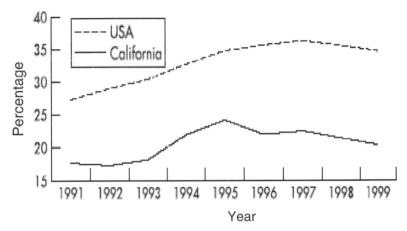

FIGURE 5-3 Smoking rates for high school seniors in California and the United States excluding California, 1991 to 1999 Monitoring the Future.
SOURCE: (Farrelly et al. 2003).

a greater percent change in the prevalence of current adult smokers than did the U.S. median.

In its last independent evaluation of the MTCP, Abt Associates Inc. similarly assessed the program by comparing state and national data. Controlling for demographic characteristics and comparing current smoking prevalence rates in Massachusetts with those in 41 states without comprehensive tobacco control programs, Abt Associates found that adult smoking prevalence rates declined more rapidly in Massachusetts than in the comparison states. According to the Abt analysis, the adjusted prevalence rate in Massachusetts declined between 1990 and 2000, from 22.7 percent to 20.5 percent (an annual rate of 0.9 percent), whereas the adjusted prevalence rate in the comparison states declined from 22.0 percent to 21.7 percent (an annual rate of 0.4 percent). Consequently, Abt Associates concluded (like Siegel and colleagues in the case of California) that the decline in the adult smoking prevalence rate in Massachusetts could be attributed to the existence of the MTCP and not to national trends or demographic changes. Abt also noted that Massachusetts experienced a drop (40 percent) in per-capita cigarette consumption from 1992 to 2001, two times greater than the drop (20 percent) experienced in the rest of the country, excluding California. Furthermore, the decline in youth smoking prevalence in Massachusetts was found to be greater than that in the rest of the United States (Hamilton et al. 2003). The results of a similar analysis that reviewed data obtained through 1999 were published in 2002 (Weintraub and Hamilton 2002).

An earlier review (the results of which were published by the CDC in 1996) sought to determine the impact of the state's excise tax and tobacco control program on per-capita cigarette consumption and adult smoking prevalence. In doing so, the authors compared the rates in Massachusetts with those in the rest of the United States during two time periods: the 3 years leading up to the passage of Question 1 on the state ballot initiative (1990 to 1992) and the years immediately following the implementation of the excise tax and establishment of the MTCP (1993 to 1996). Although they determined that smoking prevalence rates in Massachusetts required further study, they found that per capita cigarette consumption decreased significantly from the first period to the second. During the first period, consumption in Massachusetts declined by 6.4 percent, whereas that in the rest of the country declined by 5.8 percent (except for California, where consumption declined by 11.0 percent). From 1992 to 1996, however, per-capita consumption declined by 19.7 percent in Massachusetts, 15.8 percent in California, and just 6.1 percent in the remaining states and the District of Columbia. The authors reasoned that because real cigarette prices actually fell in 1993 (because of price reductions by the tobacco industry), the excise tax alone could not account for the decline in cigarette consumption that continued through 1996. Consequently, they concluded that Massachusetts's tobacco control program played a role alongside tax increases in reducing the rate of tobacco use in the years immediately following the passage of Question 1 (CDC 1996).

Biener and colleagues (2000a) confirmed and added to the findings of the 1996 CDC study. They found that although Massachusetts and 48 comparison states experienced similar declines (15 percent and 14 percent respectively) in per-capita cigarette consumption from 1988 to 1992, Massachusetts experienced a greater annual decline (more than 4 percent) than the comparison states (less than 1 percent annually) following the establishment of excise tax and the establishment of the MTCP. As the authors of the CDC study had already observed, the decline in Massachusetts occurred even though price reductions for cigarettes effectively negated the potential effects of the excise tax increase. The authors also determined that after 1992 Massachusetts experienced a greater rate of decline in adult smoking prevalence than did the comparison states. The prevalence of smoking declined by 0.43 percent per year in Massachusetts but by only 0.03 percent in the comparison states. On the basis of these findings, the authors concluded that tobacco control programs such as the MTCP can reduce the rates of tobacco use and the related health risks (Biener et al. 2000a).

Massachusetts's success in reducing the rates of tobacco use among youth has fluctuated over time, however. In its last review of the MTCP, Abt Associates reported that although the prevalence of smoking among youth in Massachusetts and the United States as a whole actually grew during the early 1990s, Massachusetts managed to reverse this trend in the second half of the decade, with the prevalence of smoking among youth falling more rapidly in Massachusetts from 1995 to 2001 (from 36 to 26 percent) than in the rest of the country (35 to 29 percent) (Hamilton et al. 2003). A separate study conducted by Soldz and colleagues (2002) identified similar trends. On the basis of data from the triennial Massachusetts Prevalence Study, Soldz and colleagues found that although the prevalence increased at both the state and national levels from 1990 to 1993, Massachusetts managed to reverse this trend in the latter half of the decade. Comparing data from the 1996 and 1999 surveys, the authors determined that over the 3-year period, the rate of cigarette use among students in grades 7 through 12 dropped from 30.7 percent to 23.7 percent. The percent decline in Massachusetts, they found, was greater than the declines seen in neighboring states and in the nation as a whole. Furthermore, the decrease in the rate of cigarette use was broad-based, occurring in numerous subsets of the youth population in Massachusetts. The prevalence rate declined among students in middle school as well as high school, boys and girls, and African Americans and whites. Soldz and colleagues concluded that the scale of this decline, especially in comparison with the smaller regional and national declines, strongly demonstrated the effectiveness of the MTCP in reducing the rate of cigarette use among Massachusetts youth (Soldz et al. 2002).

On the basis of data from the CDC's Youth Behavior Risk Survey, Figure 5-4 illustrates the progress that Massachusetts made during the mid-to-late 1990s in reducing the rate of tobacco use among youth, reflecting the conclusions reached by the independent evaluation as well as by Soldz and colleagues (2002). Figure 5-4 also shows, however, that after these two studies were conducted, the smoking prevalence rate among youth in the state began to decline at a slower rate than that among youth in the country as a whole. This slowdown coincides with the sharp reductions made to the MTCP's budget during the early part of the 2000s. Although, in light of 2005 data, the smoking prevalence rate among youth in Massachusetts once again compares favorably with that among youth in the United States at large, the prevalence of smoking among youth in the state has essentially stalled, indicating an end to the declines seen in the latter half of the 1990s.

Summary

The evidence presented and reviewed above shows that comprehensive state programs have achieved substantial reductions in the rates of tobacco use in both California and Massachusetts. This is particularly true of the early years of the CTCP and MTCP, when both states aggressively funded and implemented their tobacco control programs. Evaluations of Florida's

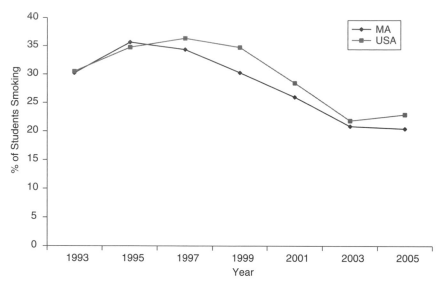

FIGURE 5-4 Comparison of the rate of current cigarette use among high school students (grades 9 to 12) in Massachusetts with the U.S. median, based on data from the Youth Risk Behavior Surveillance System.
SOURCE: (CDC 2006b).

youth-themed "truth" campaign, as well as programs in other states, such as Arizona, Oregon, and—most recently—New York, also indicate that statewide tobacco control programs can be effective in reducing the rates of tobacco use (Bauer et al. 2000; CDC 1999a; 2001; RTI International 2005; Siegel 2002; Sly et al. 2001a; Wakefield and Chaloupka 2000). In recent years, however, large budget cutbacks to many states' tobacco control programs, including that of Massachusetts, have jeopardized continued success. To effectively reduce tobacco use, states must maintain, over time, a comprehensive and integrated tobacco control strategy.

FUNDING FOR COMPREHENSIVE STATE PROGRAMS

After the end of the ASSIST program, when the responsibility for tobacco prevention shifted from NCI to OSH at CDC, OSH implemented a Tobacco Control Program to sustain comprehensive state tobacco control programs. Under that program each state can receive approximately $1 million per year for comprehensive tobacco control efforts (CDC 2003). Suggested levels of funding per capita are included to assist states in allocating funds from various sources. However, state governments are not funding such efforts at the levels that the CDC recommends for best practices (Tauras et al. 2005), either from general funds or from payments under the MSA (revenues received under the MSA have typically been siphoned off by state governments to support programs other than those for tobacco control). In this section, the committee summarizes state expenditures on tobacco control and the sources of revenues that are funding these programs.

State Tobacco Control Expenditures

Expenditures on tobacco control vary widely among states (Figure 5-5 [Prevention Spending Dollars per person] and Table 5-1). In FY 2005, per-capita state expenditures on tobacco control varied from more than $11 in Delaware ($11.87) and Maine ($11.14) to nothing (aside from the CDC grant) in the District of Columbia, Michigan, Missouri, New Hampshire, South Carolina, and Tennessee. The mean per-capita state expenditure was $2.76.

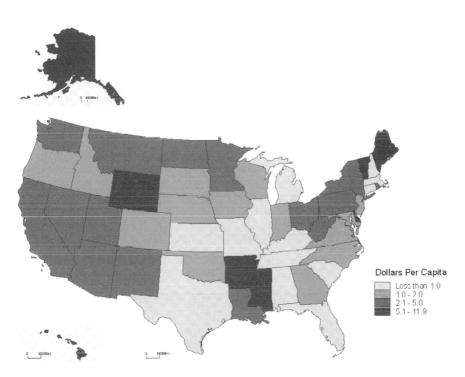

Dollars Per Capita

Less than 1.0
1.0 - 2.0
2.1 - 5.0
5.1 - 11.9

FIGURE 5-5 FY 2005 state tobacco control spending per capita (based on 2000 census data).

TABLE 5-1 Per-Capita State Tobacco Control Revenues and Expenditures, 2005

State	MSA Payment Received per Capita ($)	Net Excise Tax Revenue per Capita ($)	Prevention Spending per Capita ($)
Alabama	22.91	33.63	0.08
Alaska	34.71	77.06	6.70
Arizona	19.48	54.99	4.50
Arkansas	19.74	47.51	6.58
California	12.01	30.23	2.18
Colorado	20.31	26.74	1.00
Connecticut	34.74	74.61	0.02
Delaware	32.17	103.60	11.87
District of Columbia	66.95	35.43	0.00
Florida	24.48	27.38	0.06
Georgia	19.11	27.66	1.40
Hawaii	31.66	68.62	7.35
Idaho	17.89	34.87	1.47
Illinois	23.88	51.38	0.89
Indiana	21.38	53.94	1.78
Iowa	18.94	29.88	1.74
Kansas	19.76	43.79	0.28
Kentucky	27.77	12.35	0.67
Louisiana	32.35	31.11	2.53
Maine	38.46	72.09	11.14
Maryland	28.56	50.51	1.79
Massachusetts	40.54	65.01	0.60
Michigan	27.60	109.67	0.00
Minnesota	37.56	32.58	3.80
Mississippi	42.54	15.24	7.03
Missouri	25.91	17.74	0.00
Montana	30.01	62.72	2.77
Nebraska	22.16	39.14	1.69
Nevada	19.45	64.58	2.20
New Hampshire	34.31	75.61	0.00
New Jersey	29.29	92.84	1.31
New Mexico	20.90	33.04	2.75
New York	21.64	49.32	2.08
North Carolina	18.47	4.89	1.86
North Dakota	36.32	28.23	4.83
Ohio	28.28	48.86	4.69
Oklahoma	19.14	30.37	1.39
Oregon	21.38	63.65	1.02
Pennsylvania	29.82	83.79	3.75
Rhode Island	43.71	123.70	2.38
South Carolina	18.29	6.41	0.00
South Dakota	29.46	34.85	1.99
Tennessee	27.54	19.70	0.00
Texas	24.74	23.60	0.35
Utah	12.70	24.33	3.22

TABLE 5-1 continued

State	MSA Payment Received per Capita ($)	Net Excise Tax Revenue per Capita ($)	Prevention Spending per Capita ($)
Vermont	43.04	75.69	7.72
Virginia	18.41	15.77	1.84
Washington	22.21	55.72	4.61
West Virginia	31.24	54.21	3.26
Wisconsin	24.62	54.87	1.86
Wyoming	32.05	44.06	7.70

NOTES:
Data for states not part of the MSA from the Campaign for Tobacco-free Kids.
Figures do not reflect the $1 million given to each state by CDC (explains why some state have $0 for prevention spending).
Used Census 2000 data—not significantly different from 2005 data.
CA and NY MSA monies are only those given to the state and not the state and localities.

On average, states spend about half of CDC's recommended minimum level for comprehensive state tobacco control programs including the nine components specified in Best Practices for Comprehensive Tobacco Control Programs community programs to reduce tobacco use, chronic disease programs to reduce the burden of tobacco-related diseases, school programs, enforcement, statewide programs, countermarketing, cessation programs, surveillance and evaluation, and administration and management (CDC 1999c). In 1995, the CDC's recommended range of per-capita spending for the nation as a whole was $5.85 to $15.85. The CDC identified such an expenditure range to take into account important variations among states, including overall population (and therefore the possibility of achieving economies of scale), as well as tobacco use prevalence and demographic factors.

According to the CDC, "approximate annual costs to implement all of the recommended program components have been estimated to range from $7 to $20 per capita in smaller states (population under 3 million), $6 to $17 per capita in medium-sized states (population 3 million to 7 million), and $5 to $16 per capita in larger states (population over 7 million)" (CDC 1999c). In recommending funding ranges for each state, CDC generally works within these estimates, although it should be noted that for the states with smaller populations, CDC recommends an upper estimate higher than $20 (for example, in Delaware, the District of Columbia, Montana, North Dakota, Rhode Island, South Dakota, Vermont, and Wyoming). California has the lowest lower estimate of $5.12 per capita, and Wyoming has the highest upper estimate of $30.01.

The committee reviewed the methodology that CDC uses to calculate these estimated general ranges. The agency first identified best practices for each of the nine components of a comprehensive program and then calculated funding ranges (in millions) for each program component for each state—taking population, tobacco-use prevalence, and demographic factors into account—totaled the lower and upper estimates of each component on a state-by-state basis to find a total state program cost, and then calculated the per-capita ranges for each state. The scientific evidence that has emerged since 1999 appears to have substantiated CDC's judgment regarding best practices in each of the relevant domains, and the committee sees no reason to question the CDC's expert judgments regarding the likely costs of implementing these practices in various states. Accordingly, the committee has decided to use the CDC estimates as a template for its recommendations regarding state tobacco control expenditures.

Revenue Sources for State Tobacco Control Programs

What are the revenue sources of state funding for tobacco control? It might be expected that a certain percentage of revenues produced by tobacco excise taxes and the Master Settlement Agreement would be "earmarked" or set aside for tobacco control. However, few states have adopted this strategy, and there is very little correlation between the amounts generated by these two tobacco-related revenue streams and the amount expended on tobacco control.

State Tobacco Excise Taxes

States vary widely in their tobacco excise tax rates and in the amount of revenue that those taxes produce per capita (Table 5-1), ranging in FY 2005 from more than $80 per capita in Rhode Island ($124), Michigan ($110), Delaware ($104), New Jersey ($93), and Pennsylvania ($84) to less than $15 per capita in North Carolina ($5), South Carolina ($6), and Kentucky ($12). As these numbers suggest, and as Figure 5-6 shows, per-capita excise tax revenues are the highest in the Northeast and the lowest in the Southeast. The average per-capita excise tax revenue in all states was $47.80, and two-thirds of the states had revenues of at least $32 per capita.

In recent years, largely in response to state budget shortfalls, there has been a dramatic increase in the average tobacco excise tax rates and the number of states increasing their tax rates. According to Farrelly and colleagues (2003), in 2002 alone, 21 states raised their cigarette taxes, more states than in the past 5 years combined, and the average state cigarette excise tax rate increased significantly from 31 cents per pack (in 2002 dollars) in 1990 to 62 cents per pack in early 2003. These increases have exacerbated what were already substantial disparities in tobacco excise tax

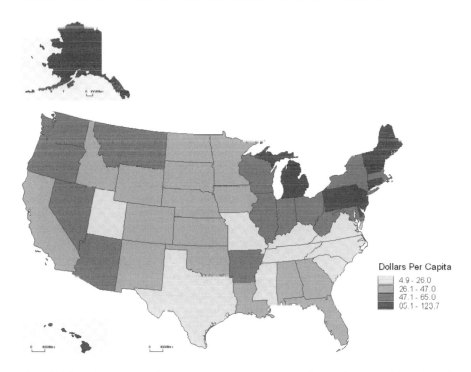

FIGURE 5-6 Per-capita tobacco excise tax revenues collected by state 2005, based on 2000 census data.

rates across the country and the attendant problems of interstate smuggling (Farrelly et al. 2003).

California was the first state to earmark a portion of its excise tax revenues for tobacco control efforts. As noted, a voter initiative, Proposition 99, increased the state tobacco tax by 25 cents per pack of cigarettes in 1988, and in 1990 the California Assembly enacted legislation distributing the revenue earned from the tobacco tax increase. The legislation directed that 20 percent of the revenues be allocated to a health education account, and funds from the health education and research accounts finance a statewide tobacco control program. Only in California, Oregon, and Utah have excise taxes served as a major designated source of funding for tobacco control.

Whether tax revenues should be earmarked for specific purposes is a controversial issue in public finance, and there is no compelling reason why tobacco control activities should be funded from any particular source of revenues (in fact, as noted above, Massachusetts was constitutionally precluded from earmarking the revenues generated by its 1992 tobacco excise tax increase to tobacco control). In addition, earmarking of a specified proportion of revenues represents a pre-commitment to prioritize tobacco control expenditures in a way that would preclude the weighing of other priorities. However, the argument for earmarking a presumptive (but reversible) portion of tobacco excise tax revenues to tobacco control does have a common-sense persuasive force (Hamilton et al. 2005), and a decision to link tobacco excise tax revenues to tobacco control efforts represents a modest political commitment to sustain these activities.

In light of the traditional political separation between decisions about revenues (including excise tax rates) and expenditure decisions, it is perhaps unsurprising that per-capita state excise tax revenues and per-capita tobacco control expenditures are only modestly correlated (Figure 5-7).

Master Settlement Agreement Allocations

Another important element in the political economy of tobacco control is the MSA. On average in 2005, the states received $27.46 per capita from the proceeds of the MSA. Because these calculations were based on projected Medicaid expenditures for tobacco-related diseases, they varied substantially (Table 5-1), from a low of $12.01 per capita in California to a high of $66.95 in the District of Columbia (Figure 5-8).

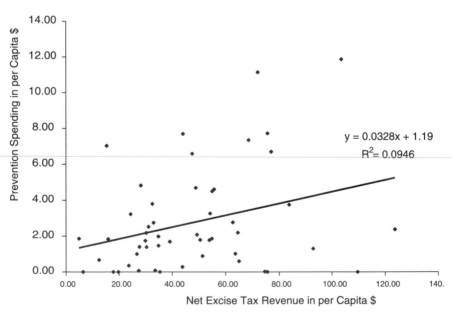

FIGURE 5-7 Correlation between per-capita tobacco control spending and per-capita excise tax revenues.

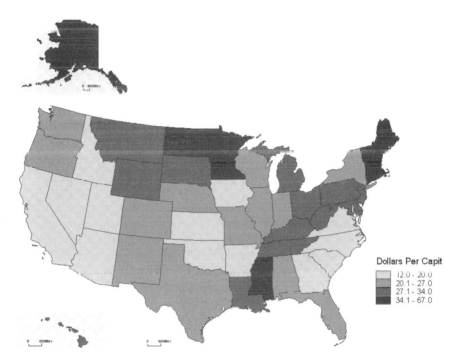

Dollars Per Capit
	12.0 - 20.0
	20.1 - 27.0
	27.1 - 34.0
	34.1 - 67.0

FIGURE 5-8 Per-capita payments received from the MSA, by state, in FY 2005 (based on 2000 census data).

The MSA does not stipulate how the states should spend the settlement funds. Consequently, the 46 states, the District of Columbia, and the five territories party to the MSA have developed various regulations, structures, and mechanisms for allocating settlement payments. A November 2005 report jointly issued by the American Cancer Society, the American Heart Association, the American Lung Association, and the Campaign for Tobacco-Free Kids illustrates the diverse approaches that the states have used to administer these funds over the past several years (AHA et al. 2005). Although some states regularly apply payments directly to their general budgets, others have established specific funds to which they direct their MSA allotments. Delaware law, for instance, mandates that all settlement payments be deposited into the Delaware Health Fund, which finances health-related programs, including the state's tobacco control efforts. Kansas law, meanwhile, directs the entirety of the state's MSA payments (after the first $70 million, which was placed into the state's general fund) into the Kansas Endowment for Youth fund, which finances a range of youth-related programs. And Michigan and Nevada direct portions of their MSA allotments to education scholarship funds. Just a few states, however, such as Nevada and Virginia, explicitly require portions of their settlement funds to be applied to tobacco control efforts.

Several tobacco-producing states apply large portions of their MSA payments to funds that assist citizens and businesses traditionally dependent on the tobacco industry. North Carolina law requires that 50 percent of the state's annual MSA receipts be placed in a fund that provides assistance to tobacco-dependent communities. An additional 25 percent is allocated to a separate fund that directly aids tobacco farmers and tobacco manufacturing workers, among others. Similarly, Virginia law allocates 50 percent of the commonwealth's MSA-derived funds to the Tobacco Indemnification and Community Revitalization Trust Fund, which provides economic assistance to tobacco growers and tobacco-dependent communities (AHA et al. 2005).

In recent years, budget shortfalls have compelled a number of states to divert MSA payments from tobacco-control–related funds and programs, such as those listed above (AHA et al. 2005). Largely to address such shortfalls, 15 states have also opted to securitize future MSA proceeds (GAO 2006). California, for instance, securitized its future settlement payments to fund its FY 2003 and FY 2004 budgets (AHA et al. 2005). In electing to securitize MSA proceeds, states receive advance income by issuing bonds backed by future MSA payments. States must pay to service the debt accrued through securitization, however; and in FY 2005 four states, including California, applied 100 percent of their MSA payments to servicing this debt (in addition, New Jersey allocated 99.9 percent of its MSA payments to debt servicing). In an April 2006 review of how states spend their MSA payments, the U.S. Government Accountability Office (GAO) calculated that servicing of securitization debt represented 24 percent of the total MSA funds allocated by states in FY 2005 (GAO 2006).

GAO also reported that between FY 2004 and FY 2005, the portion of MSA payments allocated to cover budget shortfalls decreased dramatically, from 44 to 4 percent, with states applying the largest portion of MSA-derived funds (32 percent) in FY 2005 to health-related programs (e.g., health care services, health insurance, and health research). It should be noted, however, that although the portion of funds allocated to such programs increased, the actual dollar amount decreased between FY 2004 and FY 2005, because fewer states obtained money up front through securitization. Allocations of MSA payments to tobacco control programs, meanwhile, remain extremely low, averaging just 4.7 percent of total MSA payments in FY 2005. In fact, since GAO began reviewing state allocations of MSA money, the percentage apportioned to tobacco control efforts has not exceeded 6 percent (GAO 2006). GAO does not anticipate any change in allocations to tobacco control programs for FY 2006.

Sloan and colleagues (2005) found that the mean total annual spending from settlement funds was $30.65 per capita from FY 2000 to FY 2004. Median spending was about $25 per capita. However, less than half of that money was spent on health related activities, and very little of it was spent on tobacco control efforts. Approximately one-fourth of the state budgets reported during this period allocated no money to tobacco control. Among budgets that allocated anything to tobacco control, the usual allocation was less than $2.50 per capita (see Figure 3 in the article by Sloan and colleagues 2005). States tended to spend less on tobacco control if they had more seniors, more individuals under the age of 18 years, and higher per-capita incomes. Not surprisingly, tobacco-producing states tended to spend smaller amounts of their MSA proceeds on tobacco control (Sloan et al. 2005).

In sum, only a small proportion of MSA revenues is devoted to tobacco control, and MSA revenues are specifically earmarked for this purpose in only a handful of states. In some states, however, the modest appropriations from MSA payments have accounted for a significant proportion of tobacco-control–related expenditures. Gross and colleagues (2002), for instance, determined that even though the percentage of MSA funds directed to tobacco control was very low, "when the tobacco-control-program expenditures from all 50 states were considered in aggregate, over half of the funding was derived from settlement income" (Gross et al. 2002). This proportion is probably much lower now because so many states have used their MSA funds to shore up budget gaps.

Summary and Recommendation

In the committee's view, states should adopt a funding strategy designed to provide stable support for the level of tobacco control funding recommended by the CDC. MSA payments are not a reliable source of funds in most states. The most sensible approach would be to allocate a suitable share of tobacco excise tax revenues to tobacco control efforts. History suggests that these taxes are not likely to be reduced once they have been increased; moreover, high excise taxes also serve the goal of reducing tobacco use (see below) while raising revenues for tobacco control efforts and other public purposes. In most states, the CDC's recommended expenditure target (about $16 per capita for the nation as a whole) could be achieved by setting aside about one-third of the proceeds from the tax. The committee recognizes that explicit earmarking is forbidden by some state constitutions and is presumptively unacceptable in other states. However, even if formal earmarking is unacceptable, legislators responsible for public health expenditures should embrace a political strategy of linking the amount of the tobacco control budget line to a percentage of tobacco excise tax revenues.

Recommendation 1: Each state should fund state tobacco control activities at the level recommended by the CDC. A reasonable target for each state is in the range of $15 to $20 per capita, depending on the state's population, demography, and prevalence of tobacco use. If it is constitutionally permissible, states should use a statutorily prescribed portion of their tobacco excise tax revenues to fund tobacco control programs.

EXCISE TAX

It is well established that an increase in the price of cigarettes decreases their use and that raising tobacco excise taxes is one of the most effective policies for reducing the use of tobacco. From a policy perspective, one of the unresolved questions is whether price increases act synergistically with other tobacco control interventions to decrease consumption. After a brief review of the literature on these topics, the committee addresses the proper level of excise taxation solely on the basis of tobacco control considerations and comments on the practical difficulties presented by disparate levels of state excise taxes.

Price Increases Decrease Cigarette Use

Over a period of more than three decades, economists and health policy analysts have accumulated a large body of evidence on the effect of price on cigarette consumption. The effect of price on cigarette use has also been the subject of numerous recent reviews (Chaloupka 1999, (Chaloupka and Warner 2000; Leverett et al. 2002; Pinilla 2002) and meta-analyses (Gallet and List 2003). The conclusion reached by virtually every study of every demographic group in both developed and developing countries is that an increase in cigarette price reduces the level of cigarette use. A recent cross-sectional study of 70 countries based on aggregate consumption data found a price elasticity in the range of –0.49 to –0.57 percent (Blecher and van Walbeek 2004).

Price has been found to affect virtually every measure of cigarette use, including per-capita consumption, as derived from aggregate macrolevel data, as well as smoking prevalence and the number of cigarettes smoked daily, as derived from individual microlevel data (Hu et al. 1995a). Recent studies with microlevel data have found that higher cigarette prices increase the probability that a current adult smoker will make an attempt to quit (Levy et al. 2005) and that a young adult smoker will stop smoking (Tauras 2004b). In a study of adult smokers, access to low-taxed cigarettes was found to deter cessation attempts (Hyland et al. 2005). The June 2006 National Institutes of Health (NIH) state-of-the-science panel on tobacco use (NIH 2006b) found that an increase in the unit price of tobacco products increases the rate of tobacco use cessation and reduces the level of consumption among individuals across a wide spectrum of racial and socioeconomic groups.

Just as increases in cigarette taxes deter consumption, declines in cigarette prices have been found to increase the level of consumption. In one Canadian study, for example, tax cuts in certain provinces slowed the rate of decline of smoking by inducing more smokers to start and leading fewer smokers to quit (Hamilton et al. 1997). Another study suggested that the price decrease in Canada in the early 1990s may have contributed to an increase in the rate of smoking among youth in the province of Ontario (Waller et al. 2003). In the United States, the increase in the rate of smoking among youth in the early 1990s has been attributed to declines in cigarette prices (Gruber 2001).

Cigarette Price Increases Reduce Cigarette Use by Adolescents

Although some studies have reported mixed or negative findings, the most recently published research generally supports the finding that higher cigarette prices discourage youth from smoking (Chaloupka 1999; Chaloupka and Pacula 1998; Chapman and Richardson 1990; Ding 2003; Gruber 2001; Harris and Chan 1999; Liang et al. 2003). Increased cigarette prices have been found to deter smoking among young people when investigators controlled for peer effects (Powell et al. 2005).

Some recent research has attempted to distinguish between the effects of price on adolescent experimentation with cigarettes and the effects of price on cigarette use among established adolescent smokers. One recent study, based on microlevel data from a 1993 national youth survey, found that cigarette price affects the latter group but not the former group (Emery et al. 2001). However, another study, based on the Growing Up Today Study of 1999, found that adolescents residing in states with the highest quartile of cigarette tax rates had a lower probability of experimental smoking (Thomson et al. 2004). Still another recent study suggested that cigarette prices do affect the probability that adolescent males, but not adolescent females, will initiate smoking. Adolescent female smoking initiation was found to depend on perceptions of being overweight or the desire to lose weight (Cawley et al. 2004).

Some of the inconsistencies in past research may have resulted from inaccurate measurement of the actual prices that teenagers paid for cigarettes. One study suggested that region-specific average retail prices or tax rates may incorrectly gauge the actual prices paid by youth smokers and that perceived price is a more specific measure of the smoker's actual out-of-pocket costs (Ross and Chaloupka 2003).

The June 2006 NIH state-of-the-science panel on tobacco use (NIH 2006b) determined that increases in excise taxes are effective in preventing tobacco use among adolescents and young adults, even though recent studies have found that increases in cigarette tax induce smokers to seek out tax-exempt cigarettes, to take advantage of coupon offers, and to avoid the impact of tax hikes in other ways (Hyland et al. 2004).

Do Cigarette Price Increases Act Synergistically with Other Antismoking Interventions?

Researchers have attempted to untangle the effects of price increases from those of other antitobacco policies, including informational campaigns and restrictions on public smoking, that are often carried out concurrently with governmental tax increases (Scollo et al. 2003; Stephens et al. 2001). Although many studies have established that cigarette price increases and other antismoking policies act independently to suppress demand, the question of a possible synergistic effect remains unanswered. Put differently, could antismoking policies raise the price elasticity of demand, or could price increases enhance the effectiveness of other antismoking interventions?

A number of studies have identified the independent effects of cigarette price increases and local restrictions on smoking at work sites or public places, in both the United States and Canada (Chaloupka 1999; Keeler et al. 1993; Stephens et al. 1997; Tauras 2004a; Yurekli and Zhang 2000). Other studies have identified the independent effects of tax increases and state or local tobacco control campaigns. Early research in this area was based on the antismoking campaigns in California and Massachusetts. Thus a study of quarterly cigarette sales data from 1980 to 1992 in California found that the antismoking campaign and cigarette taxation both contributed to the decline in the level of cigarette use (Hu et al. 1995b). Likewise, a study of the Massachusetts tobacco control campaign found declines in consumption greater than those expected from tax increases alone (CDC 1996).

Recent work on the interaction between price changes and other antismoking policies has extended beyond the initial experiences of California and Massachusetts. In one cross-sectional study, increases in state tobacco control funding were found to reduce smoking, even when prices are taken into account (Farrelly et al. 2003). Another study reported independent effects of cigarette price and state-level media campaigns on the probability of making a quit attempt of at least 3 months' duration (Levy et al. 2005). The combination of antismoking programs and increased tobacco taxes reduced the level of cigarette consumption among youth more than expected as a result of price increases alone (Wakefield and Chaloupka 2000).

Some studies have noted the combined effect of price increases and other antismoking measures, but made an attempt to identify specific contribution of each strategy. Thus cigarette smoking among adults declined after New York City raised local cigarette taxes, made available cessation services, distributed nicotine patches for free, and instituted legal action to ban smoking in public places in 2002 (Frieden et al. 2005). A study in the state of Oregon, reported in Morbidity and Mortality Weekly Report, found that the combination of an excise tax increase and the state's Tobacco Prevention and Education Program diminished the level of cigarette use (CDC 1999a).

A recent study focused on the impact of the 1998 MSA in the United States, specifically, the effect of the agreement on retail cigarette prices and aggregate cigarette consumption (Sloan et al. 2004). By 2002, the MSA was estimated to have reduced the rate of cigarette consumption by 13 percent among 18- to 20-year-olds, 5 percent among 21- to 65-year-olds, and 13 percent among those 65 years of age and older. The decline in consumption was mediated primarily through the effect of the MSA on cigarette prices, but there was evidence that MSA-associated policies, aside from increased prices, reduced consumption among younger smokers.

How High Should Tobacco Excise Taxes Be?

At the present time, state governments are the primary taxing authorities for tobacco products. During 2005, the consumption-weighted average state excise tax was 76.73 cents per pack (Capehart 2005). By contrast, the federal excise tax has been 39 cents per pack since 2002. Of an estimated total consumption of 388 billion cigarettes in 2004, only 5 billion (or 1.3 percent) were sold through federally tax-exempt outlets, including Indian reservations, military bases, and shipments to Puerto Rico (Capehart 2005).

Tax Evasion

When cigarette excise taxes are evaluated solely from a public health perspective (i.e., exclusively as an instrument for deterring consumption), the level to which the tax might justifiably be raised is limited only by concerns that higher taxes stimulate tax avoidance, such as by creating a demand for nontaxed or lower-taxed cigarette products or for other tobacco product substitutes. Broadly speaking, there are at least three avoidance strategies: (1) producing cigarettes at home, (2) ordering cigarettes to be shipped by mail or package delivery service from sellers who do not collect the tax, and (3) physically purchasing and importing cigarettes from a lower-tax jurisdiction.

The first cigarette tax evasion strategy, home production, has traditionally constituted a negligible fraction of the overall market and, until that situation changes, all that is required is basic monitoring to make sure that the market is not growing substantially. The second cigarette tax evasion strategy, interstate shipping, has become an increasing concern with the proliferation of internet sites selling untaxed cigarettes. The committee addresses this problem below and recommends legislation prohibiting both online tobacco sales and direct shipment of tobacco products to consumers.

The third cigarette tax evasion strategy, smuggling from states with low excise taxes to states with high excise taxes, has traditionally been the greatest concern due to the great variation in state-level excise taxes and the porosity of state borders with respect to commerce. Even if the price within the United States were uniform, policymakers would still have to consider the prospect of smuggling from other countries. International black markets could develop in which foreign cigarettes are smuggled into the country to avoid equalizing excise taxes, or U.S.-manufactured cigarettes could be exported and then illegally re-imported. International smuggling, however, does not appear to be a substantial concern at the present time. The committee will address the smuggling problem later in this chapter.

External Costs

Aside from the impact on consumption, other factors may be relevant to policymakers in selecting the proper level of an excise tax. One key concern is the "efficient" level of taxation that requires smokers to fully internalize the social costs of their smoking (Chaloupka and Warner 2000). From an economic perspective, the main purpose of excise taxes is to make the cigarette consumer who decides to buy cigarettes pay not only for the cigarettes themselves but also pay an amount equivalent to the costs that their smoking imposes on the rest of society. Such a "Pigouvian tax" raises the price of cigarettes to an economically efficient level by internalizing the external costs of consumption.

Computations of the external cost per pack of cigarettes, however, have hinged on exactly how the external costs of smoking are defined. As Chaloupka and Warner observed, "there is no complete consensus on precisely what consequences warrant inclusion, and even for those for which there is consensus, estimates of the magnitude of the true social externalities vary widely" (Chaloupka and Warner 2000, p. 1579). For example, some economists would regard the injury that a smoking mother confers on her children as an internal cost within the family, whereas others would count it as an external cost. Thus a study by Hay (1991) estimated that the costs of the long-term intellectual and physical consequences of smoking-related low-birth-weight disabilities implied a tax of $4.80 per pack (Hay 1991). Although economists would generally agree that the effects of ETS outside the family should be considered an external cost, an earlier estimate of the external costs (15 cents per pack) by Manning and colleagues (1989) was later criticized because the authors did not have full information on the consequences of ETS exposure at the time (Chaloupka and Warner 2000).

Other economists have pointed out that many smokers would like to quit and regret having made the decision to become a smoker. As discussed in Chapter 2, individuals typically become smokers when they are adolescents, at a time when the costs of smoking are not fully understood or anticipated. In this sense, the adolescent did not take into account the "costs" being imposed on the older addicted smoker who now regrets his or her earlier decision. From that standpoint, many current smokers favor higher prices, and that very fact should be taken into account in analyzing the most efficient level of taxation. In general, it takes a peculiarly strong faith in consumer rationality to apply the standard Pigouvian calculus to an inherently hazardous product to which people become addicted as teenagers.

Regressivity

Whatever the most efficient level of taxation, another concern is that higher taxes may be regressive; that is, poorer people may pay more per capita than would people with higher incomes because the prevalence of smoking is considerably higher among people with lower incomes and less education than among people with higher incomes and more education (see Chapter 1). Ordinarily, there might well be a legitimate concern when a tax increases the price of a good, simply because increases in the prices of goods particularly affect those who are the least able to pay. Tobacco is not an ordinary good, however. Its consumption is (and is perceived to be) a harm to many of its consumers. To the extent that the pool of smokers includes a disproportionate number of less educated and lower-income people, a tax may well benefit them rather than harm them. To the extent that an excise tax decreases smoking initiation and helps to spur decreases in smoking, its beneficial effects may well be concentrated among the poorer members of society. For this reason, the concern about the regressivity of any tax increase seems to the committee to be somewhat overstated, even misplaced. Nevertheless, the main implication of concern regarding the regressivity of tobacco excise taxes, in the committee's view, is that distributional concerns should be taken into account and that higher taxes should be coupled with state financing of cessation programs and services, especially for lower-income smokers.

New Measures

The states and the federal government should use tobacco excise taxes for the dual purposes of reducing consumption and funding tobacco control programs. Taking into account only tobacco control considerations, the committee believes that the ideal situation would be a uniform level of tobacco excise taxation for the entire nation at the highest feasible level. Feasibility here refers to the need to minimize cross-border smuggling and to minimize an unfair and politically unacceptable impact on current smokers, especially disadvantaged populations. A uniform tax would presumably be most efficiently administered at the federal level, although the revenues could be distributed to the states according to a mutually agreeable formula that would lead the states to refrain from exercising their own taxing authority; however, a plan under which the federal government "preempts" the field of tobacco excise taxation may be regarded as too radical at the present time.[3] Another possibility would be for the federal government to coordinate a system that creates incentives for states to reduce the disparities in state excise taxes. In Chapter 6, the committee presents the outline of a plan under which the federal government would link the availability of federal subsidies for a state's tobacco control expenditures to the amount of these tobacco control expenditures and the level of the state's tobacco excise tax. Among other purposes, this plan is designed to use federal spending leverage to induce states with lower tobacco excise taxes to raise them, reducing the disparities in state excise taxes.

Unless and until the federal government takes on such a coordinating role, cross-state smuggling is likely to remain a serious problem. For the purposes of the policy blueprint being outlined in this chapter, the committee's assumption is that the current legal structure of tobacco control will remain unchanged. On the basis of that assumption, the states will retain the responsibility to coordinate their own efforts. To help them do that, while increasing the overall level of tobacco excise taxation, the committee recommends the tobacco excise tax rates of the states in the top quintile become the target for the remaining states. (Currently, the lower bound rate for the top quintile is about $1.25 per pack. If states with lower rates were to move their tax rates toward those in the top quintile, the variation

---

[3] Congress probably has the constitutional power to adopt such a solution as part of a comprehensive plan of regulating tobacco and protecting the public health under the commerce clause. See Moorman Manufacturing Co. v. Blair, 437 U.S. 267, 280 (1978). In addition, Congress also has the authority to condition the state's receipt of federal funds for tobacco control on the states' refraining from imposing tobacco excise taxes. See South Carolina v. Dole, 483 U.S. 203 (1987). In practice, however, Congress has rarely restricted the states' taxing power. See Walter Hellerstein and Charles MacClure, Congressional Intervention in State Taxation: a Normative Analysis of Three Proposals, 2004 State Tax Today 40-3 (2004).

in state excise tax rates—and the frequency of smuggling—would be substantially lowered.) As noted earlier, all states should earmark a statutorily prescribed portion of their excise tax revenues sufficient to fund tobacco control programs at a level recommended by the CDC.

> Recommendation 2: States with excise tax rates below the level imposed by the top quintile of states should also substantially increase their own rates to reduce smuggling and tax evasion. State excise tax rates should be indexed to inflation.

The federal tobacco excise tax has traditionally served as a tool for raising revenue rather than as an instrument of tobacco control. However, for the reasons summarized above, the committee thinks that the federal tobacco excise tax rate should be increased substantially—at least on the order of $1.00 per pack—even if the federal government's overall role in tobacco control remains a supportive one. The possibility of a more substantial federal role in tobacco control is explored in Chapter 6.

> Recommendation 3: The federal government should substantially raise federal tobacco excise taxes, currently set at 39 cents a pack. Federal excise tax rates should be indexed to inflation.

SMOKING RESTRICTIONS

As noted in Chapter 3, grassroots advocacy for clean air laws was the first major achievement of contemporary tobacco control efforts. Despite continuing progress in expanding the reach of legislation restricting smoking in venues with significant public exposure, the task remains incomplete. Coverage of the existing state "smokefree indoor air" laws varies significantly. Table 5-2 summarizes the coverage of state laws as of the first quarter of 2005 (CDC 2005c). This section reviews current smoking restrictions and their effects in nonresidential indoor locations (workplaces and public accommodations), group residential locations (hospitals, nursing homes, and correctional facilities), private residences, and public outdoor areas.

Workplaces and Public Accommodations

The CDC data presented in Table 5-2 indicate that as of late 2005, most states now have some restrictions on smoking on public transportation, with 23 states banning it completely and 19 states requiring either separate ventilated areas or designated smoking areas. Similarly, 44 states have placed restrictions on smoking in government work sites. 16 of these states have enacted complete smoking bans in government workplaces.

TABLE 5-2 Scope of State Indoor Air Restrictions as of 4th Quarter, 2005

Location	Banned (100% Smoke Free)	Separate Ventilated Areas	Designated Areas	Any Restriction	No Restrictions
Bars	6	2	4	12	39[b]
Commercial day care centers	29[a]	3	6[b]	38	13
Enclosed arenas	12	3	14	29	22[b]
Government work sites	16	6	22[b]	44	7
Grocery stores	13	3	19[b]	35	16
Home-based day care centers	23[a]	3	1	27	24[b]
Hospitals	15	4	24[b]	43	8
Hotels and motels	1	1	17	19	32[b]
Malls	10	4	5	19	32[b]
Prisons	4	2	3	9	42[b]
Private work sites	11	4	16[b]	31	20
Public transportation	23[b]	3	16	42	9
Restaurants	11	2	21[b]	34	17

[a]Includes 13 states where smoking is banned when children are on the premises for commercial day care centers and 21 states for those of home-based day care centers.
[b]Includes Washington, D.C.
SOURCE: (CDC 2005c).

However, 20 states still have no restrictions at all on smoking in private-sector work sites. Of course, employers are free to adopt smoking restrictions on their own, and in 1998–1999, almost 70 percent of U.S. workers reported that their workplaces had an official policy prohibiting smoking in work areas and public or common areas, up from 46.5 percent in 1993 (CDC 2005e).

Table 5-2 also shows that 38 states either have weak regulations for restaurants (limiting smoking to designated areas) or have no restrictions at all. Bars are, of course, less regulated, with 39 states having no restrictions. In recent years, however, local governments have been more inclined to adopt comprehensive workplace restrictions that include restaurants and bars. New York City and Washington, D.C., are two prominent examples. As of October 2006, 342 municipalities ban smoking in restaurants and 252 municipalities require smoke-free bars (ANRF 2006). The trend toward coverage of restaurants and bars seems largely responsive to concerns about the plight of workers whose employment choices may be limited and to the failure of the market to respond to nonsmoker preferences for smoke-free venues.

Effects of Workplace Restrictions

Smoking restrictions serve three purposes: (1) they protect nonsmokers from the health effects and the noxious odors of secondhand smoke; (2) they help smokers quit, cut down on their smoking, and avoid relapses; and (3) they reinforce a nonsmoking social norm. Clean air laws, in fact, have done more to reduce consumption than any intervention other than price increases for cigarettes.

Effects on Nonsmokers ETS, or secondhand smoke, is a known carcinogen and has been associated with a variety of adverse health effects in nonsmokers, including lung cancer and coronary disease (EPA 1992). It is estimated that 43 percent of nonsmokers have biological evidence of secondhand smoke exposure (DHHS 2006) and that 3,000 lung cancer deaths and 35,000 to 62,000 coronary heart disease deaths in nonsmokers are attributable to such exposure (CDC 2002). In fact, for every eight smokers who die from smoking, one nonsmoker dies from secondhand smoke exposure (Schoenmarklin and Tobacco Control Legal Consortium 2004). In 2002, the International Agency for Research on Cancer (IARC) estimated that involuntary smoking increases the risk of an acute coronary heart disease event by 25 to 35 percent, and that the excess risk of lung cancer due to exposure to a spouse's secondhand smoke is approximately 20 percent for women and 30 percent for men (IARC 2002).

Involuntary smoking has been found to also have adverse effects on the respiratory system. Very strong evidence of a causal relationship exists for chronic respiratory symptoms (IARC 2002). In addition, exposure to secondhand smoke is associated with an increased risk of sudden infant death syndrome (SIDS), asthma, bronchitis, and pneumonia in young children. The CDC considers ETS exposure to be a serious public health hazard that can be effectively prevented through effective regulation designed to reduce exposure (TIPS 2006a). Furthermore, it is estimated that secondhand smoke exposure costs the United States more than $5 billion per year in direct medical costs and approximately $4.68 billion per year in lost productivity costs, although these figures are considerably lower than estimates from just 15 years ago. This difference is attributed to reductions in both the number of people smoking and the rate of ETS exposure for nonsmokers (Behan et al. 2005).

A study of hospitality workers in New York showed that the percentage of hospitality workers exposed to ETS declined by 85 percent within the 12 months after the state's smoke-free indoor ban took effect. During the same period, hospitality workers reported a 57 percent decline in sensory symptoms of ETS exposure, such as eye irritation, runny nose or sneezing, and sore or scratchy throat, and a 37 percent decline in upper respiratory symptoms, including wheezing, coughing, phlegm, and shortness of breath (Farrelly et al. 2005).

Effects on Consumption by Smokers Substantial evidence indicates that workplace smoking restrictions have been effective in decreasing cigarette consumption and increasing smoking cessation among active smokers. Various studies have shown that smoke-free workplace laws reduce smoking prevalence by amounts ranging from 3.8 percent to 6 percent and consumption among continuing users by 2 percent to 14 percent (Bonta, Appendix B). One 2002 study estimated that a smoke-free policy for all U.S. workplaces would decrease per capita cigarette consumption for the entire population by 4.5 percent (Fichtenberg and Glantz 2002). In addition, studies have shown that workplace smoking restrictions increase smoking cessation. Data collected during the Community Intervention Trial for Smoking Cessation, known as COMMIT, shows that those who reported a smoke-free work site between 1988 and 1993 were 25 percent more likely to attempt to quit smoking than those who were allowed to smoke at work (Glasgow et al. 1997). One study in California demonstrated that employees at smoke-free work sites are up to 38 percent more likely to quit smoking than those who work in areas with no workplace laws against smoking (Moskowitz et al. 2000).

Studies have shown that the prevalence of smoking is 4 percent higher in states without comprehensive clean indoor air laws and that the average annual consumption is 14 packs per person higher in such states (Emont et al. 1992). Overall, clean air laws may reduce smoking prevalence by roughly 10 percent in the general population. In addition, states with stringent smoking restrictions have an average quit rate of 50 percent, whereas states without strong smoking laws have an average quit rate of 44 percent (Bonta, Appendix B).

Ireland was the first country to institute comprehensive nationwide smoke-free workplace legislation, and initial reports indicate that the ban has been a public health success and has met with substantial public approval. In fact, survey results show, somewhat counterintuitively, that 83 percent of Irish smokers reported that they felt the ban was a "good" or a "very good" thing. Not only did the law dramatically decrease ETS in workplaces, pubs, and other public places, but also 80 percent of Irish smokers who reported quitting smoking after implementation of the ban said that the law made them more likely to quit and 88 percent said that the law helped prevent relapse. In addition, 46 percent of Irish smokers who continued smoking after the ban was implemented indicated that the law made them more likely to quit, and 60 percent reported that it decreased their overall consumption (Fong et al., in press; Fong et al. 2006).

Effects on Patronage in Restaurants and Bars Opponents of smoking bans in restaurants and bars argue that these restrictions would have a deleterious effect on business and employment in the hospitality sector. Recent research has shown, however, that this has not been the experience in jurisdictions with bans on smoking in restaurants and bars. A 2004 literature review by Scollo and Lan covering 21 studies of smoke-free policies found that there was "no negative economic impact from the introduction of smoke-free policies in restaurants and bars" (Scollo and Lal 2004). The New York City Department of Health's First Annual Independent Evaluation of New York's Tobacco Control Program reported in 2004 that after the passage of New York's Clean Indoor Air Act (CIAA), which banned smoking in all places of employment, including restaurants and bars, there was little change in the patronage of bars. The report also found that restaurants and industry employment, alcohol excise tax revenues, and bar licenses suffered no adverse effects (RTI International 2004). Additionally, a 2002 CDC report on a smoking ban in restaurants and bars in El Paso, Texas concluded that no statistically significant changes in restaurant and bar revenues occurred after the smoking ban took effect (CDC 2004b). Moreover, residents of areas that have instituted indoor smoking bans have indicated increasing support for such restrictions. Since the implementation of New York's CIAA, for instance, popular support for indoor smoking bans has grown with each passing year. By the beginning of 2005, 79 percent of adults in New York State reported that they supported the CIAA (RTI International 2005).

Recommendation 4: States and localities should enact complete bans on smoking in all nonresidential indoor locations, including workplaces, malls, restaurants, and bars. States should not preempt local governments from enacting bans more restrictive than the state ban.

Hospitals and Health Care Facilities

Implementation of smoking bans in hospitals and health care facilities increased substantially during the 1980s and early 1990s, largely because of the mandate of the Joint Commission on Accreditation of Healthcare Organizations (JCAHO) that all hospitals be smoke-free. This organization, which evaluates and accredits more than 15,000 health care organizations and programs nationwide, promulgated the nonsmoking standard effective December 31, 1993. Hospitals were quick to comply with the new standard, and by the end of 1994, more than 96 percent of hospitals had done so and more than 40 percent had enacted even stricter restrictions (Fee and Brown 2004). Hospital smoking bans were originally instituted because of a concern for the health of patients and reflected an effort to capitalize on the JCAHO restrictions by emphasizing the health risks of smoking. Studies conducted since the bans went into effect have indicated that they not only protect patient health, but also reduce smoking among hospital employees (Fee and Brown 2004). Some concern has been raised about the wisdom of a ban on patient smoking in psychiatric hospitals, but research has shown that such bans have been implemented with little adverse effect (Smith et al. 1999).

Few states have enacted bans on smoking in nursing homes, although most require designated smoking areas if smoking is permitted. However, both federal and most state laws permit a total ban. According to Bergman, in 2003 about 64 percent of nursing homes did not allow smoking inside, with the remaining 36 percent limiting smoking to designated areas (Bergman 2003).

Recommendation 5: All health care facilities, including nursing homes, psychiatric hospitals, and medical units in correctional facilities, should meet or exceed JCAHO standards in banning smoking in all indoor areas.

Correctional Facilities

Despite the substantial evidence of the effectiveness of workplace smoking bans and their widespread adoption in hospitals, correctional facilities have been reluctant to take aggressive steps to eliminate smoking. Unlike JCAHO, neither the American Jail Association nor the American

Correctional Association has mandated smoke-free policies for its institutions, although both have adopted resolutions supporting such restrictions (Hammond and Emmons 2005). According to a 2002 survey, at least 38 state correctional departments had enacted some form of ban (Bonta, Appendix B), but very few of these have instituted total bans (Hammond and Emmons 2005). However, there is a discernible trend in the direction of stricter policies. On July 15, 2004, the Federal Bureau of Prisons established a nearly total ban for employees and inmates at 105 prisons. Also, in 2004, California passed a law eliminating tobacco products from prisons and youth correctional facilities (Bonta, Appendix B).

The relatively modest level of restriction on smoking in correctional facilities is somewhat surprising, given the significant implications of secondhand smoke exposure in such facilities. First, the sheer size of the population is cause for concern, as approximately 2 million inmates are incarcerated in jails and prisons at any one time (BJS 2005). Second, the problem of secondhand smoke exposure is particularly acute in correctional facilities because about 60 percent of inmates are smokers and the mandatory enclosure and poor ventilation in many prisons can create very high levels of ETS (Hammond and Emmons 2005). Partially because of these concerns, the U.S. Supreme Court ruled in 1993 that inmates do not have a constitutional right to smoke and that exposure to unreasonable levels of ETS may constitute "cruel and unusual punishment" under certain circumstances (Helling v. McKinney, 509 U.S. 25 [1993]). Indeed, studies have shown that smoke-free prison policies have been effective in dramatically reducing ETS exposure, particularly in crowded or poorly ventilated areas (Hammond and Emmons 2005). In addition, banning smoking can improve overall inmate health and may reduce health care costs in prisons. Consequently, part of the motivation for California's recent legislation was the estimated $280 million in health care costs attributable to inmate cigarette smoking (The Monitor's View 2005).

There are practical concerns, however, about instituting smoke-free policies. Specifically, prison administrators fear that total smoking bans may lead to an increase in inmate-staff tensions and the rise of a black market for tobacco products. This concern may be somewhat overstated, though, as a 2001 survey of the 51 U.S. prison systems that had instituted bans revealed that only 2 of these systems reported any increased violence and 20 percent reported increased inmate-staff tension following the implementation of the ban (Hammond and Emmons 2005). However, these findings may be attributable to under-enforcement of the bans that have gone into effect. Patrick and Marsh report that tobacco use inside prisons often does not cease even years after universal bans are enacted (Patrick and Marsh 2001). These factors tend to mitigate the effectiveness of bans in correctional facilities. However, in the committee's view, the positive health effects of protecting staff, nonsmoking inmates, and visitors from ETS justify an indoor ban as well as the costs of meaningful enforcement.

Recommendation 6: The American Correctional Association should require through its accreditation standards that all correctional facilities (prisons, jails, and juvenile detention facilities) implement bans on indoor smoking.

Multi-Unit Residential Locations

Residents of apartment buildings are exposed to ETS entering the air from common areas and neighboring units, and these exposures have led to a steady stream of litigation, especially on behalf of children and medically vulnerable adults, aiming to force landlords to adopt smoking restrictions. The housing market is slowly beginning to respond to a growing grassroots support for smoke-free multiunit housing, particularly in California. Recent polling data reveal that 82 percent of those living in apartments in California support smoking restrictions in their buildings and 69 percent favor separate nonsmoking sections (Wilcox 2005). Several California-based organizations that promote smoke-free housing have been created. Most notable among these is an organization whose website, *www.smoke freeapartments.org*, features more than 130 apartment owners with more than 1,400 nonsmoking units, according to the most recent estimates. In addition, in 2006 the California Apartment Association, in response to member demand, began offering information on how to create smoke-free areas. However, support for apartment smoking restrictions is not limited to California. A 2003 analysis of apartment renters in Minneapolis, Minnesota, concluded that 79 percent of nonsmokers preferred that their buildings be smoke-free (Hennrikus et al. 2003). In addition, a 2003 survey of Washington State tenants found that 67 percent were interested or very interested in smoke-free housing (Tacoma-Pierce County Health Department 2003).

Despite the growing support for smoke-free housing and the fact that there is no legal impediment to legislating such a ban, virtually no legislative action has addressed smoking in multiunit residential buildings (outside common areas). No state statutes have regulated smoking in any type of private residences. For instance, in 2004, the city of Thousand Oaks, California, took an unprecedented step by adopting a resolution that one-third of the units available in every new publicly-funded apartment building in the city be designated as nonsmoking; it was the first municipality in the country to take such a step (Smokefree Apartment House Registry 2004). Similarly, in August 2005, the housing authority in Cadillac, Michigan, voted to ban smoking in an apartment complex for seniors, making it 1 of less than 10 public housing authorities nationwide that have instituted such bans (Older Americans Report 2005). Self-imposed restrictions by landlords and developers also appear to be rare.

Some occupants of multiunit residences have initiated litigation to require landlords to provide smoke-free housing. Victims of ETS exposure may pursue legal action against fellow tenants or landlords via common-law remedies, claims of safety and health code violations, or the federal Fair Housing Act. Common-law lawsuits have been the most common, although most are settled out of court, and very few cases have reached the appellate level (Schoenmarklin and Tobacco Control Legal Consortium 2004). Plaintiffs have occasionally been successful in raising common-law property or tort claims, although such cases are rare. Some of the more successful theories include breach of warranty of habitability, breach of the covenant of quiet enjoyment, or nuisance.

Legal experts have generally been skeptical regarding the prospects of victory in such lawsuits because a plaintiff must prove that living conditions have been made unbearable as a result of secondhand smoke (Osterwalder and Beeman 2005). There are indications that legal precedent may be changing, however, as a couple was recently evicted from their condominium in Boston, Massachusetts, after neighbors complained about excessive cigarette smoke. This was the first case of its kind in the United States, and some believe that this case may have a nationwide impact (Blumberg 2005).

Rather than direct regulation, the most sensible policy is to stimulate competition for smoke-free lease terms among condominium developers and owners of multiunit dwellings while encouraging landlords to make entire buildings smoke-free, perhaps with financial incentives.

> **Recommendation 7: States should enact legislation requiring leases for multiunit apartment buildings and condominium sales agreements to include the terms governing smoking in common areas and residential units. States and localities should also encourage the owners of multiunit apartment buildings and condominium developers to include nonsmoking clauses in these leases and sales agreements and to enforce them.**

To encourage the development and enforcement of nonsmoking clauses in leases and sales agreements, states and localities should modify any law that is perceived by landlords and developers to preclude nonsmoking clauses or to inhibit their enforcement.

College Campuses

The recent increase in smoking among 18–24 year olds highlights the importance of implementing smoking policies on college campuses. In 2005, the American College Health Association (ACHA) encouraged colleges and universities to move toward tobacco-free campuses, while taking a step-by-step approach to their policies. The ACHA strongly urged colleges and universities to prohibit tobacco use in all public buildings on campus (including classrooms, libraries, museums, stadiums, dormitories, building entrances, and dining facilities) and within twenty feet of these buildings. In addition, the ACHA urged colleges and universities to prohibit tobacco advertising in campus-controlled venues, and to prohibit the sale of tobacco products or provision of free sampling of tobacco products on campus (ACHA 2005).

According to the American Nonsmokers' Rights Foundation (2007), about 43 colleges and universities have adopted a completely smoke-free campus, including all indoor and outdoor spaces throughout the groups of the college or university. In a study conducted by Halperin and Rigotti (2003) of public universities' tobacco control policies, it was found that approximately half of the universities surveyed banned smoking in all residence halls and dormitories. Half of the universities also had written policies prohibiting smoking within a certain distance of all campus building entrances. However, many colleges fall well below the recommended guidelines. Halperin and Rigotti (2003) found that only 68 percent of the universities reported that no tobacco products were sold on campus, and that of the universities that did sell tobacco products, more than two-thirds (69 percent) allowed students to use their meal cards or student accounts to purchase tobacco products. Only half of the schools surveyed had written policies in place that banned the advertisement of tobacco products on campus.

Such policies restricting or prohibiting smoking on college campuses or in residential areas have been effective. For example, a study by Wechsler and colleagues (2001) found that current smoking prevalence was significantly lower among residents of smoke-free college housing as compared with residents of unrestricted housing. Cigar use was also found to be lower among students living in smoke-free residences compared to those residing in unrestricted housing. Students living in smoke-free residences were also less likely to initiate smoking (if they had not smoked regularly before age 19) compared to those living in unrestricted dorms. Borders and colleagues (2005) found that preventive education programs on campus were associated with lower odds of smoking and that designated smoking areas were associated with higher odds of smoking.

Despite the potential effectiveness of these college smoking bans, these tobacco restrictions on college campuses have been met with ambivalence. As suggested by Loukas and colleagues (2006), college officials may need to address the issue of changing student attitudes about smoke-free campuses as policies are instated.

> **Recommendation 8: Colleges and universities should ban smoking in indoor locations, including dormitories, and should consider setting a smoke-free campus as a goal. Further, colleges and universities should ban the promotion of tobacco products on campus and at all campus-sponsored events. Such policies should be monitored and evaluated by oversight committees, such as those associated with the American College Health Association.**

Residences and Privately-Owned Vehicles

The proportion of Americans living in smoke-free homes is uncertain. In 1999, more than 60 percent of U.S. homes reported having a strict smoking ban (no smoking allowed at any time or in any place in the home) (Levy et al. 2004). The most pertinent question, however, is what proportion of smokers are not allowed to smoke in their own homes. In 2006, Borland and colleagues published the results of a two-wave cohort survey that examined the prevalence of smoke-free policies in the residences and vehicles of smokers. Only 27.9 percent of U.S. smokers from the second-wave cohort reported having total smoking ban in their homes, although 57.1 percent of smokers reported that they do not smoke in their cars when nonsmokers are present (Borland et al. 2006).

The aim of the U.S. Department of Health and Human Services (DHHS), as described in Healthy People 2010, is to reduce the percentage of children regularly exposed to tobacco smoke at home to 6 percent. According to baseline data used to establish this target (from the National Health Interview Survey), 20 percent of children 5 years of age and younger lived in a home in which someone smoked at least 4 days a week in 1998 (CDC 2005a, DHHS 2001, 2006). By 2004, this rate fell to 11 percent, according to the U.S. Environmental Protection Agency's 2004 National Survey on Environmental Management of Asthma and Children's Exposure to Environmental Tobacco Smoke (EPA 2006).

Meanwhile, according to an analysis of the 1999 National Youth Tobacco Survey, 13.4 percent of middle school students and 17.0 percent of high school students reported daily exposure to cigarette smoke while they were in a car (Farrelly et al. 2001). Exposure to ETS in vehicles is an important concern, as levels of secondhand smoke in vehicles can be particularly high, even exceeding levels in bars in which smoking is permitted. Vehicles thus represent an environment in which ETS exposure can be seriously detrimental to an individual's health, particularly to that of a child or infant (OTRU 2006).

Persuading parents to adopt smoke-free policies in their homes and cars provides an opportunity for furthering the multiple goals of tobacco control in a morally compelling context. Clean air rules in homes and cars protect children from highly injurious toxic exposures, facilitate smoking cessation by parents and other family members who smoke, and reduce the rate of smoking initiation by teenagers, especially when clean air laws are combined with parental monitoring and authoritative messages (even by parents who smoke).

Protecting Children from ETS

Not surprisingly, the most important source of ETS exposure to young children is parental smoking (DHHS 2006; Jordaan et al. 1999). National data indicate that although the percentage of U.S. children exposed to sec-ondhand smoke in the home declined substantially throughout the 1990s, about 25 percent of children between the ages of 3 and 11 years still live with at least one smoker (DHHS 2006; TIPS 2006b). Furthermore, young children of smoking mothers continue to be exposed to ETS at a higher level than any other group of nonsmokers (Behan et al. 2005).

Children who are regularly exposed to ETS are at greater risk for a va-riety of respiratory ailments, including asthma, bronchitis, and pneumonia (AAP 1986; DiFranza and Lew 1996; Etzel 1997; Gortmaker et al. 1982; Mannino et al. 1996). In addition, such children are also at risk of suffer-ing cognitive impairments. Yolton and colleagues, for instance, estimated that more than 21.9 million children are at risk of reading deficits due to exposure to secondhand smoke. They also found that exposure to smoke is associated with deficits in math and visuospatial reasoning (Yolton et al. 2005). Exposure to ETS has also been linked to serious conditions in infants, such as low birth weight and SIDS (ANR 2005; DHHS 2006). The children of smokers also miss more days of school because of illness than the children of nonsmokers (Mannino et al. 1996). Overall, annual health care costs as a direct result of children's passive exposure to tobacco smoke is in the range of $5 billion (Aligne and Stoddard 1997).

The demonstrable health risks of persistent smoke exposure in the home has led many courts to take parental smoking into account in cus-tody and visitation disputes (see Pierce v. Pierce, 860 N.E.2d 1087, Ohio Ct. App. 2006). These orders typically direct smoking parents to refrain from smoking in the home when children are present and sometimes up to 48 hours before they will be present (Banzhaf 2005). Some commentators have argued that, at least under some circumstances, smoking in the home can amount to child endangerment or medical neglect warranting assertion of family court jurisdiction as a basis for mandating changes in parental behavior (Chinnock 2003). Several jurisdictions at both the local and state levels, meanwhile, have enacted or approved legislation prohibiting smoking in vehicles in which a child is present (Belluck 2007; OTRU 2006).

Reducing Smoking

Not only do household bans benefit children by reducing the adverse health effects from secondhand smoke exposure, but they also lead to reduced smoking and increased cessation by adults as well. Farkas and colleagues have conducted two studies that demonstrate this effect. Smokers who lived under a total smoking ban were more likely to report a quit attempt in the previous year, and those who made quit attempts were less likely to relapse (Farkas et al. 2000). In fact, smoke-free homes are associated with lower rates of smoking prevalence than smoke-free workplaces (Bonta, Appendix B). Similarly, a survey of Oregonians found that a full household smoking ban resulted in a doubling of the odds of a subsequent quit attempt and that for those contemplating a quit attempt (i.e., those with an intention to quit within the next month), a full ban led to a lower relapse rate (Pizacani et al. 2004). Further evidence from a survey of high school students indicates that a more restrictive home smoking policy is associated with a greater likelihood of being in an earlier stage of smoking uptake and a lower 30-day smoking prevalence (Wakefield et al. 2000). The results of studies of households with smoking bans in Australia have been even more dramatic: the odds of quitting smoking were found to be 4.5 times greater in households with a smoking ban (Siahpush et al. 2003). This evidence suggests that the social context of smoking is an important factor for smokers and that eliminating smoking from the living environment increases the rate of smoking cessation.

Reducing Initiation

Household smoking bans also have the effect of reducing smoking among youth, as the effects of parents as role models appear to be a major factor in determining children's future smoking behavior. Studies indicate that 12-year-old children of parents who smoke are roughly twice as likely to begin smoking between the ages of 13 and 21 years as those whose parents do not smoke. Also, in addition to less smoking by parents, stricter family monitoring and rules regarding smoking were related to a lower risk of smoking initiation (Hill et al. 2005). Farkas and colleagues found that adolescents age 15 to 17 years were 74 percent less likely to be smokers if they lived in houses with smoking restrictions (Farkas et al. 2000). Other studies have verified that strong home smoking bans are associated with lower rates of smoking uptake, prevalence, and consumption among teenagers (Wakefield et al. 2000). A panel convened in June 2006 by NIH found in its review of the scientific literature on tobacco use that clean indoor air policies and laws regulating exposure to tobacco smoke have indeed proven effective in preventing tobacco use among adolescents and young adults (NIH 2006b). In addition, a new Canadian study has raised the possibility that not only do parents influence their children's future smoking behavior by setting an example, but parents may also physically "prime" their children to become smokers by exposing them to nicotine. The study found that the presence of cotinine in the saliva at a young age was a significant predictor of future smoking addiction (Ubelacker 2005).

> **Recommendation 9: State health agencies, health care professionals, and other interested organizations should undertake strong efforts to encourage parents to make their homes and vehicles smoke free.**

The committee believes that a voluntary approach to reducing parental smoking in homes and vehicles is preferable to a legal prohibition. However, the committee does support otherwise appropriate legal interventions in custody or abuse cases involving parents whose smoking endangers the health of their children.

Outdoor Spaces

Smoking in outdoor spaces is the last frontier in the progressive restriction of smoking and can be expected to be controversial. Bayer and Colgrove (2002) and Chapman (2000) doubt that these restrictions can be defended on the basis of ETS exposure by nonsmokers and therefore contend that banning outdoor smoking is unambiguously paternalistic. Moreover, such bans would be difficult to enforce with an equal hand, and their enforcement would likely create a public backlash against smoke-free policies in general (Chapman 2000). Proponents of outdoor smoking restrictions, on the other hand, argue that such measures are scientifically justifiable because the nature of the atmospheric dispersion of ETS will cause nonsmokers to be exposed to equally high or higher levels of ETS in outdoor environments than they are in indoor environments (Repace 2000). Others point out that banning outdoor smoking has additional benefits, aside from reducing exposure to ETS, including reducing the fire risk, decreasing litter, and protecting the public from nuisance (Bloch and Shopland 2000). Concerns about the offensiveness of smoking are especially pronounced in crowded locations (e.g., on crowded beaches or in parks). Furthermore, the declarative effects of enacting and enforcing these restrictions are substantial because they send a powerful message about the social disapproval of smoking, a message that will not be lost on children and adolescents.

Despite the controversial nature of restrictions in outdoor places, there is a growing movement to institute such bans in California, which has been on the forefront of many innovations in tobacco control. Survey data indicate that a majority of Californians support a ban on smoking in outdoor public places such as parks, beaches, golf courses, and sports stadiums (Gilpin et al. 2004). In November 2003, Solana Beach, California became the first municipality in the county to ban smoking on beaches, and a number of other cities in California have since followed suit. Effective January 1, 2004, the California legislature enacted a ban on smoking within 20 feet of all entrances to government buildings and state university and community college buildings. In addition, on January 25, 2005, San Francisco adopted the most expansive "curb-to-curb" outdoor smoking ban in the state, prohibiting smoking in city parks, plazas, piers, gardens, and recreational fields (Bonta, Appendix B).

Given the competing values at stake, the committee believes that this is an issue that should be resolved at the community level.

Recommendation 10: States should not preempt local governments from restricting smoking in outdoor public spaces, such as parks and beaches.

YOUTH ACCESS

In 1992, Congress enacted the Synar Amendment, aimed at addressing the continuing illegal sales of tobacco to minors. The legislation required that all states enact and enforce youth tobacco access laws and prescribed loss of federal block grant substance abuse and treatment funding as a sanction for noncomplying states. Under regulations subsequently adopted by the DHSS, the states were required to reduce the rate of retailer violations of youth-access laws to 20 percent or less by 2003. In a complementary effort, the Food and Drug Administration (FDA) adopted a comprehensive set of youth-access regulations in 1996 that included a major compliance check program under the auspices of the FDA. As noted above, however, the U.S. Supreme Court invalidated the FDA program in 2000 on the grounds that tobacco regulation was outside the scope of the agency's authority.

Although every state has baseline legislation prohibiting tobacco sales to minors (usually the restriction of tobacco sales to those younger than age 18 years), both the Synar Amendment and the failed FDA effort reflected the fact that in the 1990s, states and localities were not enforcing youth-access provisions with any vigor. In 1996, once the rules promulgated by the Synar Amendment came into effect, the logical inquiry was whether the legislation would exert an independent positive influence on state and local enforcement practices. In an analysis of 1997 substance abuse block grant applications from all states, DiFranza concluded that "states and DHHS are violating the statutory requirements of the Synar Amendment rendering it ineffective" (DiFranza 1999). However, in a recent review of the experience resulting from implementation of the Synar Amendment, DiFranza and Dussault (2005) gave a more positive assessment, concluding that the Synar Amendment led to universal adoption of youth-access restrictions, that DHHS pressured some states to embrace compliance testing in lieu of retailer education alone, and that most states made considerable progress in achieving the goal of reducing retailer violation rates in random inspections to 20 percent. They reiterated, however, that some states did not implement the law aggressively and that the federal government failed to put enough pressure on these states to improve their performance (DiFranza and Dussault 2005).

Even though youth-access restrictions are taken more seriously now than they were a decade ago, there is still little evidence that increased retailer compliance has had a meaningful impact on the availability of tobacco to minors or that retailer compliance has had any independent effect in reducing the rates of youth smoking initiation or levels of cigarette consumption. In the late 1990s, a number of studies of communities that engaged in proactive enforcement were conducted. Those studies were aimed at assessing the efficacy of these efforts. Rigotti concluded that "[t]hese studies have yet to provide conclusive evidence that interventions using retailer education or law enforcement alone can change the ease with which young people obtain tobacco products" (Rigotti 2001). The June 2006 NIH state-of-the-science panel on tobacco use, however, listed youth-access restrictions as one of several effective interventions for preventing tobacco use among adolescents and young adults (NIH 2006b).

Although the available evidence does not point toward an optimal level of enforcement for youth-access restrictions, it does seem clear that a visible effort to enforce supply-side access restrictions is warranted, not necessarily because it has substantial independent value but, rather, because it is a complementary component of a comprehensive package of control initiatives. Among other reasons, meaningful enforcement is needed to demonstrate that the public commitment to reducing tobacco use in the critical early years of smoking initiation is not half-hearted (Bonnie 2001). As a previous Institute of Medicine report observed in 1994:

> In the long run, the real public health benefit of a reinvigorated youth-access policy lies not in its direct effect on consumer choices but rather in its declarative effects—that is, in its capacity to symbolize and reinforce an emerging social norm that disapproves of tobacco use. Legal restrictions often have important educative effects and thereby help to shape attitudes and beliefs. They do this best when they are congruent with an emergent social norm accompanied by a strong social consensus, precisely the conditions that now exist in the context of tobacco control. . . . Con-

versely, overt failure to implement the youth-access restrictions actually undermines the tobacco-free norm; an unenforced restriction is probably worse than no restriction at all. Unenforced laws convey the message that the intent is not to be taken seriously and thereby undermine school and community attempts to educate youth regarding the serious health consequences of tobacco use. . . . The message should be strong and unequivocal that tobacco use is unhealthful and socially disapproved. Youth-access laws are an essential part of that message (IOM 1994a).

A reasonably enforced youth-access restriction is an essential element of modern tobacco control efforts, and there is, in fact, widespread agreement among tobacco control activists and public health experts regarding the provisions that should be incorporated in a model law (IOM 1994b). The principal guideposts featured in such a program are as follows:

- Establish a minimum legal smoking age of at least 18 years
- Require that retailers establish proof of age by checking identification
- License tobacco retailers
- Require periodic assessments of retailers' compliance
- Establish administrative or civil law penalties for illegal sales
- Prohibit self-service displays of tobacco products

One important question is whether the regulation of youth access should be left exclusively to state control, which has been the traditional approach with the exception of the brief period when the FDA's Tobacco Rule was in force. In the committee's opinion, the main advantage of federal action in this area is that it provides an opportunity to establish a uniform licensing mechanism for the retail sale of tobacco products. The committee therefore endorses revival of the FDA's Tobacco Rule, which prescribes minimum requirements for retailers to prevent sales to minors and allows the states to implement more stringent requirements (see Chapter 6).

Whether or not the FDA's Tobacco Rule is revived, the states should take the following steps to reduce tobacco sales to minors:

Recommendation 11: All states should license retail sales outlets that sell tobacco products. Licensees should be required to (1) verify the date of birth, by means of photographic identification, of any purchaser appearing to be 25 years of age or younger; (2) place cigarettes exclusively behind the counter and sell cigarettes only in a direct face-to-face exchange; and (3) ban the use of self-service displays and vending machines. Repeat violations of laws restricting youth access should be subject to license suspension or revocation. States should not preempt local governments from licensing retail outlets that sell tobacco products.

A considerable number of states and localities currently license tobacco sales outlets. The weak enforcement of youth-access laws in many states, however, suggests that the potential deterrent threat of license suspension or revocation is not being realized. States should adopt a graduated penalty scheme whereby initial offenses are tied to fines but repeat violators face license suspension and revocation. Wherever possible, enforcement authority should reside in a public health agency.

The age verification requirement of the above recommendation follows the mandate contained in the FDA's 1996 Tobacco Rule and should be regarded as a baseline for effective monitoring of compliance. As recommended by the IOM committee in 1994 the FDA's 1996 Tobacco Rule set the federal minimum age requirement for the purchase of tobacco products at 18 years, but left the states free to adopt more stringent regulations, including adopting a minimum age of purchase higher than 18 years. The committee favors that approach, which would be effectuated by the proposed Family Smoking Prevention and Tobacco Control Act (discussed in Chapter 6). Although raising the minimum purchase age on a national basis would stretch the law too far from social reality, states should be permitted to experiment with a 21-year-old minimum age requirement for the purchase of tobacco products.

The remainder of the recommendation fills two gaps in the MSA. The MSA failed to adopt the behind-the-counter mandate prescribed by the FDA's 1996 Tobacco Rule. Placing product displays behind the counter not only prevents shoplifting, largely by youths, but also tends to reduce the likelihood of spontaneous impulse purchases. Similarly, the MSA failed to address the problem of youth access to vending machines, leaving it to the states to enact restrictions. This self-service mode of access to tobacco is an open invitation to violation of the proscriptions on underage sales. In view of the unlikely prospect of adult-only venues being closely policed for potential violations, the committee's strong recommendation would be for an outright ban on vending machine sales of cigarettes. The FDA's 1996 Tobacco Rule endorsed limiting such machines to adult-only facilities, and the 1994 IOM report Growing Up Tobacco Free similarly endorsed a ban and cautiously qualified an absolute prohibition by stating that "less restrictive alternatives to a complete ban should be adopted only if shown to be effective" (IOM 1994a).

The committee reaffirms all of the specific recommendations pertaining to youth access recommended by the IOM in 1994, including requiring sales units to contain at least 20 cigarettes (thereby banning so-called kiddie packs or "loosies") and making it an offense for an adult to purchase tobacco products for a minor.

RETAIL SHIPMENTS

The number of Internet tobacco retailers has increased dramatically in recent years (Ribisl, Appendix M) (Parmet and Banthin 2005), generating concerns about minors accessing tobacco products and consumers evading excise tax payments. Those concerns appear to be well founded, as research findings and anecdotal data suggest that both access by minors and avoidance of excise taxes have contributed to the popularity of Internet tobacco vendors. For example, following New York City's increase to $1.50 in excise tax per pack of cigarettes in 2002, there was an 89 percent increase in cigarettes purchased outside of the city, 18.1 percent of which were purchased over the Internet (Ribisl, Appendix M). Evasion of state excise taxes for Internet tobacco purchases is a pervasive problem. While studies suggest that few minors are now obtaining cigarettes online, researchers believe that as states adopt more restrictive approaches to retail tobacco sales, more youth may seek to purchase cigarettes from Internet retailers (Ribisl, Appendix M).

Regulation of Internet tobacco sales has presented numerous challenges for state officials, particularly because a large number of online tobacco vendors are located either outside of the United States or on Native American tribal lands (Ribisl, Appendix M). Although the federal Jenkins Act requires Native American retailers to report Internet tobacco sales to the applicable state tax administrator to facilitate collection of excise taxes from consumers (Jenkins Act, 2005), investigation and enforcement of Jenkins Act violations have been virtually nonexistent to date (GAO 2002). However, the prospects for state enforcement have recently increased by judicial decisions recognizing states' implied rights of action against online vendors under the Jenkins Act (Banthin 2004; Campaign for Tobacco-Free Kids 2003). In July 2005, a federal judge ordered a tribal Internet seller to provide Washington State officials with its list of customers within the state to facilitate the collection of excise taxes from those residents (Washington State Department of Revenue 2005).

The nature of Internet sales—conducted anonymously and in the privacy of the consumer's home—has also frustrated state efforts to police online sales, as officials have no practical way of ensuring that Internet vendors accurately verify the purchasers' ages. In fact, recent studies have revealed that most Internet tobacco vendors fail to verify their customer's age, and those that purport to do so have largely been ineffective in obtaining age verification. One study found that only 6.3 percent of Internet vendors requested that buyers submit a copy of their photo identification before a sale, and the companies that do require age verification often fulfill the orders submitted without the requested identification (Ribisl, Appendix M). Many online vendors merely require consumers to type in a valid birth date or click on a box indicating that they are 18 years or older (Ribisl,

Appendix M). Alternatively, the website may state that by submitting an order, the customer is certifying that he or she is of legal age to purchase tobacco products (Ribisl, Appendix M). Upon surveying commonly used age verification protocols, researchers have concluded that existing approaches do little to deter minors from purchasing tobacco products online (Ribisl, Appendix M) (Parmet and Banthin 2005).

Given the inadequacy of current point-of-sale age verification for Internet transactions, many states have enacted legislation to prescribe verification requirements. In 2000, Rhode Island became the first state to impose an age-verification requirement on vendors seeking to ship tobacco products into the state (Rhode Island Public Laws. Chapter 321, Section 1. Providence, RI, 1996; Rhode Island Public Laws. Chapter 210, Section 1. Providence, RI, 2000; Parmet and Banthin 2005). Before shipping any tobacco product, retailers must obtain a copy of the customer's government-issued identification, as well as a written attestation from the consumer certifying the accuracy and authenticity of the identification. In addition, the retailer must deliver the product to the address listed on the identification and must use a delivery service that requires the signature of the addressee or another adult (General Laws of Rhode Island, Chapter 392, Section 1. Section 11-9-13.11. Providence, RI, 2005). Since the passage of the Rhode Island law, a number of states have enacted similar legislation, requiring age verification at both the point of sale and the point of delivery of tobacco products, whereas others have imposed additional obligations for Internet retailers. For example, California's youth-access law requires that retailers check back with consumers via a phone call to confirm the delivery of tobacco products and ensure that the consumer's credit card statement reflects that a tobacco purchase had been made (California Business & Professions Code. Section 22963. Sacramento, CA, 2004).

In 2003, Maine imposed age-verification requirements on both retailers and delivery personnel; the law required retailers to use only carriers that deliver packages only to the actual purchaser, require the purchaser to sign for the package, and require recipients to present a valid government-issued photo identification to the delivery person as a condition of and before delivery (Maine Revised Statutes Annotated. Title 22, Sections, 1551, 1555-A et seq. Augusta, ME, 2005). This law was met with resistance by state carrier companies (Kesich 2004), and in May 2005 a federal district court enjoined enforcement of the provisions of the statute applying to carriers, and the Court of Appeals for the First Circuit affirmed a year later (N.H. Motor Transportation Association v. Rowe, 448 F.3d 66 (1st Cir. 2006). The Court of Appeals held that the provision required carriers to determine whether to impose the delivery conditions listed in the statute, thereby delaying the delivery of packages containing tobacco, as well as other packages, and was preempted by a federal law regulating cargo carriers. Although the federal courts struck down the Maine statute's applicability to carriers, the provisions requiring retailers to request and verify the purchaser's age were unaffected. These restrictions are similar to those imposed by other states, suggesting that courts will continue to uphold state laws that regulate retailers' actions but that do not impose significant requirements on carriers.

To facilitate enforcement of existing legislation regulating online tobacco transactions, state officials have forged private agreements with credit card and delivery companies to restrict Internet sales and delivery of tobacco products. In March 2005, state attorneys general and the federal Bureau of Alcohol, Tobacco, Firearms, and Explosives announced an agreement with all major credit card companies under which the companies promise to prevent their cards from being used in transactions in which Internet vendors fail to comply with age verification requirements or to register their sales with state governments (US Fed News 2005). Although the response by online tobacco companies suggests that the agreement had an initial impact on retailers (Cooper 2005; Michel 2005; Tedeschi 2005), concerns remain that tobacco vendors will circumvent the deal by accepting payments from third-party payment processing companies that will serve as intermediaries between the credit card companies and the online retailers (National Journal Group 2005).

The difficulties of enforcing age verification and tax collection requirements have led some states to prohibit Internet sales and shipments of tobacco to consumers altogether. In 2000, New York State enacted Public Health Law 1399-ll, which prohibits direct shipment of cigarettes to state residents and bans carriers from transporting such shipments (2005). Brown and Williamson challenged the constitutionality of the law, but the Second Circuit Court held that any burden on interstate commerce was significantly outweighed by the statute's benefits, and therefore the law did not violate the Commerce Clause (Brown & Williamson Tobacco Corp. v. Pataki, 320 F.3d 200, 2d Cir. 2003). Of course, the problem of enforcement remains. In July 2005, the New York attorney general announced an agreement between the state and the DHL courier company in which the carrier agreed to stop shipping cigarettes directly to residents (Times Wire Services 2006).

State attorneys general have had considerable success in forging agreements with carriers to end the shipment of tobacco products purchased over the Internet. In November, 2005, UPS announced that it would stop delivering cigarettes bought online (UPS Reviews 2005). Federal Express maintains a policy of shipping only between licensed dealers or from a distributor to a dealer and will not ship directly to consumers (Times Wire Services 2006; Tuttle 2006). However, the U.S. Postal Service declined a request by the National Association of State Attorneys General to cease shipping cigarettes directly to consumers (Kempner 2005), on the grounds that it was not able to inspect mail without a search warrant and that it would be impractical for postal clerks to decide which packages to accept or reject (Cooper 2005). In June 2005, after these failed negotiations with the U.S. Postal Service, Rep. John McHugh of New York introduced legislation that would forbid carriers from transporting cigarettes and other tobacco products and would impose a $100,000 fine for each violation (Ovarian Cancer Research and Information Amendments of 1993. H.R. 2810, 103rd Congress, 1993).

In the committee's view, given the difficulty of policing Internet tobacco transactions and constitutional barriers to additional, state-imposed delivery requirements, the only practical way to effectively regulate online tobacco retailers is through legislation prohibiting both online tobacco sales and shipment of tobacco products directly to consumers. This approach is supported not only by the states' interests in reducing sales to youth and facilitating excise tax collections, but also by the states' more general interest in reducing the convenience of tobacco purchases and thereby reducing consumption (see discussion of the goal of transforming the retail tobacco market in Chapter 6). Statutes restricting direct shipment of alcoholic beverages provide a precedent for such legislation, as most states either explicitly prohibit direct shipment of alcoholic beverages to consumers or do so practically by requiring that all transactions for alcoholic beverages take place within the state's licensed distribution system (see Kinney, Appendix I). Under a similar legislative scheme, shipment of tobacco products would be restricted to licensed wholesale or retail outlets, and consumers would be permitted to purchase these products only in face-to-face transactions in licensed retail settings.

> Recommendation 12: All states should ban the sale and shipment of tobacco products directly to consumers through mail order or the Internet or other electronic systems. Shipments of tobacco products should be permitted only to licensed wholesale or retail outlets.

PREVENTION INTERVENTIONS

The most fully developed programs for preventing tobacco use by youth have been implemented in school settings. School-based programs will remain the mainstay of group-oriented or individually-oriented prevention activities. The committee also believes, however, that investing in programs for families and health care providers is warranted, even though the evidence base remains thin. Support for these efforts should be augmented as the evidence base develops.

School-Based Interventions

Reviews and meta-analyses of school-based prevention have produced mixed results. On the one hand, meta-analyses have established that school-based prevention programs that are interactive, that teach about social influences, and that provide opportunities to learn and practice social skills have an average effect size of 0.24, which represents a 12 percent reduction in the rate of initiation of smoking among adolescents. On the other hand, some programs purporting to be of the same nature, such as Drug Abuse Resistance Education (see the meta-analysis by Ennett et al. [1994]) and the Hutchinson project (Peterson et al. 2000) have produced no significant effects.

The NIH's June 2006 state-of-the-science panel noted that previous research showed the short-term effectiveness of school-based interventions in preventing tobacco use among adolescents (NIH 2006b). Wiehe and colleagues (2005) conducted a meta-analysis of eight studies with individuals in 12th grade or age 18 years or older at follow-up and reported that only one program, Life Skills Training (Botvin and Eng 1982) produced significant long-term effects (Wiehe et al. 2005). Skara and Sussman (2003), meanwhile, found 25 studies with long-term follow-up, 15 of which reported effects 2 or more years after the intervention, with an average relative reduction of 11.4 percent (Skara and Sussman 2003). That review also indicated that program effects were less likely to decline if programs included extended programming or booster sessions in high school.

Findings from Prevention Programs That Are School-Based Only

The reviews cited above suggest that only those programs that included 15 or more interactive sessions in middle school, that taught about social influences, and that provided opportunities to learn and practice social skills are effective in the long term. In a review prepared for this report, Flay (Appendix D) found descriptions of three such school-based programs (the Tobacco and Alcohol Prevention Project [TAPP], Life Skills Training, and Project SHOUT [Students Helping Others Understand Tobacco]) that produced an average short-term (grade 8 or 9) relative reduction in smoking onset of 22 percent that increased to 28 percent at long-term follow-up (grades 10 to 12).

TAPP (Hansen et al. 1988) was a 15-session social-influences–oriented program developed in the early 1980s. The core components of the social influences approach have been employed in many evaluated programs and Hansen (1988) provides a good description of the theory and content of this approach. It has two main core elements: (1) resistance skills training to teach skills to resist the specific and general social pressures to smoke, and

(2) normative education to correct student misperceptions of prevalence and acceptability of use. Programs using this approach also often involve active learning or the use of the Socratic or dialectic teaching approaches, open discussion, the use of peers or older admired youth as instructors, and behavioral rehearsals to ensure that skills are learned well. TAPP included the above core elements plus inoculation against mass media messages, information about parental influences, information about the consequences of use, and the making of a public commitment not to smoke. Peer opinion leaders were used to assist teachers with program delivery.

TAPP was evaluated in two cohorts of seventh grade classes in a non-randomized study in Los Angeles County. Only cohort 1, conducted in two moderately-sized school districts, was followed into grade 10. Health education and social studies teachers received 2 days of training prior to delivering the program. By the end of eighth grade the relative reduction (RR) in past-month smoking was 26.2 percent. By the end of grade 10 there was a 19.1 percent RR in past-month smoking and 18.3 percent RR in ever smoking. In a secondary analysis of only those students present at all waves of the study, the RR in past-month smoking was 43 percent.

This was an early study of the social influences approach, and it demonstrated that the approach can be very effective. The use of peer leaders probably enhanced what program effects would have occurred with teacher-only delivery (Klepp et al. 1986, Tobler 1992). The whole-sample result is preferred as the initial estimate of program effects because it provides a more realistic assessment of what would happen under real-world conditions; however, note that the larger effect obtained for students present throughout the study could be obtained if all schools were to implement the program faithfully.

Life Skills Training (LST) is one of the most researched school-based smoking prevention or any other kind of substance use prevention program. Developed by Gil Botvin (Botvin and Eng 1982), LST consists of 30 classroom sessions with 15 delivered in grade 7, 10 in grade 8, and 5 in grade 9 (usually the first year of high school). The program was designed to teach students a wide array of personal and social skills. These include content similar to other smoking prevention programs that focus on social influences (Glynn 1989; Hansen 1988), including learning and practicing refusal and other assertion skills, information about the short- and long-term consequences of smoking, correction of misperceptions of the prevalence of use by same-age peers, and information about the decreasing acceptability of smoking in society. Other generic program content addresses the development of communication skills and ways to develop personal relationships.

Multiple studies over 25 years have demonstrated the effectiveness of the LST program when delivered by different providers, in different kinds of schools, and for different kinds of students (Botvin 2000; Botvin and Griffin

2002). Only one study has included medium-term follow-up through high school (Botvin et al. 1995). This was a follow-up of the largest single trial, conducted in 56 suburban and rural schools serving largely (91 percent) white students in three geographical regions of New York State (Botvin et al. 1990). Schools were assigned randomly to two experimental conditions (one day or video-taped teacher training) or a control condition. Level of implementation ranged from 27 to 97 percent by teacher reports, with about 75 percent of the students receiving 60 percent or more of the intervention. Six program schools and 18 percent of the students were excluded from the analysis of program effects because of poor implementation. At the end of grade 9 the RR was a relatively small 8.9 percent (1.63 percent versus 1.48 percent) for weekly smoking, reflecting the low prevalence of weekly smoking at this age. At the end of twelfth grade, the RRs were 19.7 percent (33 percent versus 26.5 percent) and 20.4 percent (27 percent versus 22 percent) for monthly and weekly smoking, respectively. For the high-implementation group, the medium-term RRs were both 28 percent. However, the RRs for the (almost) complete sample provide the most appropriate estimate of what effects could be obtained under real-world conditions—indeed, they may still be an overestimate of the effects that might be obtained when the program developer is not involved—although larger effects might be obtained with full, high-quality, implementation.

Independent evaluations of LST have found similar or larger short-term effects. In a nonrandomized trial in Spain, where the program was delivered by teachers to grade 9 students, a 21 percent RR in average monthly smoking at the end of grade 10 reduced to 11 percent by the end of grade 12 (Fraguela et al. 2003). Independent evaluations of LST in Midwestern states found a short-term RR of 22 percent in a randomized trial in rural Iowa (Spoth et al. 2002; Trudeau et al. 2003) and short-term RRs of 43 percent in current smoking and 9 percent in ever-use in Indianapolis (Zollinger et al. 2003). Another small-scale (three schools per condition) randomized evaluation in Pennsylvania found small immediate effects for girls only, and these had decayed by the end of grade 7 and were no longer apparent by the end of grades 8–10 (Smith et al. 2004). In a nonrandomized trial of a German adaptation of the life skills approach in 106 German-speaking elementary schools in Austria, Denmark, Luxembourg, and Germany, a 10 percent RR in ever smoking and less than 1 percent RR in past-month smoking were reported (Hanewinkel and Asshauer 2004).

Project SHOUT (Eckhardt et al. 1997; Elder et al. 1993) used trained college undergraduates to teach 18 sessions to 7th and 8th graders that included information on the health consequences of smoking, celebrity endorsements on nonuse, the antecedents and social consequences of tobacco use, decision making, resistance skills advocacy (writing letters to tobacco companies, magazines, and film producers; participating in community action projects designed to mobilize them as antitobacco activists), a public commitment to not use tobacco, and positive approaches to encouraging others to avoid tobacco or quit. A unique aspect of this program was the use of newsletters and individualized phone calls in later grades. In 9th grade, five newsletters were mailed to students and two to their parents, and each student received four phone calls from trained undergraduate counselors that were individually tailored to their tobacco use status at the end of 8th grade or the prior phone call. During 11th grade approximately half of the students received two more newsletters that focused on tobacco company tactics to recruit new smokers; information on recent city, state, or national legislation regarding tobacco; cessation advice; and information on secondhand smoke. They also received one phone call that focused on eliminating smoking in restaurants and other public places, and the rights of customers and employees in those places affected by the potential ban.

The program was evaluated in 22 schools with ethnically diverse populations in the San Diego area, some suburban and some rural. Schools were assigned randomly to program and control conditions after matching on pretest levels of tobacco use. Effects observed at the end of grade 8 (14.6 percent versus 10.8 percent, RR = 22 percent) were not statistically significant. However, by the end of grade 9 the intervention produced a relative reduction in tobacco use in the past month of 30.3 percent (19.8 percent versus 13.2 percent). By the eleventh grade, the average RR was 44.1 percent (12.6 percent versus 7 percent). For the group that did not receive the grade 11 intervention, the RR decayed to only 9.5 percent. The pattern of effects observed for this study suggests that much of the medium-term effect was due to personal attention via newsletters and phone calls in grades 9 and 11. Indeed, one has to wonder if the personal attention set up a response bias among respondents, such as those who received personalized newsletters and phone calls were motivated to tell the researchers what they wanted to hear; however, lack of a differential response rate to the surveys by condition speaks against this, at least in part. Considerable research suggests that the power of similar-age peers and the power of college-age counselors for high school students should not be underestimated. Although the cost of the intervention as studied was kept down by the use of volunteer students, it is not clear how easily this model can be disseminated. The results also strongly suggest, however, that even a brief intervention during high school was enough to actually increase the effect observed at the end of grade 9.

Results from three social influence and social competence programs with 15 or more sessions over 2–4 years, preferably with some content in high school, had significant medium-term effects (i.e., at grades 10–12): an average of a 27.6 percent (range 18.7–44.1) relative reduction in smoking. The extraordinary effects of Project SHOUT may have been due to the added content on tobacco industry activities, the teaching and encouragement of advocacy skills, and the personal attention. These results need to be replicated. The medium-term effects suggest that a minimal personal contact intervention of this kind in high school could increase the effects of any other program delivered in middle school.

Findings for School Plus Community/Media Programs

The reviews cited above (plus that of Flay [2000]) also suggest that the addition of mass media or community-based components to such programs can increase their effectiveness. Flay (Flay, Appendix D) found four such programs (North Karelia, Minnesota Class of 1989, the Midwestern Prevention Project, and the Vermont mass media and school project) and they produced a 40 percent relative reduction in smoking onset in the short term that fell to 31 percent at long-term follow-ups. The maintenance of such programs might keep their effectiveness levels as high as 40 percent.

Vartiainen and colleagues (1983, 1986, 1990, 1998) tested a 10-session social influences program delivered by trained health education teachers and peer leaders in the province of North Karelia, Finland. A community-wide heart disease prevention program and mass media campaign modeled on the Stanford three-cities project (Farquhar et al. 1977) was going on throughout North Karelia at the same time. Two schools received the 10-session program from the project health educator and trained peer leaders and two schools received a 5-session version from regular teachers. Two schools from another province, where there was no prevention program, were used as controls. At the end of grade 9 the RR (average of lifetime, monthly, and weekly) was 44.6 percent (for both program conditions), which decayed to 38.7 percent by grade 11. By 3 years beyond the end of high school, the RR had decayed to 22.9 percent in the health educator condition and 37.3 percent in the teacher condition; by 10 years beyond high school, the average RR was 20 percent with the two conditions not significantly different. These results can only be interpreted as the joint effects of the school-based smoking prevention program and the community-wide heart disease prevention campaign (which had a reduction of smoking as one of its targets). Thus these results suggest effects that are larger than those of the school-based programs reviewed above. The larger effects obtained by regular teachers suggests that programs might be more effective when delivered by regular classroom teachers than when delivered by visitors to classrooms, possibly because of the ongoing relationships that teachers establish with students. However, the long-term effects were no different.

The Minnesota Class of 1989 project was another in which a school-based prevention curriculum was tested in the context of a community-wide heart disease prevention program (Perry et al. 1989). The community program consisted of community education—including mass media—and organization activities—including screening, cessation clinics, and workplace education—designed to reduce three cardiovascular risk factors: smoking, cholesterol levels, and blood pressure (Luepker et al. 1994; Mittelmark et al. 1986). The school-based smoking prevention program (Perry et al. 1992, 1994) was based on the Minnesota Smoking Prevention Program (Arkin et al. 1981; Murray et al. 1994), one of the early social influences programs, and included material on diet and exercise as well as tobacco. Seven sessions on smoking prevention were delivered by peer leaders assisted by teachers in 7th grade. In 8th and 9th grades an additional 10 sessions concerning tobacco use were delivered by teachers. The classroom components were supplemented by the development of health councils through which students participated in other cardiovascular risk reduction projects.

The smoking prevention program was evaluated with a design in which students in all of the schools in one community received both the community-wide cardiovascular intervention and the school-based smoking prevention program, and students in all the schools in another community did not. All students in one cohort were surveyed every year from grade 6 to grade 12. As in all school-based studies, attrition occurred continuously over the 6 years, and by grade 12 only 45 percent of the original participants were surveyed. There were no differences in smoking rates at sixth grade. By the end of seventh grade, after the core smoking prevention content had been delivered, weekly smoking prevalence was about 40 percent lower in the program condition, and this effect was maintained through 12th grade, 3 years after the end of direct smoking prevention instruction and a year after the end of general community education.

Like the North Karelia project, this study demonstrates that school-plus-community programming can have substantial effects that are maintained to a large extent through the end of high school.

The Midwestern Prevention Project (also known as Project STAR, Students Taught Awareness and Resistance) tested a school-plus-community (and mass media) version of the social influences approach in eight communities in the Kansas City metropolitan area. The school-based component consisted of 10 sessions delivered by classroom teachers to 6th or 7th grade students (depending on the year of transition to middle school) and 5 sessions delivered the following year (when a parent-involvement component was also implemented). Of these schools, 8 were assigned randomly to conditions, 24 other schools elected to deliver the program and 18 others elected to wait till after the project. Mass media programming was available to all communities every year. Other community-based programming started in the third year and likewise was available in all communities. At the 2-year follow-up, the RR was 37.5 percent (Pentz et al. 1989). By grades 9–10, it was 18 percent (Johnson et al. 1990). These results are difficult to interpret because all students were exposed to the mass media and community components. The mass media programming, in particular, would be expected to reduce the difference between groups because the control group would no longer be a real control, and it might have reduced students' rate of onset relative to if they had not been exposed to the community program. This might explain the relatively fast decay.

The Vermont Mass Media Project tested the effectiveness of a mass media social influences smoking prevention program when delivered in the context of a school based program. Worden and colleagues (1988) undertook a careful development process to develop television and radio spots that would discourage cigarette smoking by adolescents. They randomly assigned two communities to the program condition (mass media plus school) and two matched communities to a school-only condition. There was no true control group. In the program communities, they purchased the time for airing the spots (734 TV spots in year 1 decreasing to 348 by year 4, and 248 radio spots in year 1 increasing to 450 by year 4) and provided schools with the school-based program (four sessions in each of grades 5–8 and three sessions in each of grades 9 and 10—each student in the study cohort was exposed to 4 years of program during grades 5–8, 6–9, or 7–10) and teacher training to deliver them. Neither schools nor students were told about the media programming, and the mass media programming never mentioned the school program. Thus, as far as students were concerned, there was no linkage between the two programs.

The RRs in weekly smoking among the school plus mass media program group compared to the school-only program group were 36.6 percent (14.8 percent versus 9.1 percent) at the end of the program (grades 9–11) and 28.8 percent 2 years later at grades 10–12 (Flynn et al. 1992, 1994, 1995). Larger effects were observed for daily smoking—44 percent RR at the end of the program and 36 percent a year later. It is difficult to estimate what the effects of the school-only program might have been, and, therefore, the relative contributions of the school and mass media programming. Nevertheless, this study demonstrates that well-designed media programming can produce large effects above those of the school-only program, about 80 percent of which are maintained for at least 2 years.

Summary Regarding School-Based Prevention

Flay (Appendix D) suggested, in part on the basis of the results described above, and after making adjustments for levels of adoption and implementation, that the implementation of effective school-based programs in the nation's schools could reduce smoking onset by age 24 by 10 percent, and that effective school-based programs combined with coordinated complementary mass media or community programming could reduce the rate of smoking onset by age 24 by 20 percent.

> **Recommendation 13: School boards should require all middle schools and high schools to adopt evidence-based smoking prevention programs and implement them with fidelity. They should coordinate these in-school programs with public activities or mass media programming, or both. Such prevention programs should be conducted annually. State funding for these programs should be supplemented with funding from the U.S. Department of Education under the Safe and Drug-Free School Act or by an independent body administering funds collected from the tobacco industry through excise taxes, court orders, or litigation agreements.**

Parent- or Family-Based Interventions

Extensive research shows that youths reared in homes in which parents have authoritative parenting styles characterized by warmth and involvement, clear and firm boundaries, and active monitoring are less likely to engage in health risk behaviors, including tobacco use (Andersen et al. 2004; Chassin et al. 2005; Clark et al. 1999; Cohen et al. 1994; Kerr and Stattin 2000; O'Byrne et al. 2002; Simons-Morton et al. 2004; Stattin and Kerr 2000; Steinberg et al. 1994). Research also shows that youth are more likely to smoke if their parents or others in the household smoke. Despite compelling evidence showing associations between parent smoking and adolescent smoking (Chassin et al. 1996; Fagan et al. 2005; Flay et al. 1998; Jackson and Henriksen 1997; Simons-Morton et al. 2004; Tilson et al. 2004), few adolescent tobacco interventions include a parent or family component and little research has evaluated the effects of parent- or family-based interventions. Moreover, the available intervention studies have serious methodological limitations, including the fact that they have small sample sizes that typically include parents who are already motivated, they have little likelihood of being faithfully replicated, and they assess only short-term outcomes.

Some interventions have been successful at increasing parent-child communication about the risks associated with tobacco and the reasons not to smoke. Programs have also had some success at changing attitudes toward smoking among youth and knowledge about tobacco through parental influences and communication between parents and their children. Few interventions and evaluations have been aimed at increasing parental monitoring of health risk behaviors, and even fewer studies have examined whether changes in parental behaviors and increased parent-child communication about tobacco use results in changes in actual youth smoking behaviors.

Those few studies that have been conducted, however, have shown mixed results, with most showing no positive effect of these activities on smoking initiation or cessation rates.

Part of the explanation for the relative lack of parental interventions is that research has not focused on identifying the causal mechanisms and processes by which parents influence their children's tobacco use to produce practical applications. It is plausible that parents can directly prevent their children from smoking by monitoring and restricting their activities, restricting their access to tobacco, and discouraging or disallowing their children from associating with peers who use tobacco. Alternatively, parents might have an indirect effect on adolescent tobacco use by spending time discussing tobacco-related risks with their children and suggesting alternative activities in which their children might engage (Halpern-Felsher, Appendix G).

In the absence of more substantial evidence, the committee is reluctant to include any definitive recommendation on parental and family interventions in this blueprint, aside from recommending that increasing the proportion of smoke-free homes be included as a marker of progress in tobacco control efforts. Instead, the committee emphasizes the need for more evaluation of parent interventions and their effects on youth smoking behaviors. The committee also recommends more research on how and why parental monitoring of their children's activities and other means of involvement in their children's lives might influence youth behavior. Such mechanistic information will allow determination of the most proximal influences on youth behavior that can be translated into parental interventions.

Health Care-Based Interventions

In addition to providing primary health care for children, adolescents, and families, the annual health visit provides a potentially pivotal opportunity for physicians to provide clinical preventive services that can reduce children's and adolescents' engagement in health risk behaviors, including tobacco use. As such, a number of national guidelines concerning physicians' provision of preventive services have been developed (e.g., Guidelines for Adolescent Preventive Services; Bright Futures; Guidelines for Health Supervision of Infants, Children, and Adolescents; Health Supervision Guidelines; The Clinician's Handbook of Preventive Services: Put Prevention into Practice; and Guide to Clinical Preventive Services).

In general, these guidelines recommend that all children and adolescents have an annual health care visit during which all patients receive confidential preventive services, including screening, education, and counseling in a number of areas such as the biomedical, emotional, and sociobehavioral aspects of their lives (e.g., alcohol and tobacco use, sexual behavior, violence, and safety). Furthermore, the guidelines recommend that pediatricians discuss substance use as part of routine health care during prenatal visits (Kulig 2005). The guidelines suggest that, in addition to inquiring about tobacco use in general, physicians should specifically query youth about the extent to which they use tobacco; about the settings in which they use tobacco; and whether their tobacco use has had a negative impact on their social, educational, or vocational activities (Kulig 2005). Furthermore, physicians should ask their patients about tobacco use in the home, including whether the child's parents, siblings, or other members of the household use tobacco (Kulig 2005). Health care providers need to encourage smoke-free homes and provide guidance and assistance to parents and youth on the various means of smoking cessation, including counseling and the use of nicotine replacement products and other pharmacological treatments.

Despite these guidelines, research shows that physicians' rates of patient screening, educating, and counseling on tobacco use during routine visits are less than optimal. Physicians cite a number of barriers to their provision of clinical preventive services such as (1) their large number of patients, resulting in constraints on the amount of time that they may spend with each patient; (2) inadequate reimbursement relative to the time and effort required to provide such services; (3) fear of alienating patients and their families; (4) insufficient education and training; (5) a lack of dissemination to physicians of research supporting positive tobacco treatment outcomes and the negative effects of the failure to intervene; and (6) a lack of information about how to access referral and treatment resources (Kulig 2005). Research also suggests that whether physicians do, in fact, screen their adolescent patients about their tobacco use may be related to their overall willingness to deliver preventive services (Ozer et al. 2004).

Recent research indicates that the rates of screening, educating, and counseling of youth about tobacco use during routine medical exams can be significantly increased through skills-based training of health care providers and the implementation of clinical administrative tools, such as reminders and charting forms. Little research has been conducted, however, on whether increased rates of screening, educating, and counseling by physicians result in reduced rates of tobacco initiation or greater rates of cessation (Halpern-Felsher, Appendix F).

In addition to primary health care visits, another time in which health care providers can be effective in screening for tobacco use and referring smoking cessation is during an emergency room (ER) visit. Smokers are disproportionately more likely to visit an ER compared with nonsmokers, accounting for 40 percent of adult patients attending ERs (Boudreaux et al. 2005; Lowenstein et al. 1995). Children and adolescents raised by caregivers who smoke are also more likely to visit an ER, especially for respiratory-related illnesses such as asthma or bronchitis. Beyond acute or emergency care needs, ERs are increasingly used by adults as their primary source of health care (Bernstein et al. 1997; Lowenstein et al. 1995). Therefore, the ER visit provides a timely and convenient opportunity, as well as the relevant patient population, for smoking screening and cessation efforts. Bernstein and Cannata (2006) showed that smokers who visit an ER have at least some interest in quitting, and that the motivation to quit is highest among patients who believe that their purpose for the ER visit is due to a smoking-related illness.

Citing these and other statistics on tobacco use among ER patients, guidelines (e.g., a joint task force comprised of individuals from the American College of Emergency Physicians, Council of Emergency Medicine Residency Directors, Emergency Medicine Residents Association, and Emergency Nurses Association; see Bernstein et al., in press) have been developed, and recommend that emergency room health care providers screen, council, and refer patients who smoke to cessation programs, with particular emphasis placed on referring patients to the national smokers' Quitline. Despite these recommendations, tobacco screening and referral among ER health care providers is low. While ER providers are more likely to inquire about tobacco use, they are much less likely to inquire about their patients' desire to quit or to advise or refer smoking cessation. For example, Vokes et al. (2006) showed that only 56 percent of ER patients were screened about their smoking status, with higher rates of screening for patients who had a tobacco-related illness. While 56 percent of patients who smoke were advised to quit, only 13 percent were provided with a smoking cessation referral.

Tobacco-related preventive services in the ER setting may be met with some resistance in part because ER providers do not believe that they are the correct source for initiating smoking cessation efforts. Instead, ER providers view primary health care providers as responsible for screening, counseling, and treatment concerning tobacco use (Bernstein and Cannata 2006). ER providers also feel reluctant to provide tobacco-related intervention because of perceptions that such brief interventions are not efficacious or that they have limited time for such provision of care (Bernstein et al. 2006). Nevertheless, Schroeder and other researchers argue that smoking prevention and cessation should take place for all smokers during all ER visits, and can be accomplished in a brief, 30-second intervention in which ER providers "ask, advise, and refer" their patients, with referral being to the national Quitline (Bernstein et al. 2006; Schroeder 2006; Vokes et al. 2006).

Tobacco-related screening and intervention efforts are not limited to the physician, nor do they need to be conducted solely through direct patient-provider communication. Triage or treatment nurses, social workers, health educators, and trained peer counselors can also deliver the messages. Tobacco screening, advice, and referral can be conducted through direct communication or through computerized self-assessments, kiosks in the waiting rooms, or brochures provided throughout the ER departments (see Bernstein et al., in press, for a review). These efforts can also be extended to pediatric emergency rooms, in which screening and cessation efforts can take place directly with youths who might be smoking as well as with their caregivers. Providing the clear message about the effects of second-hand smoke on children, especially when a child presents to the ER with respiratory illness, is likely to be a powerful deterrent.

Empirical data showing the efficacy of providing tobacco screening, counseling, and referral in the ER setting is limited and an inadequate number of studies have been conducted to inform the development of ER interventions. Nonetheless, evidence is accumulating suggesting that ER visits can indeed be a source of public health interventions (e.g., injury prevention), and that this public health message can be extended to tobacco cessation as well.

Notwithstanding the absence of evaluation research, the committee is persuaded by the uniform endorsement of clinical guidelines and by the general literature on physician interventions that the increased use of preventive interventions by physicians and other primary care providers during routine, acute, and ER visits for youth and adults is a worthwhile investment. For this reason, the committee believes that physicians, dentists, and other health care providers should screen and counsel their patients about their tobacco use, not only during annual health visits, but also in any other clinical context in which health screening is being undertaken, such as in emergency rooms.

> Recommendation 14: All physicians, dentists, and other health care providers should screen and educate youth about tobacco use during their annual health care visits and any other visit in which a health screening occurs. Physicians should refer youth who smoke to counseling services or smoking cessation programs available in the community. Physicians should also urge parents to keep a smoke-free home and vehicles, to discuss tobacco use with their children, to convey that they expect their children to not use tobacco, and to monitor their children's tobacco use. Professional societies, including the American Medical Association, the American Nursing Association, the American Academy of Family Physicians, the American College of Physicians, and the American Academy of Pediatrics, should encourage physicians to adopt these practices.

MEDIA CAMPAIGNS TO PREVENT SMOKING

Media campaigns have recently been used as an important measure to reduce initiation of tobacco use. Before we review them and the evidence of effectiveness, we comment on the Fairness Doctrine campaign, one of the first and one of the most effective tobacco control interventions, which focused on adult smokers.

The Fairness Doctrine Campaign

In the early decades of television broadcasting, media outlets allotted little airtime to educating the public about the health risks of tobacco use, whereas cigarette advertisements appeared on the airwaves with great regularity (Warner 1985). In 1967, however, the Federal Communications Commission (FCC) issued a ruling that required stations airing cigarette commercials to also provide airtime for antismoking messages. The FCC based its decision on the so-called Fairness Doctrine, which required broadcasters to offer balanced coverage of controversial issues of public importance (Cummings and Clarke 1998a; Farrelly et al. 2003).

The FCC's ruling resulted in the implementation of television's first major antismoking campaign. Between 1967 and 1970, public service announcements (PSAs) on the health consequences of tobacco use appeared on television, often during prime time viewing hours, which was a rarity for non-revenue–producing spots (Cummings and Clarke 1998a). Advocates of antismoking media campaigns have pointed to the leveling off of cigarette sales during that time period and to television viewers' increased knowledge of the health risks of tobacco use as evidence of the PSAs' effectiveness (Cummings and Clarke 1998b; Farrelly et al. 2003; Warner 1979, 1985). According to Warner, between 1967 and 1970 (when the antismoking messages mandated by the Fairness Doctrine appeared on the airwaves), per-capita cigarette consumption decreased with each successive year. This represents the first 4-year decline in per-capita cigarette consumption in the 20th century (Warner 1979, 1985). In comparing the actual annual per-capita cigarette consumption to predictions of what the level of consumption would have been if the antismoking initiatives of the 1960s and early 1970s had not taken place, Warner found that the antismoking PSAs that aired from 1968 to 1970 were associated with a significant decline in the level of cigarette consumption. He concluded that had the FCC not mandated antismoking messages, the predicted level of consumption would have been 19.5 percent greater than the actual level of consumption (Warner 1977).

By January 1971, however, federal laws banning the advertisement of cigarettes on television and radio had come into effect, and the FCC could no longer require media outlets to donate airtime for antismoking PSAs under the Fairness Doctrine. Consequently, the number of PSAs addressing tobacco use declined drastically over the next two decades (Cummings and Clarke 1998b; Dorfman and Wallack 1993). In the end, no other large-scale national antismoking media campaign would occur for almost 30 years (Farrelly et al. 2005).

State Campaigns

During the 1990s, the antismoking media campaign emerged as a key component of many states' tobacco control efforts. California, Florida, and Massachusetts organized some of the earliest and most prominent statewide media campaigns (Pechmann and Reibling 2000), with a number of other states following suit in the latter part of the decade. Noting the importance of these state-funded antismoking media campaigns in preventing tobacco use, in 2005 the CDC reported the estimated monthly exposure of adolescents to anti-tobacco advertisements in 37 states and the District of Columbia between 1999 and 2003. The CDC study found that exposure to the media campaigns among adolescents increased considerably between 1999 and 2002, but then dropped in 2003 when states across the country, facing serious budget crises, scaled back or eliminated their antismoking media campaigns. Noting that the lack of substantial change in youth smoking prevalence between 2002 and 2004 might have been attributable to reduced exposure to antismoking media campaigns, the CDC called on states to better ensure that adolescents are exposed to state-funded antitobacco advertisements. In its review, the CDC study highlighted the discouraging declines in expenditures in Florida and Massachusetts, and to a lesser extent California, given these three states' early dedication to funding antismoking media campaigns (CDC 2005f).

California

California launched its media campaign in April 1990 as one part of the newly established CTCP. Californians voted in November 1998 to increase the tax on cigarette sales by 25 cents per pack, and approximately 20 percent of the revenue earned from that tax was allotted to the Health Education Account to fund the media campaign and other educational initiatives (Stevens 1998). At the time of its inception, the campaign was the largest and most expensive statewide antismoking media campaign in the United States and featured paid advertisements in a wide variety of media, including television, radio, billboards, and newspapers (Popham et al. 1993, 1994a; Stevens 1998).

During the campaign's initial phase (April 1990 through June 1991),

CDHS spent more than $28.6 million and produced more than 50 television spots, 50 radio announcements, 20 outdoor advertisements, and 40 newspaper advertisements (Popham et al. 1994a). The campaign initially focused on achieving two main goals: (1) increasing general awareness of the dangers of secondhand smoke and (2) convincing the public that the tobacco industry had employed manipulative strategies in marketing its products (Stevens 1998). To achieve the second goal, CDHS developed advertisements holding the tobacco industry responsible for smoking-related deaths and disease. "Industry Spokesperson," one of the first ads aired in the campaign, portrayed a group of tobacco industry executives discussing the need to recruit new smokers to replace those that had either quit or died from smoking. The advertisement closes with the cynical declaration, "We're not in this business for our health" (Stevens 1998). Another advertisement, "Testifiers," exposed the industry's attempts to minimize the public's knowledge about the health consequences of smoking. Representatives of the tobacco industry were shown giving circuitous testimony and denying the adverse health effects of smoking (Dorfman and Wallack 1993). The strategy of exposing the tobacco industry's marketing methods has since emerged as a central theme in other state and national media campaigns (Farrelly et al. 2005).

Despite the large financial investment that the state made during the first 15 months of the media campaign, funding levels fluctuated throughout the rest of the 1990s. Per-capita annual expenditures stood at about 50 cents between 1990 and 1993, fell to about 35 cents between 1994 and 1996, and then rose to about 90 cents from 1997 to 1998 (Friend and Levy 2002). Furthermore, in the latter half of the decade, California's media campaign lost one of its most effective tools when the state prohibited the airing of advertisements that attacked the tobacco industry. In 2001, however, a newly integrated media campaign once again featured the failings of the industry (Givel et al. 2001).

Because antismoking media campaigns generally constitute just one element of statewide comprehensive tobacco control programs, evaluating the direct effects of such campaigns can be difficult. The studies that have looked specifically at California's media campaign, however, have indicated that it has proven somewhat effective in altering tobacco-related attitudes and behavior. In evaluating the first year of the campaign (1990–1991), Popham and colleagues (1994) collected and analyzed data from the campaign's two main target groups, students in grades 4 through 12 and adult smokers. Although they reported some mixed results, Popham and colleagues pointed to increased levels of campaign awareness and desired changes in attitudes relating to health and smoking among youth as evidence of the campaign's beneficial impact (Popham et al. 1994b). In a

1995 study, Hu and colleagues (1995) sought to disentangle the effects of the media campaign from the effects of other factors that may have played a role in reducing tobacco use in California in the early 1990s. Controlling for increased cigarette prices and the tobacco industry's own advertising efforts, they found that the media campaign's antismoking messages reduced aggregate cigarette sales (Hu et al. 1995b). In addition, upon reviewing the empirical literature on the effectiveness of state-funded media campaigns, including results from the aforementioned studies, Friend and Levy determined that the California campaign, in conjunction with other tobacco control efforts, could be associated with decreases in smoking rates. They noted, however, that the evidence indicated that California's media campaign proved most effective during its first few years of implementation (Friend and Levy 2002).

Massachusetts

Massachusetts's media campaign closely mirrored California's in both its origins and scope. Like California, Massachusetts organized its media campaign within the broader framework of a comprehensive tobacco control program. In early 1993, having increased the per-pack cigarette tax by 25 cents, the state established the MTCP. The MTCP unveiled the country's second statewide antismoking media campaign in October of that year (CDC 1996; Friend and Levy 2002; Miller 1998).

Massachusetts's campaign focused on three main themes: (1) ETS, (2) smoking cessation, and (3) the health risks (Friend and Levy 2002). Under the tagline "It's time we made smoking history," the campaign featured a wide variety of stylistic approaches. Several studies have indicated that the most effective spots in Massachusetts's campaign were those that evoked feelings of outrage, sadness, and fear (Biener 2000, 2002; Biener et al. 2000b). One series of ads portrayed real people suffering from smoking-related diseases, including Janet Sackman, a cigarette model who lost her vocal cords to cancer; Victor Crawford, a tobacco lobbyist who died from throat cancer; and Wayne McClarren, a former Marlboro Man who was shown dying from lung cancer (Biener 2000). Like California, Massachusetts also highlighted the practices of the tobacco industry. The state's 1999 media campaign, under the slogan "Where's the Outrage?," presented statistics on smoking-related deaths and exposed efforts by the tobacco industry to recruit young smokers (Biener 2002).

From 1993 to 2000, MTCP spent approximately $13 million per year on antitobacco advertising (Biener et al. 2000b), representing one-third of MTCP's total expenditures (Biener et al. 2000a). Much of that investment, however, was made in the first 3 years of the campaign (CDC 1996). The state, in fact, repeatedly cut the campaign's budget throughout the latter half of the 1990s (Friend and Levy 2002), and in FY 2001 effectively eliminated the campaign, as the state began to reduce the scale of the tobacco program in general (Hamilton et al. 2003).

Several researchers have sought to determine the impact of Massachusetts's media campaign on tobacco use in the state. In a 2000 study, Siegel and Biener reported the results of a 4-year longitudinal study of a cohort of Massachusetts youth, concluding that exposure to television antismoking advertisements had a significant effect on younger adolescents. Although they could not identify a significant effect among 14- to 15-year-olds, they found that 12- to 13-year-olds who had reported exposure to antismoking advertisements at the baseline were significantly less likely to be established smokers by the time that follow-up interviews were conducted (Siegel and Biener 2000). In another 2000 study, Biener and colleagues analyzed Massachusetts adults' level of exposure and receptivity to antismoking television advertisements. With 88 percent of the cohort reporting some exposure to the advertisements, and 56 percent reporting seeing an advertisement at least once a week, Biener and colleagues concluded that the Massachusetts media campaign had achieved a high level of penetration among adults. Finding that only 12 percent of the cohort held a negative opinion of at least one advertisement, Biener and colleagues determined that the media campaign was well received by Massachusetts adults in general. They also found that the most effective advertisements for adults who had quit smoking or who were preparing to quit were those that elicited strong negative emotions (Biener et al. 2000b). In a separate study, Biener determined that Massachusetts youth responded to antitobacco television advertisements in a manner similar to adults (Biener 2002). Finally, based on their review of the empirical literature, Friend and Levy determined that Massachusetts's antismoking media campaign, like California's, could be associated with decreased smoking rates, specifically in conjunction with a comprehensive tobacco control program. They concluded, however, that Massachusetts's efforts, like California's, were most successful in the earliest years of the media campaign (Friend and Levy 2002).

Florida

Unlike California and Massachusetts, Florida did not initiate a statewide antismoking media campaign until the end of the decade, nor did Florida fund its program with excise tax revenues (Friend and Levy 2002). Instead, the state used funds from a settlement that it reached with the tobacco industry in August 1997, which provided the state with $11.3 billion over the course of 25 years (Givel and Glantz 2000; Sly et al. 2001b).

After establishing the Florida Tobacco Pilot Program (FTPP) in early

1998, state officials immediately set out to develop and implement a large-scale antitobacco media campaign (Givel and Glantz 2000). Unique to Florida, this campaign would focus exclusively on youth (Sly et al. 2002). While performing background research, FTPP staff determined that the program's target audience perceived traditional PSAs as preachy and severe. Consequently, FTPP incorporated efforts to work with youth representatives in developing a media campaign that would be better received by younger viewers. Industry manipulation emerged as a theme of particular resonance. At the March 1998 Teen Tobacco Summit, youth participants, angered by the tobacco industry's marketing practices, selected "truth" as the campaign's brand name. The state and its partners would continue to solicit youth input even after the campaign's initiation (Givel and Glantz 2000; Zucker et al. 2000).

During the campaign's first 10 months, 12 advertisements appeared on the airwaves statewide (Sly et al. 2001b). The campaign also included outdoor signage, print ads, and posters. T-shirts, baseball caps, and other merchandise featuring the "truth" brand complemented the advertisements. In addition, in the summer of 1998, youths, politicians, and celebrities participated in a cross-state train tour that promoted the "truth" campaign and its message (Zucker et al. 2000).

Initially, the 1997 settlement forbade Florida from attacking the industry and limited the antitobacco campaign to 2 years. In September 1998, however, Florida reached a new agreement with the tobacco industry that lifted the ban on industry attacks as well as the 2-year time limit. Subsequently, the "truth" campaign turned to exposing the industry's manipulative tactics. To capture the attention of young and savvy viewers, the campaign produced advertisements in a range of styles, from high-tech to home video. One advertisement that appeared in the wake of the 1998 settlement renegotiation portrayed the tobacco industry as the villain in a mock film trailer. Another, "Demon Awards," showed the tobacco industry accepting an award for the amount of deaths it has caused; fellow attendees included Hitler and Stalin (Givel and Glantz 2000; Zucker et al. 2000).

Data from Florida indicate that the "truth" campaign quickly succeeded in reducing tobacco use among youth. In their review of the literature on the effectiveness of statewide antismoking media campaigns, Farrelly and colleagues point to the results of the Florida Youth Tobacco Survey, which indicate that after the first year of the campaign, the rate of smoking among middle school and high school students dropped by 18 percent and 8 percent, respectively (Farrelly et al. 2003). The CDC declared the drop in teen smoking following the first year of the campaign to be "the largest annual reported decline observed in this nation since 1980" (CDC 1999b). Several studies, meanwhile, have established the "truth" campaign's success in generating high levels of message and campaign awareness (Sly et al.

2001a; Zucker et al. 2000), and a 2001 study, based on longitudinal survey results, associated exposure to the media campaign with a lower likelihood of youth smoking initiation (Sly et al. 2001b). Finally, in comparing the effectiveness of Florida's media campaign with a similar national effort (see below), Niedereppe and colleagues found that Florida teenagers were less likely than teenagers in the rest of the United States to have smoked in the previous 30 days. Moreover, that study determined that Florida teenagers had higher levels of antitobacco awareness and held less favorable opinions of the tobacco industry than their national counterparts (Niederdeppe et al. 2004).

American Legacy Foundation's National truth® Campaign

As already described, antismoking media campaigns have, in recent years, primarily been implemented at the state level. In February 2000, however, the American Legacy Foundation (Legacy) launched the first comprehensive national antismoking media campaign in the United States since the Fairness Doctrine era (Farrelly et al. 2005).

Modeled closely after Florida's program, Legacy's own truth® campaign promoted a similar counterindustry message (Niederdeppe et al. 2004). In an effort to appeal to the campaign's target audience (youth between the ages of 12 and 17 years), Legacy featured trendy teenagers in its truth® advertisements and (borrowing another element from Florida's campaign) marketed its message as an integrated brand, complementing the television spots with promotional items, street marketing, and a website (Farrelly et al. 2002).

Unlike the directive-oriented "Just Say No" antismoking PSAs of the 1970s and 1980s, the Legacy-produced advertisements vividly delivered stark facts on industry marketing practices and the health consequences of smoking. One prominent ad from the truth® campaign, "Body Bags," portrayed a group of youth piling bags outside the headquarters of a tobacco company. They announced through a megaphone, that the bags represented the 1,200 people killed by tobacco each day (Farrelly et al. 2002, 2005).

Between 2000 and 2002, Legacy spent approximately $100 million per year on the truth® campaign (Farrelly et al. 2005). To evaluate the effectiveness of this substantial investment, in 1999, it began sponsoring the Legacy Media Tracking Surveys, which, among other indicators, measured exposure to ETS, access to tobacco products, knowledge and attitudes regarding tobacco use, intention to quit, and awareness of the truth® campaign and its messages among 12- to 17-year-olds and 18- to 24-year-olds. Survey results showed significant increases in campaign awareness among youth, as well as growing support for campaign-sponsored messages just 10 months into the campaign (Farrelly et al. 2002). Data have also revealed an accelerated national decline in youth smoking following the initiation of Legacy's national truth® campaign (Farrelly et al. 2005).

Effectiveness of Media Campaigns

National or statewide media campaigns intended largely or primarily to discourage the uptake of smoking by youth appear to be, in most cases, reasonably effective in achieving their goal. This finding was reaffirmed by the NIH's June 2006 state-of-the-science panel, which identified mass media campaigns as one of three effective approaches to reaching the general population and preventing tobacco use among adolescents and young adults (NIH 2006b).

Effect sizes, as noted in the technical appendix (Slater, Appendix N), appear to average about 6 percent relative to the preexisting rate—that is, the rate of smoking among youth in the particular population being studied falls about 6 percent. These effects appear to be reasonably consistent in studies that use a variety of different evaluation designs within regional and national field intervention contexts.

Although these effect sizes are modest and cost of achieving them is high, the reach of television and other media-based campaigns is exceptionally broad; a 6 percent relative effect size in the context of a media campaign represents a substantial number of young people, especially in a national campaign. Slater (Appendix N) suggests that the absolute prevalence of smoking among American youth is probably about 2 percent less than it would be in the absence of such campaigns and that further efforts might make that prevalence another 1 percent lower. In other words, if such media campaign efforts were to end and their effects to date were to dissipate, the prevalence of smoking in each succeeding cohort of youth might be expected to be 3 percent higher than it would be if such campaigns were to continue. This means that millions more American youth will begin smoking over the next twenty years than would otherwise be the case. It should also be noted that the effects of campaigns to discourage the uptake of smoking by youth are probably conservative, in that they do not take into account the possible effects on uptake among youth younger or older than the target age or the likely reinforcement of public support for local, regional, or national tobacco control policy efforts.

It also should be noted that most evaluations of such campaigns have taken place in contexts in which a variety of other community or regional education or control efforts are taking place. In most cases it is not possible to distinguish the extent to which the effects of media campaigns are facilitated by such efforts or, conversely, to identify the extent to which such local efforts are supported by media campaigns. (There is some empirical evidence regarding the reinforcing effects of media efforts on in-school smoking prevention curricula, see Appendix D for information on such curricula.) Some evaluations, however, (Farrelly et al. 2005) have examined the independent effects of potential media exposure, suggesting that the effects that they find are attributable to the media campaign. Given these uncertainties, it is probably best to assume that it is preferable, whenever possible, to run such campaigns simultaneously with more comprehensive, community-based efforts.

Finally, media campaigns do have various effects, and it is entirely possible for an expensive campaign to have no effect or even effects that result in the rates of smoking moving in the wrong direction. It is essential to ensure that media interventions be research-based, with rigorous testing of the messages and periodic evaluation of their effects, and that they be independent from political pressures that might lead to efforts being driven by political agendas rather than by data (Pechmann and Slater 2005). Finally, it should be noted that it is considerably more cost-effective to purchase media time and space nationally than on a state-by-state basis.

Recommendation 15: A national, youth-oriented media campaign should be funded on an ongoing basis as a permanent component of the nation's strategy to reduce tobacco use. State and community tobacco control programs should supplement the national media campaign with coordinated youth prevention activities. The campaign should be implemented by an established public health organization with funds provided by the federal government, public-private partnerships, or the tobacco industry (voluntarily or under litigation settlement agreements or court orders) for media development, testing, and purchases of advertising time and space.

CESSATION INTERVENTIONS

An estimated 44.5 million adults in the United States are smokers, and these individuals comprise about 20.9 percent of the adult population (CDC 2005g). If nothing is done to help them stop smoking, almost half of them will die prematurely of tobacco-related diseases. On the basis of projections of future smoking prevalence by use of current smoking trends among adults in the United States, there will be at least 33 million smokers 20 years from now, regardless of how well the next generation of young people is prevented from initiating tobacco use and becoming addicted to tobacco.

Abundant epidemiological evidence demonstrates that populations who quit smoking have improved health status and lower rates of morbidity and mortality compared with those of populations that do not quit. Increased population smoking cessation rates will likely decrease cigarette smoking prevalence rates more quickly than an approach focusing exclusively on reducing initiation rates. Accelerating cessation among current smokers will produce immediate benefits, saving millions of lives and billions of dollars over the next decade (see work of Levy, Appendix J and Mendez, Appendix K, and later in this chapter "Projected Impact of Strengthening Measures").

In general, the committee favors a comprehensive, coordinated system of care management for cessation treatment. Such a comprehensive system of care management has five key components: (1) motivating more smokers to make more frequent quit attempts; (2) educating smokers to use evidence-based interventions when they do try to quit; (3) reducing the extraordinarily high rates of relapse after cessation; (4) ensuring that all smokers receive continuity of care management and follow-up, including access to the best care available and full insurance reimbursement; and (5) structuring the comprehensive system of care to provide additional levels of more intensive/specialized treatment (i.e., stepped-care) for smokers that need them (i.e., those who fail to quit with lesser levels of care). Stepped-care is especially important for smokers who are hardest to reach and hardest to treat, such as those at disproportionate risk of treatment failure (e.g., underserved, low-income, uninsured smokers and those with comorbid psychiatric/substance abuse and medical disorders—see also Wallace, Appendix P). The overriding challenge is to educate and motivate more smokers to try to quit and to provide suitable access to effective cessation interventions for as many smokers as possible.

Effective Interventions Exist

A large number of randomized clinical trials and other research studies confirm the efficacy of smoking cessation interventions (Fiore et al. 2000; Hopkins et al. 2001; Task Force on Community Preventive Services 2005) (see Abrams, Appendix A). Interventions can be categorized in terms of the type of intervention, the venue, the intensity, the duration, and the cost. Interventions may be behavioral, pharmacological, or both. They can be administered by health care or other professionals, lay volunteers, or they can be self-administered. They can be guided interventions available in print media, on the telephone, via the Internet, or through purchase of over-the-counter treatments. They may be administered incidentally to other activities, such as at the workplace, during health care visits, and during educational activities. Interventions may include brief episodes of counseling or prolonged programs addressing both cessation and cessation maintenance.

In general, greater intensity of treatment (duration and number of contacts, more modalities of intervention) improves cessation outcomes (for details see Abrams, Appendix A). At the risk of oversimplification, the committee believes that intervention intensity can be classified into three broad categories: (1) minimal, (2) moderate, and (3) maximal. Abstinence at a minimum of 6 months follow-up is related to the intensity of the intervention in a dose-response fashion. Abstinence rates range from (1) about 5–10 percent for smokers quitting on their own or using self-help materials; (2) 10–20 percent for brief, moderate intensity interventions; (3) 20 percent to over 30 percent for maximally intensive individual or combined pharmacological and behavioral interventions (Fiore et al. 2000).

Along with behavioral therapy, pharmacotherapy is an important adjunct to smoking cessation treatments. Currently marketed pharmacotherapies include nicotine replacement products (gums, patches, nasal sprays, inhalers, and lozenges), bupropion, and other recent agents such as Varenicline—a novel $\alpha_4\beta_2$ nicotinic receptor partial agonist pharmacotherapy. In clinical trials, existing pharmacotherapies can improve cessation rates by 1.2 to 2.5 times, on average, compared with those achieved with a placebo (Fiore et al. 2000). Combined behavioral and pharmacological treatment can triple to quadruple cessation rates but these results are not as consistent across studies. The limitations of the pharmacotherapies are that their effectiveness is moderate (achieving cessation rates of 10 to 20 percent, depending on the population of smokers and whether concomitant behavioral therapies are used) and the fact that many dependent smokers have already tried these therapies and failed to quit smoking when they have used them. Most studies of re-treatment with the same medication find that cessation rates are very low.

Thus it is imperative that new medications and other new psychosocial treatments or modes of delivery be developed to aid smoking cessation. Such medications might be more effective than existing medications, which is particularly important for highly nicotine-dependent smokers. Even if new medications are not more effective than the currently available medications, new medications would provide an alternative to current medications and would encourage more smokers who failed cessation in the past to consider making another quit attempt using the new medication. In addition to medications, helping smokers who have repeatedly failed to quit may require more intensive and specialized treatments such as a stepped-care approach (for details see Abrams et al. 1996, 2003). Services might also include a comprehensive system of care management that enables smokers to obtain better continuity of care and follow-up. Smokers with higher levels of nicotine dependence and those with comorbid psychiatric/substance abuse disorders might especially benefit from new pharmacotherapy and a new systems of care management (for details see Abrams, Appendix A and Wallace, Appendix P).

In moving from clinical trials to large-scale community dissemination research, intervention strategies generally shift from treating highly motivated volunteers to reaching out to a more diverse, less-motivated population of smokers. In this community-wide effort, interventions with different types, modes, methods, and channels of delivery are used to reach defined subpopulations on the basis of geography, demography (e.g., age, gender, race, ethnicity, or impoverishment), clinical status (e.g., the presence of a psychiatric comorbidity or pregnancy), health plan, insurance status, or other group status (e.g., youth smokers in secondary schools). Each high-prevalence group represents special challenges to community-based tobacco control efforts. Interventions that are translated from clinical to community settings reveal considerable variability in outcome effectiveness and effect sizes are therefore more difficult to calculate with confidence.

The Limitations of Cessation Programs

Although cessation programs have much to offer, they also have limitations and shortcomings. Less than 50 percent of the 44.5 million current smokers make a quit attempt each year. Of those that try to quit, over 70 percent do so on their own without use of evidence-based programs, and, of those, over 90 percent will relapse. Most programs are evaluated for a maximum of only 6 to 12 months, and efficacy beyond that point may not be well understood; long-term relapse rates have also been documented. Furthermore, randomized trials of interventions are often conducted with smokers who are motivated to quit and who are free of many impediments to program participation; such trials possibly yield higher cessation rates than would occur in general community settings (for details see Abrams, Appendix A).

Less intensive, less costly, and less specialized programs, however, can reach more smokers, with the most intensive interventions being reserved for those that require them. (Abrams et al. 1996, 2003; Orleans 1993). For example, a two-tiered intervention based on intensity and cost might consist of (1) standard care, such as brief behavioral therapy and over-the-counter nicotine replacement therapy; and (2) intensive specialized care, such as the use of multiple clinical sessions and prescription medications, and treatment delivery by addiction specialists. Smokers who either fail standard care or have comorbid complications can be placed on more advanced specialized care. An explicit clinical trial of stepped-care has not yet been published, but many delivery systems implicitly use some form of stepped-care in their intervention programs, in addition to the minimal levels of care recommended by U.S. Public Health Service Guidelines (Fiore et al. 2000).

The Challenge: Increasing Rates of Smoking
Cessation at the Population Level

Despite the presence of many successful interventions, the impact of smoking cessation efforts on reducing population smoking prevalence is currently small and falls far short of its potential. The NIH's June 2006 state-of-the-science panel on tobacco use summarized this challenge as follows: "Most adult smokers want to quit, and effective interventions exist. However, only a small proportion of tobacco users receive intervention. This gap represents a major national quality-of-care problem" (NIH 2006b, p. 11). Interventions are underused for a variety of reasons pertaining to the individual consumer (a lack of knowledge of or demand for cessation programs) as well as to systems and organizational barriers, such as the failure to provide accessible, comprehensive, convenient, continuous, and affordable treatments. Achieving higher cessation rates can be attained by increasing the demand for and use of existing evidence-based cessation interventions by (1) reaching more smokers with cessation messages—including education about the quitting process—as well as the availability and the safety of smoking cessation modalities and products for tobacco use cessation, such as nicotine replacement therapies; (2) motivating more quit attempts among people who now make none, and more frequent quit attempts among those who now try by providing meaningful incentives to quit; (3) increasing the use of evidence-based interventions when smokers are attempting to quit; (4) providing continuity of care, tailored and targeted interventions, and a stepped-care model for those with smoking histories and other individual susceptibility characteristics (e.g., comorbidity) who need more intensive and specialized treatments; and (5) providing adequate and aligned financial, political, and policy initiatives to fully integrate all the effective components into a comprehensive, multilevel system of care, commensurate with the need to address the nation's largest preventable cause of disease and death.

Currently, the demand among smokers for cessation programs and services remains modest, despite the desire of most smokers to quit (NIH 2006b) and the increasingly restrictive environmental and normative social climate against smoking. A multifaceted approach to increasing the demand for smoking cessation programs can include increasing restrictions on smoking, mass media campaigns, financial incentives, and efforts to create a strong consumer-driven demand for attractive smoking cessation products and services. These same strategies were identified by the NIH's state-of-the-science panel as effective methods of increasing the use of cessation interventions (NIH 2006b).

Data addressing the demand for cessation services among smokers are available. For example, Zhu and colleagues (2000) reported that 78 percent of smokers believed that they were just as likely to quit on their own as with assistance, but smokers who believed that cessation assistance was effective were twice as likely to intend to quit or make a quit attempt and more than three times as likely to use intervention assistance when quitting (Zhu et al. 2000). Hammond and colleagues (2004) surveyed smokers' perceived effectiveness of cessation methods and found that the great majority of respondents said they wanted additional information on where to get help quitting (87 percent), how to quit (86 percent), the benefits of quitting (85 percent), and toll-free quitlines (70 percent), and that they wanted access to a website that would provide more information about cessation (68 percent). Respondents had inadequate awareness of the availability and utility of clinical cessation intervention methods, such as counseling (Hammond et al. 2004). Yong and colleagues (2005) reported that older smokers (those older than age 60 years) perceived themselves to be less vulnerable to harm (self-exempting beliefs), less concerned about the health effects of smoking, less confident about being able to quit (self-efficacy), and less willing to try to quit. However, respondents' knowledge of cigarette prices, health providers' advice, inexpensive medications, and health risk information was associated with a greater intent to quit and more quit attempts (Yong et al. 2005).

Although the best mix of smoking cessation strategies remains unclear, the overarching objective is readily apparent: In order to enhance program use and population cessation rates, smokers must know that safe, effective, and accessible cessation programs—including medications—are available. It is important to point out that from an population perspective, overall impact is a product of "reach × efficacy" (Abrams et al. 1996). Thus reaching a larger number of smokers with a somewhat less effective intervention can produce a greater number of people who quit than reaching a small number of people with a more effective intervention. Getting more smokers to use even a minimal intensity cessation program generally doubles the likelihood of success and therefore makes an important contribution to the overall impact on population smoking prevalence rates.

> Recommendation 16: State tobacco control agencies should work with health care partners to increase the demand for effective cessation programs and activities through mass media and other general and targeted public education programs.

Disseminating Cessation Programs

Well-performed studies on the ability to disseminate smoking cessation programs to the community provide reasonable and reliable data as a basis for projecting the impact, on a populationwide basis, of the efficient implementation of the best available practices. An important example is the use of quitlines, which can increase smoking abstinence by as much as 30 to 50 percent over the rate achieved under control conditions (Fiore et al. 2000). On the basis of the growing body of evidence from smoking cessation program dissemination research trials and the extensive deliberations of an expert panel, Fiore and colleagues recommended funding a national telephone quitline as a means of reaching more smokers, achieving an additional 5 million quitters per year, and saving 3 million lives over the next two decades (Fiore et al. 2004).

Quitlines have proven to be an effective smoking cessation intervention. Recognizing their value in helping individuals to stop smoking and acknowledging recommendations for a more robust, countrywide quitline, DHHS established a national quitline network in 2004. The network increased funding to states with existing quitlines, offered grants for the creation of quitlines in states that did not yet provide the service, and made available smoking cessation counselors in states without quitlines (DHHS 2004).

Given the demonstrated success of smoking quitlines and the ease by which most Americans can now access them, the national quitline network is an important cessation tool that should be maintained with adequate funding. Other emerging technologies are also beginning to show promise such as the use of tailored evidence-based cessation programs delivered on a 24/7/365 basis via the internet, either alone or in combination with quit lines, or brief primary care interventions in physician's offices (for details see Abrams Appendix A).

Recommendation 17: Congress should ensure that stable funding is continuously provided to the national quitline network.

The quitline is a highly useful intervention because advertising the availability of the quitline helps to stimulate demand and accessing it provides a low-cost service for facilitating cessation. What other steps should be taken to stimulate awareness of and demand for cessation technologies? Would a large-scale social marketing campaign be cost-effective? Unfortunately, important gaps in knowledge on how to expand cessation awareness and demand remain, particularly for some large and important smoking populations, such as youth. Some evidence indicates that mediated communication efforts can be effective in facilitating smoking cessation (Snyder et al. 2004), but expanding the use of cessation technologies will require improved communication, education, and marketing.

At present, the evidence on how best to combine media interventions, other social marketing techniques, and innovative strategies for disseminating cessation technologies is inconclusive. Without such evidence it is premature to endorse a major national media and social marketing effort intended to accelerate smoking cessation rates. The immediate goal should be to identify successful combined strategies, with the intent of implementing them on a national scale with public funding, with resources provided by public-private partnerships, or with funds provided under court orders or litigation settlements with tobacco companies.

> **Recommendation 18: The Secretary of the U.S. Department of Health and Human Services, through the National Cancer Institute, the Centers for Disease Control and Prevention, and other relevant federal health agencies, should fund a program of developmental research and demonstration projects combining media techniques, other social marketing methods, and innovative approaches to disseminating smoking cessation technologies.**

If such projects show success, future efforts should be national in scope and should be implemented by a public health organization with no ties to the tobacco industry and with funds provided by the federal government, public-private partnerships, or the tobacco industry (whether voluntarily or under litigation settlement agreements or court orders) for media development, testing, and purchases of advertising time and space. Regional, state, or local funding should be provided to supplement the national campaign with coordinated cessation activities.

Delivering Cessation Services

Targeting populations with a high smoking prevalence at the community level is part of any important tobacco control program (for a discussion on these populations, see Wallace, Appendix P). However, for the general delivery of cessation services within the health care system, the adoption of an integrated, multilevel, systems approach is needed to maximize the potential for carrying out all the components of effective cessation programs in an organized, evidence-based manner. It is important to align clinical policies and delivery system structures to support and finance tobacco cessation as a chronic, refractory, addictive condition and to approach it as one might approach the chronic management of hypertension, diabetes, or asthma. Such an approach would ensure continuous engagement with smokers and provide coordinated, tailored interventions before, during, and after they quit smoking. Smokers must be supported in their cessation efforts at every level of the infrastructure of health care delivery systems through the use of aligned policies, financial incentives, and full reimbursement for the costs that they incur in their cessation efforts.

Ideally, health care delivery systems, such as managed care organizations and mental health clinics, not only should foster comprehensive smoking cessation management but also should track the type and extent of care delivered within that system over time as a matter of quality assurance. For example, a managed health care organization may have a policy that requires all providers in all settings (e.g., emergency rooms, primary care, and specialty care settings) to screen for smokers and to develop, document, and implement an individualized treatment plan for each smoking member of the health plan. Surveillance and measurement of key performance and quality indicators will improve accountability, fidelity, and adherence to best practices. Such activities are already in place in quality assurance programs, such as those promoted by the National Committee for Quality Assurance.

Recommendation 19: Public and private health care systems should organize and provide access to comprehensive smoking cessation programs by using a variety of successful cessation methods and a staged disease management model (i.e. stepped care), and should specify the successful delivery of these programs as one criterion for quality assurance within those systems.

All health care delivery organizations should have in place a comprehensive care management system for smoking cessation that includes continuity of care, appropriate tracking systems and quality indicators and properly aligned structural and financial incentives to support providers' and smokers' efforts to treat their condition in much the same manner as other chronic conditions like diabetes. They should also target populations with high rates of comorbidity and high smoking prevalences.

Reimbursement for Smoking Cessation Services

Evidence suggests that institutions investing in comprehensive smoking cessation programs or services (e.g., health care facilities and worksites) will receive a substantial return on their investment within 2 to 3 years (AHIP 2004). Warner and colleagues (2004) simulated the financial impact and cost effectiveness of a smoking cessation program in a hypothetical managed care organization (MCO) using data from three large MCOs (Warner et al. 2004). Quitters gained an average of 7.1 years of life, with a direct coverage cost of $3,417 for each year of life saved. The net cost to the MCO was $0.41 per patient per month. With the costs of health care expenditures for smokers and productivity losses from smoking estimated to be more than $167 billion per year (CDC 2005d) the expected savings from the implementation of effective cessation programs could be substantial.

In recent years, there has been significant improvement in private, federal, and state insurance coverage for some components of the evidence-based treatments recommended in the U.S. Public Health Service clinical guidelines (Fiore et al. 2000; Task Force on Community Preventive Services 2001). For example, Medicare announced that as of March 2005 it will cover up to two cessation attempts per year, and that each attempt may include four counseling sessions, for a total of eight sessions per year. Pharmacotherapy for smoking cessation is also covered by the new Medicare prescription drug benefit. The NIH's state-of-the-science panel on tobacco use found "strong evidence" supporting the effectiveness of reducing out-of-pocket costs and reimbursing providers for cessation services (NIH 2006b). However, in the United States overall, insurance coverage remains spotty, and covered cessation treatment programs typically invest only in the minimum recommended level of coverage. A 2002 national survey of MCOs found that 30 percent had no written policy on coverage for tobacco cessation services and 42 percent provided no coverage for behavioral interventions (McPhillips-Tangum et al. 2004). In 1998, only half of the 5 million Medicaid recipients nationwide who were current smokers were eligible for any type of smoking cessation treatment benefit (Schauffler et al. 2001).

States purchase health insurance for more than 5 million employees and retirees. In a survey of state employee insurance plans conducted in 2002 and 2003, only 6 of 45 states required smoking cessation coverage that was fully consistent with the U.S. Public Health Service guidelines for all employees (Fiore et al. 2000). To capture the demonstrable benefits of cessation programs, various public and private health insurance programs available in the United States should provide reimbursement for a broad range of effective smoking cessation interventions.

In sum, insurance and benefit coverage for smoking cessation programs remains an important problem. Identifying funds for these programs is always a challenge, but two important sources of additional revenues for cessation services that have been used in some venues are tobacco excise taxes and court-ordered litigation settlements from tobacco companies.

Recommendation 20: All insurance, managed care, and employee benefit plans, including Medicaid and Medicare, should cover reimbursement for effective smoking cessation programs as a lifetime benefit.

For a smoker, it is long journey from starting to smoke and enjoying smoking to wanting to stop and successfully stopping. For much of that journey the smoker is not actively attempting to quit. Thus there are many opportunities to enhance cessation success rates at many points along the smoker's journey. Opportunities range from becoming more aware of the risks of smoking and the benefits of cessation to learning about the tools available for cessation, understanding the process of cessation and what to expect, becoming motivated to make frequent and serious quit attempts, not becoming discouraged by relapse, and eventually quitting for good. There is substantial room to improve the overall cessation outcome rate at every step of the way during this journey. This extraordinary opportunity can only be fully realized by strengthening and developing policies that support a comprehensive smoking cessation care management system that addresses each and every step in the journey from current smoker to lifetime ex-smoker.

COMMUNITY MOBILIZATION

Community coalitions played a central role in the acceleration of successful tobacco control efforts from 1988 to 2000. The scientific literature bearing on the effects of coalition activity is reviewed by Sparks in Appendix O and the following discussion is drawn from the information presented.

The most important functions of these community coalitions were that they mobilized organized grassroots support for tobacco control activities, gave a voice to the community in policymaking, and held governments and businesses accountable for their decisions. Mobilizing communities for advocacy has become a mainstream public health tool over the past generation. One area in which success has been documented is alcohol policy, specifically, in relation to drunk driving and underage drinking (IOM/NRC 2004). Ironically, one of the ingredients of success in the alcohol policy domain has been participation in local coalitions by some segments of the alcohol industry. This experience poses a stark contrast to the efforts of the tobacco industry to terminate community action in the smoking domain, in which the tobacco industry uses the false claim that community action and advocacy amount to "lobbying," which is often limited by federal and state laws. The value at stake in these disputes with the tobacco industry is not only public health but also local self-determination.

From the beginning, public policy advocacy was an integral part of comprehensive state tobacco control programs because they emphasized population-level changes, including changes in legislation and public policy. For example, the ASSIST program promoted three types of interventions (program services, policy, and mass media) and the guidelines stated that "efforts to achieve priority public policy objectives should take precedence over efforts to support service delivery" (NCI 2005, p. 23). Mass media initiatives were intended to support those policy changes, which meant that media advocacy that engaged the news media in support of prevention policies was the focus of media initiatives, whereas social marketing played a secondary role. The four ASSIST program priority policy areas were eliminating ETS, raising tobacco taxes, limiting tobacco advertising and promotion, and reducing youth access.

The CDC identifies governmental and voluntary policies that promote clean indoor air and restrict access to tobacco products as well as other policy objectives as best practices, citing the successes of the California, Massachusetts, and Oregon community coalitions in achieving policy and program objectives (CDC 1999c). Statewide programs that promote media advocacy and countermarketing campaigns are also cited among the best practices, based on the CDC's review of core documents from the California and Massachusetts campaigns.

There have been few efforts to analyze the contributions of the state tobacco control coalitions to comprehensive state programs, and it has been especially difficult to measure the impacts of their advocacy initiatives. Most investigators who have evaluated state programs observe that state coalitions have played a key role in the achievement of policy changes that reduce tobacco consumption; yet, those investigators have also commented on the difficulty of measuring the extent to which coalition activities at the state or local level were responsible for either policy change or health outcomes. One reason that the link between community action and reductions in tobacco use is difficult to document is that public health methodology for measuring complex community and population-based social and policy changes is not as well developed as it is for measuring individual and small group changes (Sparks, Appendix O). However, evidence from the domain of alcohol policy convincingly demonstrates the effects of mobilizing community coalitions, both on the enactment of new policies to reduce underage drinking and alcohol-impaired driving and on the actual changes in the prevalence of consumption as well as the targeted alcohol problems (IOM/NRC 2004).

Even without quantitative studies of the efficacy of policy advocacy, most people in the tobacco control community assume that without citizen advocacy, it is doubtful that the changes in tobacco taxes, smoke-free workplace laws, restrictions on smoking in public accommodations, and restrictions on sales to youth would have occurred. This assumption is reasonable because decision makers do not decide to strengthen tobacco control policies unless an active citizenry demands such change. In this sense, tobacco control policies are the end point of coalition advocacy initiatives, and their effectiveness can be measured by counting the hundreds, possibly thousands, of local and state tobacco control policies adopted during the 1990s (Gerlach and Larkin 2005). The Surgeon General's report, Reducing Tobacco Use, called the emergence of statewide coalitions the most important advance in comprehensive programs and concluded that comprehensive state programs, such as those in California and Massachusetts, provide evidence that such programs reduce smoking (Public Health Service 2000).

Tobacco Industry Reaction to Successful Public Policy Advocacy

The tobacco industry immediately recognized the potential power of an advocacy strategy by state coalitions when such coalitions began to be formed. The industry attacked the ASSIST program from its inception (NCI 2005; Trochim et al. 2003; White and Bero 2004) to reduce the threat of citizen action. Analysis of internal documents from members of the tobacco industry indicates that the tobacco industry deliberately pursued a campaign to equate citizen advocacy efforts with lobbying and to limit those activities (NCI 2005; White and Bero 2004). Congress eventually prohibited anyone receiving federal funds from lobbying state and local governments (Federal Acquisition Streamlining Act of 1994 Pub. L. No. 103-355, 108 Stat. 3243). The tobacco industry used the Freedom of Information Act to divert state health department resources and threatened lawsuits against state health departments and individual state employees for violating the lobbying restriction (NCI 2005). The MSA also prohibits the American Legacy Foundation from engaging in any political activities or lobbying. The industry's position equates advocacy with lobbying and cites Internal Revenue Service regulations that forbid public agencies from using public money for lobbying (White and Bero 2004).

In reaction to the tobacco industry's position, federal agencies and many state health departments have severely limited advocacy activities that were—and that still are—perfectly legal. Lobbying, a well-understood term in various legal contexts, such as in the statutes governing tax-exempt foundations, refers to direct communication to a legislator on specific legislation or grassroots communication to the members of the general public urging them to take action on specific legislation (Gerlach and Larkin 2005; IOM 1988; Wallack et al. 1993). As the term is used in public health, however, "advocacy" refers to a much broader concept and set of activities, such as organized social action aiming to create a shift in public opinion and to mobilize resources and forces to support an issue, policy, or constituency (Wallack et al. 1993), or the process of educating policymakers and members of the community about certain health-related issues and the measures that can be taken to address them (Gerlach and Larkin 2005).

Gerlach and Larkin point out that as early as the first year of the SmokeLess States program, the RWJF's support of the Coalition for Tobacco-Free Colorado was challenged as lobbying by the tobacco industry (Gerlach and Larkin 2005). In response, the RWJF was careful to make a distinction between lobbying, (which the SmokeLess States program would not fund) and advocacy (which it would). Coalitions were free to use their own funds for such activities; indeed, the Foundation encouraged and finally insisted that coalitions find such funds. Both the RWJF and the NCI ASSIST program held training workshops for state coalitions on policy advocacy. As the report on the ASSIST program from NCI makes clear policy advocacy and lobbying are not the same thing (NCI 2005, p. 352).

The tobacco industry's strong opposition to public health advocacy is a good indication of how important advocacy initiatives should be in any blueprint for future tobacco control efforts. The industry attacks have weakened federal and state willingness to fund advocacy programs. The potential for future gains is thus endangered if state health departments, foundations, and community organizations become hesitant to openly acknowledge how critical citizen advocacy is to successful policy change.

States and local communities should not be barred from using federal funds for tobacco control advocacy efforts at the state or local levels, as long as such activities do not involve lobbying (i.e., contacting legislators about a specific bill or urging constituents to do so). Advocating policies that would promote the public health and education of the public or legislators about the effects of adopting new policies (or of failing to do so) does not constitute lobbying. The CDC should encourage citizen participation in the democratic process and should clarify the distinction between legitimate citizen advocacy and restricted lobbying.

Maintaining Momentum

Recent evidence of the impact of advocacy by mobilized communities lies in the continuing adoption of smoke-free cities and towns across the United States. As of October 2006, 519 municipalities have enacted local smoke-free laws, including some localities that have banned smoking in restaurants and bars (ANRF 2006). Smoke-free movements' success has also accelerated at the state level; 19 states and Washington, D.C., have now enacted smoke-free state laws, many of which include workplaces, restaurants, and bars (Table 5-3). Even as funding for coalitions has become less secure, these policy successes continue to occur with a momentum that was unanticipated in the late 1990s. The success of smoke-free policies in the past 5 years shows the importance of continued federal and state support for community-level strategies for tobacco control efforts as well as the need for broad demonstration programs.

The evidence reviewed above indicates that the comprehensive approach used in the 1990s, including policy advocacy, has resulted in many policy changes for tobacco control efforts that, in turn, have had an effect on the prevalence of tobacco use. There are two main reasons to continue such a comprehensive approach and a focus on policy advocacy. The first, which is specific to tobacco control, is that, if all state and local policies for

TABLE 5-3 Summary of Smoke Free State Laws

State	Enactment Date	Provisions (Effective Date)
California	July 1994	Restaurants (01/01/95) and bars (01/01/98)
Utah	1994, March 2006	Workplaces (05/01/06), restaurants (01/01/95), and bars (01/07/09)
South Dakota	February 2002	Workplaces (07/01/02)
Delaware	May 2002	Workplaces, restaurants, and bars (11/27/02)
Florida	November 2002	Workplaces and restaurants (07/01/03)
New York	March 2003	Workplaces, restaurants, and bars (07/24/03)
Connecticut	May 2003	Restaurants (10/01/03) and bars (04/01/04)
Maine	June 2003	Restaurants and bars (01/01/04)
Idaho	April 2004	Restaurants (07/01/04)
Massachusetts	June 2004	Workplaces, restaurants, and bars (07/05/04)
Rhode Island	April 2005	Workplaces and restaurants (03/10/05), bars (03/31/05)
North Dakota	June 2005	Workplaces (08/01/05)
Vermont	June 2005	Restaurants and bars (09/01/05)
Montana	April 2005	Workplaces and restaurants (10/01/05), bars (10/01/09)
Washington	November 2005	Workplaces, restaurants, and bars (12/08/05)
New Jersey	January 2006	Workplaces, restaurants, and bars (04/15/06)
District of Columbia	January 2006	Workplaces (04/03/06), restaurants and bars (01/01/07)
Colorado	March 2006	Restaurants and bars (07/01/06)
Louisiana	June 2006	Workplaces and restaurants (01/01/07)
Hawaii	July 2006	Workplaces, restaurants, and bars (11/16/06)

NOTE: Workplaces includes both public and private nonhospitality workplaces, including, but not limited to, offices, factories, and retail stores. Restaurants includes any attached bar in the restaurant. Bars include freestanding bars without separately ventilated rooms.

SOURCE: See http://www.no-smoke.org/pdf/SummaryUSPopList.pdf.

tobacco control are counted, policy advocacy has had its greatest effect in altering the normative environment supporting tobacco use. Even though formal evaluation data for a meta-analysis may be scant, state health departments have broadened the scope of their tobacco control activities. Accordingly, state officials can document changes in social norms that support tobacco-free environments and public support for tobacco control efforts, and they can also list changes in public policy that limit tobacco use. A cadre of public health advocates was trained intensively through the ASSIST, IMPACT, and SmokeLess States program coalition initiatives. Not only should this cadre be maintained, but funding and resources also should be available so that these advocates may provide training for the next generation of tobacco control workers in the 50 states and the other territories in the United States. The momentum of public advocacy should not be lost.

The second, and even more crucial, reason to continue to support a comprehensive approach is that continuing to implement and evaluate comprehensive social and environmental interventions is essential to the continued development of effective public health promotion efforts. Understanding of how to implement such interventions, as well as how to develop methods for evaluating the effectiveness of such interventions, cannot advance if the federal government, state governments, and national nonprofit foundations do not take the lead in advancing the public's health through such initiatives. Involvement in broad initiatives is critical to the training of future public health professionals who need practice in population-based solutions to public health problems. Such initiatives, with their national focus, are so costly, however, that they require federal coordination and support. As an example of the kind of advances that the field needs, OSH's recent release of Key Outcome Indicators for Evaluating Comprehensive Tobacco Control Programs (CDC 2005b) illustrates how program evaluation of complex initiatives can be enhanced. The OSH tobacco control program requires that states receiving funds for tobacco control efforts develop action plans based on logic models, in which community mobilization and policy and regulatory actions lead to defined short-, intermediate-, and long-term outcomes for tobacco control efforts. Detailed outcome indicators then make it possible to measure success quantitatively.

> Recommendation 21: While sustaining their own valuable tobacco control activities, state tobacco control programs, CDC, philanthropic foundations, and voluntary organizations should continue to support the efforts of community coalitions promoting, disseminating, and advocating for tobacco use prevention and cessation, smoke-free environments, and other policies and programs for reducing tobacco use.

SPECIAL POPULATIONS WITH HIGHER
RATES OF CIGARETTE SMOKING

As Chapter 1 illustrates, tobacco use and tobacco-related diseases impact segments of society differentially. Prevention and cessation problems need to be attentive to the special circumstances and outreach needs of these subgroups. For example, Native-American and Alaska Native adults are more likely to smoke than white, Asian-American, or Hispanic-American adults.[4] Not surprisingly, members of subgroups with a high smoking prevalence are more likely to experience tobacco-related morbidity and mortality such as from heart disease or lung cancer, thereby contributing significantly to health disparities. Although African Americans have a similar smoking prevalence to whites, African Americans are more susceptible to developing and dying from lung cancer and are less likely to quit smoking than white smokers. At least one study shows that Hispanic-American smokers are less likely than white smokers to receive cessation advice from health care providers (Levinson et al. 2004).

Attention should also be given to the special circumstances and needs of recent immigrants from countries where smoking is socially acceptable. For example, smoking rates among Southeast Asian adults, Korean men in particular, have been shown to be significantly higher (34–43 percent) than in the U.S. male population (Kandula et al. 2004; Ma et al. 2004). For new immigrant populations and populations for whom English is a second language, access to culturally competent and linguistically appropriate interventions could be a key requirement for engaging them in prevention and cessation programs (Baezconde-Garbanati and Garbanati 2000; Orleans and Fishman 2000). Research into the design and impact of culturally sensitive intervention programs, however, is limited. Such research should be further developed to enhance the evidence base on how to best address the needs of an increasingly diverse population (NIH 2006a).

Other populations at increased risk for tobacco use are described by Wallace in Appendix P. These groups include individuals with psychiatric disorders and a history of substance abuse, among others. Typical approaches to smoking cessation in populations with comorbidities and risk behaviors can help individuals to stop smoking, but long-term abstinence has been shown to be more difficult to achieve. Research is also needed on how best to design smoking cessation intervention and their effectiveness in the treatment of individuals with co-occurring conditions.

Wallace (Appendix P) also notes, that "the themes of poverty, lower socioeconomic status and health and social disparities pervade many of the high risk groups for tobacco use" (Wallace, Appendix P). The rate of smok-

---

[4]There are wide gender differences within each ethnic category, with male adults having higher rates than female adults.

ing among adults who are below the poverty level is about 32.9 percent (CDC 2004a). Persons with low socioeconomic status may have less access to health care that might be needed to address smoking-related morbidities. While data on the prevalence of smoking among homeless individuals is difficult to obtain, reports from international studies indicate that prevalence rates can range from 75 to 85 percent (Folsom and Jeste 2002). Identifying and eliminating disparities in tobacco use and related morbidity and mortality is an important part of the CDC's goal for ensuring success in tobacco control programs, leading many state programs to include a stated emphasis on disparities in their strategic plans. State- and locally-supported prevention and treatment programs need to assess the proportion of their population who fall into these categories and to consider modifying prevention and treatment programs to ensure that they reach these populations effectively.

Military personnel are another population at high risk of tobacco use. Following a significant decline in cigarette smoking from 51 percent in 1980 to 30 percent in 1998, cigarette smoking rates have begun to increase (Hamlett-Berry 2004). More recently, a 2005 Department of Defense Survey of Health-Related Behaviors Among Active Duty Military Personnel found that about one third of military personnel reported smoking in the past month across all branches of service (Bray et al. 2006). The prevalence of smoking in the past month was highest (38.2 percent) among army personnel. Veterans who have separated from active duty also show higher smoking rates than those found in the general civilian population. Reporting data from a 1999 health survey of veterans who received care from the Veterans Health Administration, (Miller et al. 2001) found the prevalence of smoking to be 33 percent compared to 23 percent in the adult civilian population. Military service has been suggested by some researchers as a risk factor for smoking (Klevens et al. 1995). Veterans could benefit from cessation services from the Veterans Administration or from state and locally provided treatment programs. Active duty military personnel could also benefit from prevention and cessation services from the Department of Defense.

> Recommendation 22: Tobacco control programs should consider populations disproportionately affected by tobacco addiction and tobacco-related morbidity and mortality when designing and implementing prevention and treatment programs. Particular attention should be paid to ensuring that health communications and other materials are culturally-appropriate and that special outreach efforts target all high-risk populations. Standard prevention or treatment programs that are modified to reach high-risk populations should be evaluated for effectiveness.

PROJECTED IMPACT OF STRENGTHENING
EXISTING TOBACCO CONTROL MEASURES

This chapter has outlined a blueprint for how the country can strengthen and intensify current tobacco control policies and programs, assuming that the current legal structure of tobacco control efforts remains unchanged. What would be the impact on national tobacco use prevalence of following, or not following, this blueprint, relative to prevalence based on the baseline projections outlined at the end of Part I of the committee's report?

Table 5-4 (from Table 3 of Levy, Appendix J) shows that the SimSmoke model projects considerable potential benefit if the policies outlined in this chapter are pursued aggressively. Specifically, the policies modeled by the SimSmoke model are as follows:

- Tax increases of $1 and $2 per pack
- Nationwide implementation of clean air laws for all work sites (including bars)
- Comprehensive media campaigns targeting youth and adults and funded at the levels recommended by the CDC (i.e., beyond the levels that have been used in the past) to prevent initiation and to increase quit attempts, heighten consumer demand for proven cessation programs and to increase smoker's health literacy about the value of using evidence-based treatments when trying to quit
- Comprehensive cessation policies (full coverage of pharmacotherapy and behavioral therapy, training and coverage for tobacco brief interventions, multisession quit lines, internet interventions, and free nicotine replacement therapy)
- Universal implementation of school-based prevention sufficient to

TABLE 5-4 Projected Adult Smoking Prevalence Through 2025 Under Status Quo and Best-Case Policy Scenarios

Policy Scenario	2005	2010	2015	2020	2025
Status quo	20.6%	19.3%	18.1%	16.9%	15.5%
$1.00 tax increase	20.6%	18.4%	17.1%	15.9%	14.5%
$2.00 tax increase	20.6%	17.8%	16.4%	15.1%	13.7%
Clean air laws	20.6%	18.6%	17.4%	16.3%	14.9%
Media campaign	20.6%	18.1%	16.9%	15.8%	14.4%
Cessation treatment	20.6%	18.2%	16.7%	15.3%	13.8%
Education programs	20.6%	19.2%	17.6%	16.1%	14.6%
Youth-access policies	20.6%	19.1%	17.6%	16.2%	14.7%
All policies with $1.00 tax	20.6%	15.5%	13.4%	11.8%	10.2%
All policies with $2.00 tax	20.6%	14.9%	12.9%	11.2%	9.7%

cut the rate of smoking initiation by 10 percent
- Heavy enforcement of youth-access laws, accompanied by publicity and high penalties
- All of these things being done together with $1- or $2-per-pack tax increases

Empirical data concerning interactions among multiple policy interventions implemented simultaneously are sparse. The SimSmoke model makes the reasonable but still untested assumption that "when more than one policy is in effect, the percentage reductions are multiplicatively applied," implying that "the relative effect is independent of other policies but the absolute effect is smaller when another policy is in effect" (Levy, Appendix J). For example, if two policies that would each reduce a model flow by 10 percent are both implemented together, they reduce that flow by 19 percent since (1–10 percent) × (1–10 percent) = 81 percent, which is a 19 percent reduction. Hence the results of an estimated "all-policies" analysis are less certain than those of an analysis of individual policies.

The individual policies, particularly the cessation interventions and tax increases, could have a substantial effect on tobacco use prevalence over time. Indeed, collectively they are projected to meet the Healthy People 2010 smoking prevalence target of 12 percent in about 2020, with a 10 percent prevalence reached in 2025. The potential impact of full implementation of the blueprint presented in this chapter is depicted in Figure 5-9, which compares the SimSmoke model projections under the best-case conditions with the status-quo and worst-case projections presented in Chapter 3.

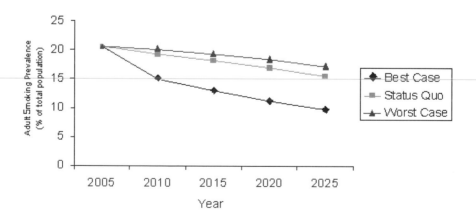

FIGURE 5-9 Comparison of SimSmoke model estimates of adult smoking prevalence, 2005 to 2025, under the best-case, status-quo, and worst-case scenarios.

Overall, however, the committee finds these model projections only modestly encouraging. On the positive side, the actions outlined in this chapter seem to be powerful and effective. Implementing this set of recommendations fully might allow the important goal of a 10 percent smoking prevalence to be achieved, albeit 15 years later than envisioned in Healthy People 2010. On the other hand, removing any single one of the comprehensive policy's components would prevent the modeled prevalence from hitting the 10 percent target in 2025. Hence, the success of these strategies is, in some sense, fragile, requiring absolute commitment to full implementation. Given the recent retrenchment in tobacco control efforts described in Chapter 3, one might worry whether that level of commitment can be achieved and sustained. Nevertheless, any major initiatives undertaken to reduce tobacco use, including those outlined in the blueprint described in this chapter, should be carefully evaluated both for their levels and integrity of delivery and for their effectiveness.

It is not literally true that the only way that the 10 percent smoking prevalence target can be reached in 2025 is by implementing this particular combination of actions. Any set of actions, whether they are produced by policy interventions or by exogenous events, that sufficiently reduces initiation or increases the rate of smoking cessation would enable the country to meet that 10 percent target. This point is illustrated in Figure 5-10, which was created by running the System Dynamics Model in reverse to determine the break-even changes in initiation and cessation that are needed to achieve

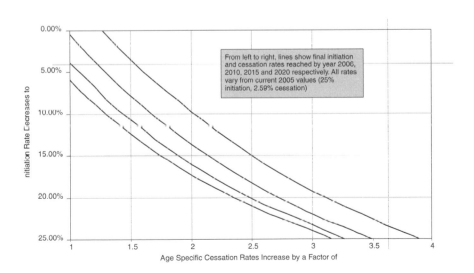

FIGURE 5-10 Combination of initiation and cessation rates required to reach a smoking prevalence of 10 percent by 2025.

a smoking prevalence of 10 percent by 2025. The figure shows four different break-even lines, each corresponding to different rates of change. The line farthest to the left shows the initiation and cessation that would be required if those changes took place more or less instantly. The line farthest to the right shows the changes that would be needed if such changes were phased in between now and 2020.

Figure 5-10 presents a lot of information into one display, so it is worth pausing to explain exactly how to read it. Note that the line farthest to the right essentially crosses the point (2, 10 percent) corresponding to a doubling in the cessation rate (horizontal axis) and a 10 percent rate of initiation (vertical axis). That means that if, between now and 2020 (2020 is used because this is the fourth line from the left), initiation rates fell from the current rates of 25 percent down to 10 percent, and cessation rates doubled over the same time period, then by 2025 those changes would be enough to drive the smoking prevalence to 10 percent by 2025. Any combination of changes to the lower left of that line would not be enough. Any combination of changes to the upper right, if effective by 2020, would be enough to drive the smoking prevalence below 10 percent by 2025.

Reductions in initiation and increases in cessation are complements, or alternative ways to reach the target (hence the lines slope from upper left to lower right). The general impression that the committee takes away from this chart is that the 10 percent smoking prevalence in 2025 target is attainable, but it will require rather potent actions sustained over a long period of time.

One way to achieve the goal would be full implementation of the actions described in this chapter. However, these proposals have been selected within two substantial constraints: they are known to be effective, and they can be implemented within the existing legal structure of tobacco control.

Chapter 6 describes proposals that relax these two constraints. The ideas presented go beyond implementation of the tried and trusted methods that have been subject to extensive experimentation and peer review. Rather, they are policy strategies that hold great potential but that are relatively untried and that therefore have been relatively unexamined empirically. One overall lesson that can be taken from the modeling exercises is this: if the country is serious about attaining 10 percent smoking prevalence by 2025, then unless the country has great confidence that the plan outlined in this chapter will be rapidly, faithfully, and continuously implemented in its entirety, other approaches should be considered.

Realistically, the committee is doubtful that the prevalence of smoking among adults will drop significantly below 15 percent, or that the rate of smoking initiation will permanently fall below 15 percent if the basic legal structure of the tobacco market, and the tobacco control community's responses to that market, remain unchanged. Although achieving these levels would be a major improvement, they are not satisfactory from a public health standpoint, simply because of the large numbers of premature deaths and other serious harmful consequences that would inevitably follow. The steps outlined in this chapter are surely necessary in the short run, but we should be prepared to do more over the long run.

REFERENCES

AAP (American Academy of Pediatrics). 1986. Involuntary smoking: a hazard to children. *Pediatrics* 77:755-757.

Abrams DB, Niaura R, Brown RA, Emmons KM, Goldstein MG, Monti PM. 2003. *The Tobacco Dependence Treatment Handbook: A Guide to Best Practices*. New York: The Guilford Press.

Abrams DB, Orleans CT, Niaura RS, Goldstein MG, Prochaska JO, Velcer W. 1996. Integrating individual and public health perspectives for treatment of tobacco dependence under managed health care: a combined stepped-care and matching model. *Annals of Behavioral Medicine* 18(4):290-303.

ACHA (American College Health Association). 2005. *Position Statement on Tobacco on College and University Campuses*. Web Page. Available at: http://www.acha.org/info_resources/tobacco_statement.pdf; accessed June 12, 2007.

AHA (American Heart Association), American Cancer Society, Campaign for Tobacco-Free Kids, and American Lung Association. 2005. *A Broken Promise to Our Children: The 1998 State Tobacco Settlement Seven Years Later*. Web Page. Available at: http://www.tobaccofreekids.org/reports/settlements/2006/fullreport.pdf; accessed May 30, 2006.

AHIP (America's Health Insurance Plans). 2004. *Making the Business Case for Smoking Cessation*. Web Page. Available at: http://www.businesscaseroi.org/roi/default.aspx; accessed July 26, 2006.

Aligne CA, Stoddard JJ. 1997. Tobacco and children: an economic evaluation of the medical effects of parental smoking. *Archives of Pediatric and Adolescent Medicine* 151(7):648-653.

Andersen MR, Leroux BG, Bricker JB, Rajan KB, Peterson AV Jr. 2004. Antismoking parenting practices are associated with reduced rates of adolescent smoking. *Archives of Pediatric and Adolescent Medicine* 158(4):348-352.

ANR (Americans for Nonsmokers' Rights). 2005. *Health Effects of Secondhand Smoke on Children*. Web Page. Available at: http://www.no-smoke.org/document.php?id=212; accessed July 11, 2006.

ANRF (American Nonsmokers' Rights Foundation). 2006. *Municipalities with Local 100% Smokefree Laws*. Web Page. Available at: http://www.no-smoke.org/pdf/100ordlisttabs.pdf; accessed August 11, 2006.

ANRF. 2007. *Colleges and Universities with Smokefree Air Policies*. Web Page. Available at: http://www.no-smoke.org/pdf/smokefreecollegesuniversities.pdf; accessed June 12, 2007.

Arkin RM, Roemhild HF, Johnson CA, Luepker RV, Murray DM. 1981. The Minnesota smoking prevention program: a seventh-grade health curriculum supplement. *Journal of School Health* 51(9):611-616.

Baezconde-Garbanati L, Garbanati JA. 2000. Tailoring tobacco control messages for Hispanic populations. *Tobacco Control* 9(Suppl I):i51.

Bal DG. 1998. Designing an effective statewide tobacco control program—California. *Cancer* 83(12 Suppl Robert):2717-2721.

Banthin C. 2004. Cheap smokes: state and federal responses to tobacco tax evasion over the internet. *Health Matrix* 14:325-356.

Banzhaf JF. 2005. *17th State Bans Smoking in Home to Protect Children.* Web Page. Available at: http://www.no-smoking.org/august05/08-05-05-1.html; accessed July 14, 2006.

Bauer UE, Johnson TM, Hopkins RS, Brooks RG. 2000. Changes in youth cigarette use and intentions following implementation of a tobacco control program: findings from the Florida Youth Tobacco Survey, 1998–2000. *Journal of the American Medical Assocation* 284(6):723-728.

Bayer R, Colgrove J. 2002. Science, politics, and ideology in the campaign against environmental tobacco smoke. *American Journal of Public Health* 92(6):949-954.

Behan DF, Eriksen MP, Lin Y. 2005. *Economic Effects of Environmental Tobacco Smoke.* Schaumburg, IL: Society of Actuaries.

Belluck P. 2007, January 19. Maine city bans smoking in cars with children. *The New York Times.*

Bergman J. 2003. *Smoking Policies in Long-Term Care and Residential Facilities Serving Older Persons.* Web Page. Available at: www.tcsg.org/powerpoint7/index.htm; accessed February 23, 2005.

Bernstein E, Bernstein J, Levenson S. 1997. Project ASSERT: an ED-based intervention to increase access to primary care, preventative services, and the substance abuse treatment system. *Annals of Emergency Medicine* 30(2):181-189.

Bernstein SL, Boudreaux ED, Cydulka RK, Rhodes KV, Lettman NA, Almeida SL, McCullough LB, Mizouni S, Kellermann AL. 2006. Tobacco control interventions in the emergency department: a joint statement of emergency medicine organizations. *Annals Emergency Medicine* 48(4):e417-e426.

Bernstein SL, Cannata M. 2006. Nicotine dependence, motivation to quit, and diagnosis in emergency department patients who smoke. *Addictive Behavior* 31(2):288-297.

Biener L. 2000. Adult and youth response to the Massachusetts anti-tobacco television campaign. *Journal of Public Health Management and Pracicet* 6(3):40-44.

Biener L. 2002. Anti-tobacco advertisements by Massachusetts and Philip Morris: what teenagers think. *Tobacco Control* 11 (Suppl 2):ii43-ii46.

Biener L, Harris JE, Hamilton W. 2000a. Impact of the Massachusetts tobacco control programme: population based trend analysis. *British Medical Journal* 321(7257):351-354.

Biener L, McCallum-Keeler G, Nyman AL. 2000b. Adults' response to Massachusetts anti-tobacco television advertisements: impact of viewer and advertisement characteristics. *Tobacco Control* 9(4):401-417.

BJS (Bureau of Justice Statistics). 2005. *Summary Findings: Prisons.* Web Page. Available at: http://www.ojp.usdoj.gov/bjs/prisons.htm; accessed May 11, 2007.

Blecher EH, van Walbeek CP. 2004. An international analysis of cigarette affordability. *Tobacco Control* 13(4):339-346.

Bloch M, Shopland DR. 2000. Outdoor smoking bans: more than meets the eye. *Tobacco Control* 9(1):99.

Blumberg DL. 2005, June 22. Even home isn't haven for smokers. *Christian Science Monitor.* P. 16.

Bonnie RJ. 2001. Tobacco and public health policy: A youth centered approach. Slovic PE, Ed. *Smoking: Risk, Perception, and Policy.* Thousand Oaks, CA: Sage Publications.

Borders TF, K Tom Xu, Bacchi D, Cohen L, SoRelle-Miner D. 2005. College campus smoking policies and programs and students' smoking behaviors. *BioMed Center Public Health* 5(74).

Borland R, Yong HH, Cummings KM, Hyland A, Anderson S, Fong GT. 2006. Determinants and consequences of smoke-free homes: findings from the International Tobacco Control (ITC) Four Country Survey. *Tobacco Control* 15(Suppl 3):iii42-iii50.

Botvin GJ. 2000. Preventing drug abuse in schools: social and competence enhancement approaches targeting individual-level etiologic factors. *Addictive Behavior* 25(6):887-897.

Botvin GJ, Baker E, Dusenbury L, Botvin EM, Diaz T. 1995. Long-term follow-up results of a randomized drug abuse prevention trial in a white middle-class population. *Journal of the American Medical Association* 273(14):1106-1112.

Botvin GJ, Baker E, Dusenbury L, Tortu S, Botvin EM. 1990. Preventing adolescent drug abuse through a multimodal cognitive behavioral approach: results of a 3-year study. *Journal of Consulting and Clinical Psychology* 58(4):437-446.

Botvin GJ, Eng A. 1982. The efficacy of a multicomponent approach to the prevention of cigarette smoking. *Preventative Medicine* 11(2):199-211.

Botvin GJ, Griffin KW. 2002. Life skills training as a primary prevention approach for adolescent drug abuse and other problem behaviors. *The International Journal of Emergency Mental Health* 4(1):41-47.

Boudreaux ED, Kim S, Hohrmann JL, Clark S, Camargo CA. 2005. Interest in smoking cessation among emergency department patients. *Health Psychology* 24(2):220-224.

Bray RM, Hourani LL, Rae Olmsted KL, Witt M, Brown JM, Pemberton MR, Marsden ME, Marriott, Scheffler, Vandermaas-Peeler R, Weimer B, Calvin S, Bradshaw M, Close K, Hayden D. 2006. *2005 Department of Defense Survey of Health Related Behaviors Among Active Duty Military Personnel*. Washington, DC: Department of Defense/RTI International.

Cady B. 1998. History of successful ballot initiatives—Massachusetts. *Cancer* 83(12 Suppl Robert):2685-2689.

Campaign for Tobacco-Free Kids. 2003. *State of Washington V. Dirtcheapcig.Com, Inc.* Web Page. Available at: http://tobaccofreekids.org/reports/internet/WARuling.pdf; accessed May 29, 2007.

Capehart T. 2005. *Tobacco Outlook: Leaf Production Plummets with End of Program*. Washington, DC: Economic Research Service, U.S. Department of Agriculture.

Cawley J, Markowitz S, Tauras J. 2004. Lighting up and slimming down: the effects of body weight and cigarette prices on adolescent smoking initiation. *Journal of Health Economics* 23(2):293-311.

CDC (Centers for Disease Control and Prevention). 1996. Cigarette smoking before and after an excise tax increase and an antismoking campaign—Massachusetts, 1990–1996. *MMWR (Morbidity and Mortality Weekly Report)* 45(44):966-970.

CDC. 1999a. Decline in cigarette consumption following implementation of a comprehensive tobacco prevention and education program—Oregon, 1996–1998. *MMWR (Morbidity and Mortality Weekly Report)* 48(7):140-143.

CDC. 1999b. Ten great public health achievements—United States, 1900–1999. *MMWR (Morbidity and Mortality Weekly Report)* 48(12):241-243.

CDC. 1999c. *Best Practices for Comprehensive Tobacco Control Programs—August 1999*. Atlanta, GA: U.S. Department of Health and Human Services, Centers for Disease Control and Prevention, National Center for Chronic Disease Prevention and Health Promotion, Office on Smoking and Health.

CDC. 2001. Tobacco use among adults—Arizona, 1996 and 1999. *MMWR (Morbidity and Mortality Weekly Report)* 50(20):402-406.

CDC. 2002. Annual smoking-attributable mortality, years of potential life lost, and economic costs—United States, 1995–1999. *MMWR (Morbidity and Mortality Weekly Report)* 51(14):300-303.

CDC. 2003. *Chronic Disease. Grants and Funding: Consolidating and Streamlining Program Announcements*. Web Page. Available at: http://www.cdc.gov/nccdphp/grants_funding/consolidating.htm; accessed August 15, 2006.

CDC. 2004a. Prevalence of cigarette use among 14 racial/ethnic populations—United States, 1999–2001. *MMWR (Morbidity and Mortality Weekly Report)* 53(3):49-52.

CDC. 2004b. Impact of a smoking ban on restaurant and bar revenues—El Paso, Texas, 2002. *MMWR (Morbidity and Mortality Weekly Report)* 53(7):150-152.

CDC. 2005a. *CDC Wonder: DATA 2010 . . . The Healthy People 2010 Database.* Web Page. Available at: http://wonder.cdc.gov/data2010/focus.htm; accessed July 10, 2006.

CDC. 2005b. *Key Outcome Indicators for Evaluating Comprehensive Tobacco Control Programs.* Atlanta, GA.

CDC. 2005c. *State Tobacco Activities Tracking and Evaluation (STATE) Stysystem.* Web Page. Available at: http://apps.nccd.cdc.gov/statesystem/; accessed June 8, 2007.

CDC. 2005d. Annual smoking-attributable mortality, years of potential life lost, and productivity losses—United States, 1997–2001. *MMWR (Morbidity and Mortality Weekly Report)* 54(25):625-628.

CDC. 2005e. State smoking restrictions for private-sector worksites, restaurants, and bars—United States, 1998 and 2004. *MMWR (Morbidity and Mortality Weekly Report)* 54(26):649-653.

CDC. 2005f. Estimated exposure of adolescents to state-funded anti-tobacco television advertisements—37 states and the District of Columbia, 1999–2003. *MMWR (Morbidity and Mortality Weekly Report)* 54(42):1077-1080.

CDC. 2005g. Cigarette smoking among adults—United States, 2004. *MMWR (Morbidity and Mortality Weekly Report)* 54(44):1121-1124.

CDC. 2006a. *Behavioral Risk Factor Surveillance System.* Web Page. Available at: http://www.cdc.gov/brfss/; accessed July 19, 2006.

CDC. 2006b. *YRBSS: Youth Risk Behavior Surveillance System.* Web Page. Available at: http://www.cdc.gov/HealthyYouth/yrbs/index.htm; accessed July 19, 2006.

CDHS (California Department of Health Services). 1998. *A Model for Change: The California Experience in Tobacco Control.* Sacramento, CA: California Department of Health Services.

CDHS. 2002. *California Tobacco Control Update.* Web Page. Available at: http://www.dhs.ca.gov/tobacco/documents/pubs/TCSupdate.pdf; accessed February 1, 2006.

CDHS. 2005. *Prevalence: Youth Smoking.* Sacramento, CA.

Celebucki C, Biener L, Koh HK. 1998. Evaluation: methods and strategy for evaluation—Massachusetts. *Cancer* 83(12 Suppl Robert):2760-2765.

Chaloupka FJ. 1999. Macro-social influences: the effects of prices and tobacco-control policies on the demand for tobacco products. *Nicotine and Tobacco Research* 1(Suppl 1):105-109 .

Chaloupka FJ, Pacula RL. 1998. *An Examination of Gender and Race Differences in Youth Smoking Responsiveness to Price and Tobacco Control Policies, Working Paper 6541.* Web Page. Available at: http://www.impacteen.org/fjc/PublishedPapers/w6541.pdf; accessed June 8, 2007.

Chaloupka FJ, Warner KE. 2000. The Economics of Smoking. *Handbook of Health Economics.* Vol. 1B. Pp. 1541-1612.

Chapman S. 2000. Banning smoking outdoors is seldom ethically justifiable. *Tobacco Control* 9(1):95-97.

Chapman S, Richardson J. 1990. Tobacco excise and declining tobacco consumption: the case of Papua New Guinea. *American Journal of Public Health* 80(5):537-540.

Chassin L, Presson CC, Rose JS, Sherman SJ. 1996. The natural history of cigarette smoking from adolescence to adulthood: demographic predictors of continuity and change. *Health Psychology* 15(6):478-484.

Chassin L, Presson CC, Rose J, Sherman SJ, Davis MJ, Gonzalez JL. 2005. Parenting style and smoking-specific parenting practices as predictors of adolescent smoking onset. *Journal of Pediatric Psychology* 30(4):333-344.

Chinnock WF. 2003. No smoking around children: the family courts' mandatory duty to restrain parents and other persons from smoking around children *Arizona Law Review* 453.

Clark PI, Scarisbrick-Hauser A, Gautam SP, Wirk SJ. 1999. Anti-tobacco socialization in homes of African-American and white parents, and smoking and nonsmoking parents. *Journal of Adolescent Health* 24(5):329-339.

Cohen DA, Richardson J, LaBree L. 1994. Parenting behaviors and the onset of smoking and alcohol use: a longitudinal study. *Pediatrics* 94(3):368-375.

Connolly G, Robbins H. 1998. Designing an effective statewide tobacco control program— Massachusetts. *Cancer* 83(12 Suppl Robert):2722-2727.

Cooper M. 2005, June 9. Bill would ban delivery of cigarettes in mail. *The New York Times.* B. p. 4.

Cummings KM, Clarke H. 1998a. *The Use of Counter-Advertising as a Tobacco Use Deterrent.* Web Page. Available at: http://www.advocacy.org/publications/mtc/counterads.htm; accessed September 12, 2005.

Cummings KM, Clarke H. 1998b. *Health Science Analysis Project—Policy Analysis No. 8.* Washington, DC: Advocacy Institute.

DHHS (U.S. Department of Health and Human Services). 2000. *Reducing Tobacco Use: A Report of the Surgeon General.* Atlanta, GA: U.S. Department of Health and Human Services.

DHHS. 2001. *Healthy People 2010, Volume II: 27 Tobacco Use.* Web Page. Available at: http://www.healthypeople.gov/Document/HTML/Volume2/27Tobacco.htm#_Toc489766224; accessed July 20, 2006.

DHHS. 2004. *HHS Announces National Smoking Cessation Quitline Network.* Web Page. Available at: http://www.hhs.gov/news/press/2004pres/20040203.html; accessed July 17, 2006

DHHS. 2006. *The Health Consequences of Involuntary Exposure to Tobacco Smoke: A Report of the Surgeon General.* Atlanta, GA: U.S. Department of Health and Human Services, Centers for Disease Control and Prevention, Coordinating Center for Health Promotion, National Center for Chronic Disease Prevention and Health Promotion, Office on Smoking and Health.

DiFranza JR. 1999. Are the federal and state governments complying with the Synar Amendment? *Archives of Pediatric and Adolescent Medicine* 153(10):1089-1097.

DiFranza JR, Dussault GF. 2005. The federal initiative to halt the sale of tobacco to children— the Synar Amendment, 1992-2000: lessons learned. *Tobacco Control* 14(2):93-98.

DiFranza JR, Lew RA. 1996. Morbidity and mortality in children associated with the use of tobacco products by other people. *Pediatrics* 97(4):560-568.

Ding A. 2003. Youth are more sensitive to price changes in cigarettes than adults. *Yale Journal of Biological Medicine* 76(3):115-124.

Dorfman L, Wallack L. 1993. Advertising health: the case for counter ads. *Public Health Reports* 108(6):716-726.

Eckhardt L, Woodruff SI, Elder JP. 1997. Related effectiveness of continued, lapsed, and delayed smoking prevention intervention in senior high school students. *American Journal of Health Promotion* 11(6):418-421.

Elder JP, Edwards CC, Conway TL, Kenney E, Johnson CA, Bennett ED. 1996. Independent evaluation of the California Tobacco Education Program. *Public Health Reports* 111(4):353-358.

Elder JP, Wildey M, de Moor C, Sallis JF Jr, Eckhardt L, Edwards C, Erickson A, Golbeck A, Hovell M, Johnston D, et al. 1993. The long-term prevention of tobacco use among junior high school students: classroom and telephone interventions.[see comment]. *American Journal of Public Health* 83(9):1239-1244.

Emery S, White MM, Pierce JP. 2001. Does cigarette price influence adolescent experimentation? *Journal of Health Economics* 20(2):261-270.

Emont S, Choi W, Novotny T, Giovino G. 1992. Clean indoor air legislation, taxation, and smoking behaviour in the United States: an ecological analysis. *Tobacco Control* 2:13-17.

Ennett ST, Tobler NS, Ringwalt CL, Flewelling RL. 1994. How effective is drug abuse resistance education? A meta-analysis of Project DARE outcome evaluations. *American Journal of Public Health* 84(9):1394-1401.

EPA (Environmental Protection Agency). 1992. *Respiratory Health Effects of Passive Smoking: Lung Cancer and Other Disorders*. Washington, DC: Office of Health and Environmental Assessment, Office of Research and Development, U.S. Environmental Protection Agency.

EPA. 2006. *Health Effects of Exposure to Secondhand Smoke*. Web Page. Available at: http://www.epa.gov/smokefree/healtheffects.html; accessed July 7, 2006.

Etzel RA. 1997. Active and passive smoking: hazards for children. *Central European Journal of Public Health* 5(2):54-56.

Fagan P, Brook JS, Rubenstone E, Zhang C. 2005. Parental occupation, education, and smoking as predictors of offspring tobacco use in adulthood: a longitudinal study. *Addictive Behavior* 30(3):517-529.

Farkas AJ, Gilpin EA, White MM, Pierce JP. 2000. Association between household and workplace smoking restrictions and adolescent smoking. *Journal of the American Medical Association* 284(6):717-722.

Farquhar JW, Maccoby N, Wood PD, Alexander JK, Breitrose H, Brown BW Jr, Haskell WL, McAlister AL, Meyer AJ, Nash JD, Stern MP. 1977. Community education for cardiovascular health. *Lancet* 1(8023):1192-1195.

Farrelly MC, Chen J, Thomas KY, Healton CJ. 2001. *Legacy First Look Report 6: Youth Exposure to Environmental Tobacco Smoke*. Washington, DC: American Legacy Foundation.

Farrelly MC, Davis KC, Haviland ML, Messeri P, Healton CG. 2005. Evidence of a dose—response relationship between "truth" antismoking ads and youth smoking prevalence. *American Journal of Public Health* 95(3):425-431.

Farrelly MC, Healton CG, Davis KC, Messeri P, Hersey JC, Haviland ML. 2002. Getting to the truth: evaluating national tobacco countermarketing campaigns.[erratum appears in *American Journal of Public Health* 2003 May;93(5):703]. *American Journal of Public Health* 92(6):901-907.

Farrelly MC, Niederdeppe J, Yarsevich J. 2003. Youth tobacco prevention mass media campaigns: past, present, and future directions. *Tobacco Control* 12(Suppl 1):i35-i47.

Farrelly MC, Nonnemaker JM, Chou R, Hyland A, Peterson KK, Bauer UE. 2005. Changes in hospitality workers' exposure to secondhand smoke following the implementation of New York's smoke-free law. *Tobacco Control* 14(4):236-241.

Farrelly MC, Pechacek TF, Chaloupka FJ. 2003. The impact of tobacco control program expenditures on aggregate cigarette sales: 1981-2000. *Journal of Health Economics* 22(5):843-859.

Fee E, Brown TM. 2004. Hospital smoking bans and their impact. *American Journal of Public Health* 94(2):185.

Fichtenberg CM, Glantz SA. 2000. Association of the California Tobacco Control Program with declines in cigarette consumption and mortality from heart disease. *New England Journal of Medicine* 343(24):1772-1777.

Fichtenberg CM, Glantz SA. 2002. Effect of smoke-free workplaces on smoking behaviour: systematic review. *BMJ* 325(7357):188.

Fiore MC, Bailey WC, Cohen SJ. 2000. *Treating Tobacco Use and Dependence (Clinical Practice Guideline)*. Rockville, MD: U.S. Department of Health Human Services, Public Health Service.

Fiore MC, Croyle RT, Curry SJ, Cutler CM, Davis RM, Gordon C, Healton C, Koh HK, Orleans CT, Richling D, Satcher D, Seffrin J, Williams C, Williams LN, Keller PA, Baker TB. 2004. Preventing 3 million premature deaths and helping 5 million smokers quit: a national action plan for tobacco cessation. *American Journal of Public Health* 94(2):205-310.

Flay BR. 2000. Approaches to substance use prevention utilizing school curriculum plus social environment change. *Addictive Behavior* 25(6):861-885.

Flay BR, Hu FB, Richardson J. 1998. Psychosocial predictors of different stages of cigarette smoking among high school students. *Preventive Medicine* 27(5 Pt 3):9-18.

Flynn BS, Worden JK, Secker-Walker RH, Badger GJ, Geller BM. 1995. Cigarette smoking prevention effects of mass media and school interventions targeted to gender and age groups. *Journal of Health Education* 26(2):S45-S51.

Flynn BS, Worden JK, Secker-Walker RH, Badger GJ, Geller BM, Costanza MC. 1992. Prevention of cigarette smoking through mass media intervention and school programs. *American Journal of Public Health* 82(6):827-834.

Flynn BS, Worden JK, Secker-Walker RH, Pirie PL, Badger GJ, Carpenter JH, Geller BM. 1994. Mass media and school interventions for cigarette smoking prevention: effects 2 years after completion. *American Journal of Public Health*. 84(7):1148-1150.

Folsom D, Jeste DV. 2002. Schizophrenia in homeless persons: a systematic review of the literature. *Acta Psychiatrica Scandinavica* 105(6):404-413 .

Fong GT, Hyland A, Borland R, Hammond D, Hastings G, McNeill A, Anderson S, Cummings KM, Allwright S, Mulcahy M, Howell F, Clancy L, Thompson ME, Connolly G, Driezen P. 2006. Reductions in tobacco smoke pollution and increases in support for smoke-free public places following the implementation of comprehensive smoke-free workplace legislation in the Republic of Ireland: findings from the ITC Ireland/UK Survey. *Tobacco Controll* 15(Suppl 3):iii51-iii58.

Fraguela J, Martin A, Trinanes E. 2003. Drug-abuse prevention in the school: four-year follow-up of a programme. *Psychology in Spain* 7(1):29-38.

Frieden TR, Mostashari F, Kerker BD, Miller N, Hajat A, Frankel M. 2005. Adult tobacco use levels after intensive tobacco control measures: New York City, 2002–2003. *American Journal of Public Health* 95(6):1016-1023.

Friend K, Levy DT. 2002. Reductions in smoking prevalence and cigarette consumption associated with mass-media campaigns. [Review] [63 refs]. *Health Education Research*. 17(1):85-98.

Gallet CA, List JA. 2003. Cigarette demand: a meta-analysis of elasticities. *Health Economics* 12(10):821-835.

GAO (General Accounting Office). 2002. *Internet Cigarette Sales: Giving ATF Investigative Authority May Improve Reporting and Enforcement*. Washington, DC: GAO.

GAO. 2006. *Tobacco Settlement: States' Allocations of Fiscal Year 2005 and Expected Fiscal Year 2006 Payments*. Washington, DC: GAO.

Gerlach KK, Larkin MA. 2005. *To Improve Health and Health Care, Vol. VIII*. San Francisco, CA: Jossey-Bass.

Gilpin EA, Lee L, Pierce JP. 2005. How have smoking risk factors changed with recent declines in California adolescent smoking? *Addiction* 100(1):117-125.

Gilpin E, Lee L, Pierce JP, Tang H, Lloyd J. 2004. Support for protection from second hand smoke: California 2002. *Tobacco Control* 13(1):96.

Givel M, Glantz S. 2000. Failure to defend a successful state tobacco control program: policy lessons from Florida. *American Journal of Public Health* 90(5).

Givel S, Dearlove J, Glantz S. 2001. *Tobacco Policy Making in California 1999-2001: Stalled and Adrift.* San Francisco, CA: Center for Tobacco Research and Education (University of California).

Glantz S, Balbach E. 2000. *Tobacco War: Inside the California Battles.* Berkeley: University of California Press.

Glasgow RE, Cummings KM, Hyland A. 1997. Relationship of worksite smoking policy to changes in employee tobacco use: findings from COMMIT. Community Intervention Trial for Smoking Cessation. *Tobacco Control* 6(Suppl 2):S44-S48.

Glynn TJ. 1989. Essential elements of school-based smoking prevention programs. *Journal of School Health* 59(5):181-188.

Gortmaker SL, Walker DK, Jacobs FH, Ruch-Ross H. 1982. Parental smoking and the risk of childhood asthma. *American Journal of Public Health* 72(6):574-579.

Gross CP, Soffer B, Bach PB, Rajkumar R, Forman HP. 2002. State expenditures for tobacco-control programs and the tobacco settlement. *New England Journal of Medicine* 347(14):1080-1086.

Gruber J. 2001. Tobacco at the crossroads: the past and future of smoking regulation in the United States. *The Journal of Economic Perspectives* 15(2):193-212.

Halperin AC, Rigotti NA, Rothstein WG, Rajapaksa S. 2003. US public universities' compliance with recommended tobacco-control policies. *Journal of American College Health* 51(5):181.

Hamilton VH, Levinton C, St-Pierre Y, Grimard F. 1997. The effect of tobacco tax cuts on cigarette smoking in Canada. *Canadian Medical Association Journal* 156(2):187-191.

Hamilton W, Norton G, Weintraub J. 2002. *Independent Evaluation of the Massachusetts Tobacco Control Program, 7th Annual Report—January 1994 to June 2000.* Cambridge, MA: Abt Associates Inc.

Hamilton WL, Biener L, Rodger CN. 2005. Who supports tobacco excise taxes? Factors associated with towns' and individuals' support in Massachusetts. *Journal of Public Health Management and Practice* 11(4):333-340.

Hamilton WL, Rodger CN, Chen X, Njobe TK, Kling R, Norton G. 2003. *Independent Evaluation of the Massachusetts Tobacco Control Program. Eighth Annual Report: January 1994–June 2001.* Cambridge, MA: Abt Associates Inc.

Hamlett-Berry K. 2004. Smoking cessation policy in the VA health care system: Where have we been and where are we going? In: Isaccs S, ed. *VA in the Vanguard: Building on Sucess in Smoking Cessation: Proceedings of a Conference Held September 21, 2004 in San Francisco, California.* Washington, DC: Department of Veterans Affairs. Pp. 7-40.

Hammond D, McDonald PW, Fong GT, Borland R. 2004. Do smokers know how to quit? Knowledge and perceived effectiveness of cessation assistance as predictors of cessation behaviour. *Addiction* 99(8):1042-1048.

Hammond SK, Emmons KM. 2005. Inmate exposure to secondhand smoke in correctional facilities and the impact of smoking restrictions. *Journal of Exposure Analysis and Environmental Epidemiology* 15(3):205-211.

Hanewinkel R, Asshauer M. 2004. Fifteen-month follow-up results of a school-based life-skills approach to smoking prevention. *Health Education Research* 19(2):125-137.

Hansen W. 1988. Theory and Implementation of the Social Influence Model of Primary Prevention. *Prevention Research Findings: 1988. OSAP Prevention Monograph-3.* Washington, DC: Office of Substance Abuse Prevention (U.S. HHS).

Hansen WB, Malotte CK, Fielding JE. 1988. Evaluation of a tobacco and alcohol abuse prevention curriculum for adolescents. *Health Education Quarterly* 15(1):93-114.

Harris JE, Chan SW. 1999. The continuum-of-addiction: cigarette smoking in relation to price among Americans aged 15-29. *Health Economics* 8(1):81-86.

Hay JW. 1991. The Harm They Do to Others: A Primer on the External Costs of Drug Abuse. *Searching for Alternatives: Drug Control Policy in the United States.* Stanford, CA: Hoover Institution Press. Pp. 200-225.

Hennrikus D, Pentel PR, Sandell SD. 2003. Preferences and practices among renters regarding smoking restrictions in apartment buildings. *Tobacco Control* 12(2):189-194.

HEW (Department of Health, Education, and Welfare). 1964. *Smoking and Health: Report of the Advisory Committee to the Surgeon General of the Public Health Service.* Washington, DC: U.S. Department of Health, Education, and Welfare; Public Health Service.

Hill KG, Hawkins JD, Catalano RF, Abbott RD, Guo J. 2005. Family influences on the risk of daily smoking initiation. *J Adolesc Health* 37(3):202-210.

Hopkins DP, Briss PA, Ricard CJ, Husten CG, Carande-Kulis VG, Fielding JE, Alao MO, McKenna JW, Sharp DJ, Harris JR, Woollery TA, Harris KW. 2001. Reviews of evidence regarding interventions to reduce tobacco use and exposure to environmental tobacco smoke. *American Journal of Preventive Medicine* 20(2 Suppl):16-66.

Hu TW, Ren QF, Keeler TE, Bartlett J. 1995a. The demand for cigarettes in California and behavioural risk factors. *Health Economics* 4(1):7-14.

Hu TW, Sung HY, Keeler TE. 1995b. The state antismoking campaign and the industry response: the effects of advertising on cigarette consumption in California. *American Economic Review* 85(2):85-90.

Hyland A, Higbee C, Li Q, Bauer JE, Giovino GA, Alford T, Cummings KM. 2005. Access to low-taxed cigarettes deters smoking cessation attempts. *American Journal of Public Health* 95(6):994-995.

Hyland A, Li Q, Bauer JE, Giovino GA, Steger C, Cummings KM. 2004. Predictors of cessation in a cohort of current and former smokers followed over 13 years. *Nicotine and Tobacco Research* 6(Suppl 3):S363 S369.

IARC (International Agency for Research on Cancer). 2002. *Volume 83 Tobacco Smoke and Involuntary Smoking.* Web Page. Available at: http://monographs.iarc.fr/ENG/Monographs/vol83/volume83.pdf; accessed June 8, 2007.

Independent Evaluation Consortium. 2002. *Final Report. Independent Evaluation of the California Tobacco Control Prevention and Education Program: Waves 1, 2, and 3 (1996–2000).* Rockville, MD: The Gallup Organization.

IOM (Institute of Medicine). 1988. *The Future of Public Health.* Washington, DC: National Academy Press.

IOM. 1994a. *Growing Up Tobacco Free: Preventing Nicotine Addiction in Children and Youth.* Washington, DC: National Academy Press.

IOM. 1994b. *Growing Up Tobacco Free: Preventing Nicotine Addiction in Children and Youth.* Washington, DC: National Academy Press.

IOM/NRC (National Research Council). 2004. *Reducing Underage Drinking: A Collective Responsibility.* Washington, DC: The National Academies Press.

Jackson C, Henriksen L. 1997. Do as I say: parent smoking, antismoking socialization, and smoking onset among children. *Addictive Behavior* 22(1):107-114.

Jemal A, Cokkinides VE, Shafey O, Thun MJ. 2003. Lung cancer trends in young adults: an early indicator of progress in tobacco control (United States). *Cancer Causes Control* 14(6):579-585.

Johnson CA, Pentz MA, Weber MD, Dwyer JH, Baer N, MacKinnon DP, Hansen WB, Flay BR. 1990. Relative effectiveness of comprehensive community programming for drug abuse prevention with high-risk and low-risk adolescents. *Journal of Consulting and Clinical Psychology* 58(4):447-456.

Jordaan ER, Ehrlich RI, Potter P. 1999. Environmental tobacco smoke exposure in children: household and community determinants. *Archives of Environmental Health* 54(5):319-327.

Kandula NR, Kersey M, Lurie N. 2004. Assuring the health of immigrants: what the leading health indicators tell us. *Annual Review of Public Health* 25:357-376.

Keeler TE, Hu TW, Barnett PG, Manning WG. 1993. Taxation, regulation, and addiction: a demand function for cigarettes based on time-series evidence. *Journal of Health Economics* 12(1):1-18.

Kempner M. 2005, June 6. UPS reviews cigarette shipments. *The Atlanta Journal-Constitution*. Business.

Kerr M, Stattin H. 2000. What parents know, how they know it, and several forms of adolescent adjustment: further support for a reinterpretation of monitoring. *Developmental Psychology* 36(3):366-380.

Kesich GD. 2004, November 18. UPS, others sue over Maine tobacco law; the suit challenges the rewuirement that delivery driver verify age, identity of tobacco recipients. *Portland Press Herald*. Local & State.

Klepp KI, Halper A, Perry CL. 1986. The efficacy of peer leaders in drug abuse prevention. *Journal of School Health* 56(9):407-411.

Klevens RM, Giovino GA, Peddicord JP, Nelson DE, Mowery P, Grummer-Strawn L. 1995. The Association Between Veteran Status and Cigarette-Smoking Behaviors. *American Journal of Preventive Medicine* 11(4):245-250.

Kuiper N, Nelson D, Schooley M. 2005. *Evidence of Effectiveness: A Summary of State Tobacco Control Program Evaluation Literature*. Atlanta, GA: U.S. Department of Health and Human Services, Centers for Disease Control and Prevention, National Center for Chronic Disease Prevention and Health Promotion, Office on Smoking and Health.

Kulig JW. 2005. Tobacco, alcohol, and other drugs: the role of the pediatrician in prevention, identification, and management of substance abuse. *Pediatrics* 115(3):816-821.

Leverett M, Ashe M, Gerard S, Jenson J, Woollery T. 2002. Tobacco use: the impact of prices. *Journal of Law, Medicine and Ethics* 30(3 Suppl):88-95.

Levinson A, Pérez-Stable E, Espinoza P, Flores E, Byers TE. 2004. Latinos report less use of pharmaceutical aids when trying to quit smoking. *American Journal of Prevtive Medicine* 26(2):105-111.

Levy DT, Romano E, Mumford E. 2005. The relationship of smoking cessation to sociodemographic characteristics, smoking intensity, and tobacco control policies. *Nicotine & Tobacco Research* 7(3):387-396.

Levy DT, Romano E, Mumford EA. 2004. Recent trends in home and work smoking bans. *Tobacco Control* 13(3):258-263.

Liang L, Chaloupka F, Nichter M, Clayton R. 2003. Prices, policies and youth smoking, May 2001. *Addiction* 98(Suppl 1):105-122.

Loukas A, Garcia M, Gottlieb NH. 2006. Texas college students' opinions of no-smoking policies, secondhand smoke, and smoking in public places. *Journal of American College Health* 1(55):27-32.

Lowenstein S, Tomlinson D, Koziol-McLain J, Prochazka A. 1995. Smoking habits of emergency department patients: an opportunity for disease prevention. *Academic Emergency Medicine* 2:165-171.

Luepker RV, Murray DM, Jacobs DR Jr, Mittelmark MB, Bracht N, Carlaw R, Crow R, Elmer P, Finnegan J, Folsom AR, et al. 1994. Community education for cardiovascular disease prevention: risk factor changes in the Minnesota Heart Health Program. *American Journal of Public Health* 84(9):1383-1393.

Ma GX, Tan Y, Toubbeh JI, Su X, Shive SE, Lan Y. 2004. Acculturation and smoking behavior in Asian-American populations. *Health Education Research* 19(6):615-625.

Manning WG, Keeler EB, Newhouse JP, Sloss EM, Wasserman J. 1989. The taxes of sin: do smokers and drinkers pay their way? *Journal of the American Medical Assocation* 261(11):1604-1609.

Mannino DM, Siegel M, Husten C, Rose D, Etzel R. 1996. Environmental tobacco smoke exposure and health effects in children: results from the 1991 National Health Interview Survey. *Tobacco Control* 5(1):13-18.

McPhillips-Tangum C, Bocchino C, Carreon R, Erceg C, Rehm B. 2004. Addressing tobacco in managed care: results of the 2002 survey. *Preventing Chronic Disease* 1(4): 1-11

MDPH (Massachusetts Department of Public Health). 2002a. *MTCP Background*. Web Page. Available at: http://www.mass.gov/dph/mtcp/background/background.htm; accessed June 23, 2006.

MDPH. 2002b. *MTCP Statewide Services*. Web Page. Available at: http://www.mass.gov/dph/mtcp/programs/statewide.htm; accessed July 20, 2006.

MDPH. 2006, June 22. *Massachusetts Tobacco Control Program Accomplishments*. Web Page. Available at: http://www.mass.gov/dph/mtcp/reports/accomplishments.pdf; accessed June 22, 2006.

Michel L. 2005, April 4. Internet cigarette sales take hit. *Buffalo News*. News.

Miller A. 1998. Designing an effective counteradvertising campaign—Massachusetts. *Cancer* 83(12 Suppl Robert):2742-2745.

Miller DR, Kalman D, Ren XS, Lee AF, Niu Z, Kazis LE. 2001. *Health Behaviors of Veterans in the VHA: Tobacco Use*. Washington, DC: U.S. Department of Veterans Affairs Veterans Health Administration Office of Quality and Performance and VHA Health Assessment Project Center for Health Quality, Outcomes, and Economic Research.

Mittelmark MB, Luepker RV, Jacobs DR, Bracht NF, Carlaw RW, Crow RS, Finnegan J, Grimm RH, Jeffery RW, Kline FG, et al. 1986. Community-wide prevention of cardiovascular disease: education strategies of the Minnesota Heart Health Program. *Preventive Medicine* 15(1):1-17.

The Monitor's View. 2005, July 7. Snuffing out tobacco in prisons. *Christian Science Monitor*. P. 8.

Moskowitz JM, Lin Z, Hudes ES. 2000. The impact of workplace smoking ordinances in California on smoking cessation. *American Journal of Public Health* 90(5):757-761.

Murray DM, Hannan PJ, Jacobs DR, McGovern PJ, Schmid L, Baker WL, Gray C. 1994. Assessing intervention effects in the Minnesota Heart Health Program. *American Journal of Epidemiology* 139(1):91-103.

Najera AP. 1998. History of successful ballot initiatives—California. *Cancer* 83(12 Suppl Robert):2680-2684.

National Journal Group. 2005, June 20. Efforts to regulate internet tobacco sales may be revived. *National Journal's Congress Daily*.

NCI (National Cancer Institute). 2005. ASSIST: shaping the future of tobacco prevention and control. NCI. *Tobacco Control Monograph Series*. Vol. 8, No. NIH Publication Number 05-5645. Bethesda, MD: National Institutes of Health.

Nicholl J. 1998. Tobacco tax initiatives to prevent tobacco use: a study of eight statewide campaigns. *Cancer* 83(12 Suppl Robert):2666-2679.

Niederdeppe J, Farrelly MC, Haviland ML. 2004. Confirming "truth": more evidence of a successful tobacco countermarketing campaign in Florida. *American Journal of Public Health* 94(2):255-257.

NIH (National Institutes of Health). 2006a. *Final Statement: National Institutes of Health State-of-the-Science Conference Statement, Tobacco Use: Prevention, Cessation, and Control.* Web Page. Available at: http://consensus.nih.gov/2006/TobaccoStatement Final090506.pdf; accessed January 18, 2007a.

NIH. 2006b. *National Institutes of Health State-of-the-Science Conference Statement.* Web Page. Available at: http://consensus.nih.gov/2006/2006TobaccoSOS029html.htm; accessed July 26, 2006.

O'Byrne KK, Haddock CK, Poston WS. 2002. Parenting style and adolescent smoking. *Journal of Adolescent Health* 30(6):418-425.

Older Americans Report. 2005, August 5. City's housing authority bans smoking in senior apartments. *Older Americans Report.*

Orleans CT. 1993. Treating Nicotine Dependence in Medical Settings: A Stepped-Care Model. Orleans CT, Slade J, Editors. *Nicotine Addiciton: Principles and Management.* New York: Oxford University Press. Pp. 145-161.

Orleans CT, Fishman J. 2000. Tailored communications for smoking cessation. *Tobacco Control* 9(Suppl I):i49.

Osterwalder J, Beeman DE. 2005, April 13. Fresh air: officials to consider tougher rules; no vacancy for smokers; smoke-free housing debate forces leaders to pit personal rights vs. health concerns. *The Press Enterprise.* A. p. 1.

OTRU (Ontario Tobacco Research Unit). 2006. *The Smoke-Free Ontario Act: Extend Protection to Children in Vehicles.* Web Page. Available at: http://www.otru.org/pdf/updates/update_aug2006.pdf; accessed January 19, 2007.

Ozer EM, Adams SH, Gardner LR, Mailloux DE, Wibbelsman CJ, Irwin CE Jr. 2004. Provider self-efficacy and the screening of adolescents for risky health behaviors. *Journal of Adolescent Health* 35(2):101-107.

Parmet WE, Banthin C. 2005. Public health protection and the commerce clause: controlling tobacco in the Internet Age. *New Mexico Law Review* 35:81-122.

Patrick S, Marsh R. 2001. Current tobacco policies in U.S. adult male prisons. *The Social Science Journal* 38:27-37.

Pechmann C, Reibling ET. 2000. Planning an effective anti-smoking mass media campaign targeting adolescents. *Journal of Public Health Management and Practice* 6(3):80-94.

Pechmann C, Slater MD. 2005. Social Marketing Messages That May Motivate Irresponsible Behavior. Ratneshwar S. *Inside Consumption: Consumer Motives, Goals, and Desires.* New York: Routledge.

Pentz MA, MacKinnon DP, Dwyer JH, Wang EY, Hansen WB, Flay BR, Johnson CA. 1989. Longitudinal effects of the midwestern prevention project on regular and experimental smoking in adolescents. *Preventive Medicine* 18(2):304-321.

Perry C, Kelder S, Klepp K. 1994. Community-wide cardiovascular disease prevention in young people. *European Journal of Public Health* 4:188-194.

Perry CL, Kelder K-I, Siller C. 1989. Community-wide strategies for cardiovascular health: the Minnesota heart health program youth program. *Health Education Research* 4: 87-101.

Perry CL, Kelder SH, Murray DM, Klepp KI. 1992. Communitywide smoking prevention: long-term outcomes of the Minnesota Heart Health Program and the Class of 1989 Study. *American Journal of Public Health* 82(9):1210-1216.

Peterson AV Jr, Kealey KA, Mann SL, Marek PM, Sarason IG. 2000. Hutchinson Smoking Prevention Project: long-term randomized trial in school-based tobacco use prevention—results on smoking. *Journal of the National Cancer Institute* 92(24):1979-1991.

Pierce J, Gilpin E, Emery S, Farkas A, Zhu S, Choi W, Berry C, Distefan J, White M, Soroko S, Navarro A. 1998. *Tobacco Control in California: Who's Winning the War? An Evaluation of the Tobacco Control Program, 1989–1996*. La Jolla, CA: University of California, San Diego.

Pierce JP, White MM, Gilpin EA. 2005. Adolescent smoking decline during California's tobacco control programme. *Tobacco Control* 14(3):207-212.

Pinilla J. 2002. [Tobacco taxes, prices and demand for tobacco products: a comparative analysis]. *Gaceta Sanitaria* 16(5):425-435.

Pizacani BA, Martin DP, Stark MJ, Koepsell TD, Thompson B, Diehr P. 2004. A prospective study of household smoking bans and subsequent cessation related behaviour: the role of stage of change. *Tobacco Control* 13(1):23-28.

Popham WJ, Potter LD, Bal DG, Johnson MD, Duerr JM, Quinn V. 1993. Do anti-smoking media campaigns help smokers quit?. *Public Health Report.* 108(4):510-513.

Popham WJ, Potter LD, Hetrick MA, Muthen LK, Duerr JM, Johnson MD. 1994a. Effectiveness of the California 1990-1991 Tobacco Education Media Campaign. *American Journal of Preventive Medicine* 10(6):319-326.

Popham WJ, Potter LD, Hetrick MA, Muthen LK, Duerr JM, Johnson MD. 1994b. Effectiveness of the California 1990–1991 tobacco education media campaign. *American Journal of Preventive Medicine* 10(6):319-326.

Powell LM, Tauras JA, Ross H. 2005. The importance of peer effects, cigarette prices and tobacco control policies for youth smoking behavior. *Journal of Health Economics* 24(5):950-968.

Public Health Service. 2000. *Reducing Tobacco Use: A Report of the Surgeon General*. Public Health Service Pub.

Repace J. 2000. Banning outdoor smoking is scientifically justifiable. *Tobacco Control* 9(1):98.

Rigotti N. 2001. Chapter 6—reducing the supply of tobacco to youths. *Regulating Tobacco*. New York: Oxford University Press. Pp. 143-175.

Ross H, Chaloupka FJ. 2003. The effect of cigarette prices on youth smoking. *Health Economics* 12(3):217-230.

RTI International. 2004. *First Annual Independent Evaluation of New York's Tobacco Control Program*. Research Triangle Park, NC: RTI International.

RTI International. 2005. *Second Annual Independent Evaluation of New York's Tobacco Control Program*. Research Triangle Park, NC: RTI International.

Russell CM. 1998. Evaluation: methods and strategy for evaluation—California. *Cancer* 83(12 Suppl Robert):2755-2759.

Schauffler HH, Barker DC, Orleans CT. 2001. Medicaid coverage for tobacco-dependence treatments. *Health Affairs (Millwood)* 20(1):298 303.

Schoenmarklin S, Tobacco Control Legal Consortium. 2004. *Infiltration of Secondhand Smoke into Condominiums, Apartments and Other Multi-Unit Dwellings*. St. Paul, MN: Tobacco Control Legal Consortium.

Schroeder SA. 2006. Should emergency physicians help smokers quit? *Annals of Emergency Medicine* 48(4):415-416.

Scollo M, and Lal A. 2004. *Summary of Studies Assessing the Economic Effects of Smoke-Free Policies in the Hospitality Industry*. Web Page. Available at: http://www.vctc.org.au/tc-res/Hospitalitysummary.pdf; accessed February 23, 2005.

Scollo M, Younie S, Wakefield M, Freeman J, Icasiano F. 2003. Impact of tobacco tax reforms on tobacco prices and tobacco use in Australia. *Tobacco Control* 12(Suppl 2):ii59-ii66.

Siahpush M, Borland R, Scollo M. 2003. Factors associated with smoking cessation in a national sample of Australians. *Nicotine and Tobacco Research* 5(4):597-602.

Siegel M. 2002. The effectiveness of state-level tobacco control interventions: a review of program implementation and behavioral outcomes. *Annual Review of Public Health* 23:45-71.

Siegel M, Biener L. 2000. The impact of an antismoking media campaign on progression to established smoking: results of a longitudinal youth study. *American Journal of Public Health* 90(3):380-386.

Siegel M, Mowery PD, Pechacek TP, Strauss WJ, Schooley MW, Merritt RK, Novotny TE, Giovino GA, Eriksen MP. 2000. Trends in adult cigarette smoking in California compared with the rest of the United States, 1978–1994. *American Journal of Public Health* 90(3):372-379.

Simons-Morton B, Chen R, Abroms L, Haynie DL. 2004. Latent growth curve analyses of peer and parent influences on smoking progression among early adolescents. *Health Psychology* 23(6):612-621.

Skara S, Sussman S. 2003. A review of 25 long-term adolescent tobacco and other drug use prevention program evaluations. *Preventive Medicine* 37(5):451-474.

Sloan FA, Carlisle ES, Rattliff JR, Trogdon J. 2005. Determinants of states' allocations of the master settlement agreement payments. *Journal of Health and Political Policy Law* 30(4):643-86.

Sloan FA, Mathews CA, Trogdon JG. 2004. Impacts of the Master Settlement Agreement on the tobacco industry. *Tobacco Control* 13(4):356-361.

Sly DF, Heald GR, Ray S. 2001a. The Florida "truth" anti-tobacco media evaluation: design, first year results, and implications for planning future state media evaluations.[see comment]. *Tobacco Control* 10(1):9-15.

Sly DF, Hopkins RS, Trapido E, Ray S. 2001b. Influence of a counteradvertising media campaign on initiation of smoking: the Florida "truth" campaign. *American Journal of Public Health* 91(2):233-238.

Sly DF, Trapido E, Ray S. 2002. Evidence of the dose effects of an antitobacco counteradvertising campaign. *Preventive Medicine*. 35(5):511-518.

Smith CM, Pristach CA, Cartagena M. 1999. Obligatory cessation of smoking by psychiatric inpatients. *Psychiatric Service*. 50(1):91-94.

Smith E, Swisher J, Vicary J, et al. 2004. Evaluation of life skills training and infused-life skills training in a rural setting: outcomes at two years. *Journal of Alcohol and Drug Education* 48(1):51-70.

Smokefree Apartment House Registry. 2004. *News Release: City Creates Non-Smoking Sections in New Affordable Housing*. Web Page. Available at: http://www.smokefree apartments.org/T.O.%20News%20Release.pdf; accessed July 14, 2006.

Snyder LB, Hamilton MA, Mitchell EW, Kiwanuka-Tondo J, Fleming-Milici F, Proctor D. 2004. A meta-analysis of the effect of mediated health communication campaigns on behavior change in the United States. *Journal of Health Communication* 9(Suppl 1):71-96.

Soldz S, Clark TW, Stewart E, Celebucki C, Klein Walker D. 2002. Decreased youth tobacco use in Massachusetts 1996 to 1999: evidence of tobacco control effectiveness. *Tobacco Control* 11(Suppl 2):ii14-ii19.

Spoth RL, Redmond C, Trudeau L, Shin C. 2002. Longitudinal substance initiation outcomes for a universal preventive intervention combining family and school programs. *Psychology of Addictive Behavior* 16(2):129-134.

State of California. 2004. *Proposition 99 and the Legislative Mandate for the California Tobacco Control Program*. Web Page. Available at: http://www.dhs.ca.gov/tobacco/html/about.htm; accessed May 22, 2006.

Stattin H, Kerr M. 2000. Parental monitoring: a reinterpretation. *Childhood Development* 71(4):1072-1085.

Steinberg L, Fletcher A, Darling N. 1994. Parental monitoring and peer influences on adolescent substance use. *Pediatrics* 93(6 Pt 2):1060-1064.

Stephens T, Pederson LL, Koval JJ, Kim C. 1997. The relationship of cigarette prices and no-smoking bylaws to the prevalence of smoking in Canada. *American Journal of Public Health* 87(9):1519-1521.

Stephens T, Pederson LL, Koval JJ, Macnab J. 2001. Comprehensive tobacco control policies and the smoking behaviour of Canadian adults. *Tobacco Control* 10(4):317-322.

Stevens C. 1998. Designing an effective counteradvertising campaign—California. *Cancer* 83(12 Suppl Robert):2736-2741.

Stillman FA, Hartman AM, Graubard BI, Gilpin EA, Murray DM, Gibson JT. 2003. Evaluation of the American Stop Smoking Intervention Study (ASSIST): a report of outcomes. *Journal of the National Cancer Institute* 95(22):1681-1691.

Tacoma-Pierce County Health Department. 2003. *Fresh Air Everywhere*. Web Page. Available at: http://www.tpchd.org/files/library/fb76d4134077b3c4.pdf; accessed July 11, 2006.

Task Force on Community Preventive Services. 2001. Recommendations regarding interventions to reduce tobacco use and exposure to environmental tobacco smoke. *American Journal of Preventive Medicine* 20(2 Suppl):10-15.

Task Force on Community Preventive Services. 2005. *The Guide to Community Preventive Services (Community Guide): What Works to Promote Health?* Oxford, England: Oxford University Press.

Tauras JA. 2004a. Public policy and smoking cessation among young adults in the United States. *Health Policy* 68(3):321-332.

Tauras JA. 2004b. Public policy and smoking cessation among young adults in the United States. *Health Policy* 68(3):321-332.

Tauras JA, Chaloupka FJ, Farrelly MC, Giovino GA, Wakefield M, Johnston LD, O'Malley PM, Kloska DD, Pechacek TF. 2005. State tobacco control spending and youth smoking. *American Journal of Public Health* 95(2):338-344.

Tedeschi B. 2005, April 4. Now That Credit Card Companies Won't Handle Online Tobacco Sales, Many Merchants Are Calling It Quits. *The New York Times*. C. p. 5.

TEROC (Tobacco Education and Research Oversight Committee). 2000. *Toward a Tobacco-Free California: Strategies for the 21st Century, 2000-2003*. Web Page. Available at: http://www.dhs.ca.gov/tobacco/documents/pubs/TEROCReport99.pdf; accessed February 1, 2006.

TEROC. 2003. *Toward a Tobacco-Free California, 2003-2005: The Myth of Victory*. Web Page. Available at: http://www.dhs.ca.gov/tobacco/documents/pubs/TobaccoMasterPlan 2003.pdf; accessed February 1, 2006.

Thomson CC, Fisher LB, Winickoff JP, Colditz GA, Camargo CA Jr, King C 3rd, Frazier AL. 2004. State tobacco excise taxes and adolescent smoking behaviors in the United States. *Journal of Public Health Management and Practice* 10(6):490-496.

Tilson EC, McBride CM, Lipkus IM, Catalano RF. 2004. Testing the interaction between parent-child relationship factors and parent smoking to predict youth smoking. *Journal of Adolescent Health* 35(3):182-189.

Times Wire Services. 2006, July 6. DHL to Restrict Cigarette Shipments. *Los Angeles Times*. Business. P. 3.

TIPS (Tobacco Information and Prevention Source). 2006a. *Exposure to Environmental Tobacco Smoke and Nicotine Levels—Fact Sheet*. Web Page. Available at: http://www.cdc.gov/tobacco/research data/environmental/factsheet ets.htm; accessed July 14, 2006.

TIPS. 2006b. *Secondhand Smoke: Fact Sheet*. Web Page. Available at: http://www.cdc.gov/tobacco/factsheets/secondhand_smoke_factsheet.htm; accessed July 10, 2006.

Tobler NS. 1992. Drug prevention programs can work: research findings. *Journal of Addictive Disorders* 11(3):1-28.

Trochim WM, Stillman FA, Clark PI, Schmitt CL. 2003. Development of a model of the tobacco industry's interference with tobacco control programmes. *Tobacco Control* 12(2):140-147.

Trudeau L, Spoth R, Lillehoj C, Redmond C, Wickrama KA. 2003. Effects of a preventive intervention on adolescent substance use initiation, expectancies, and refusal intentions. *Prevention Science* 4(2):109-122.

Tuttle R. 2006, July 6. DHL Agrees to Stop Shipping Cigarettes Sold Via Internet. *Newsday.*

Ubelacker S. 2005, August 15. Kids' exposure to second-hand smoke may lead to smoking as teens: study. *Canadian Press NewsWire.* Web page. Available at: http://www.nexis.com; accessed July 11, 2006.

UPS reviews cigarette shipments. 2005. *Atlanta Journal Constitution.* July 6, D3.

U.S. Fed News. 2005, March 17. Attorneys General, ATF Announce Joint Initiative with Credit Card Companies to Prevent Illegal Cigarette Sales Over Internet. *U.S. Fed News.*

Vartiainen E, Fallonen U, McAlister AL, Puska P. 1990. Eight-year follow-up results of an adolescent smoking prevention program: the North Karelia Youth Project. *American Journal of Public Health* 80(1):78-79.

Vartiainen E, Paavola M, McAlister A, Puska P. 1998. Fifteen-year follow-up of smoking prevention effects in the North Karelia youth project. *American Journal of Public Health* 88(1):81-85.

Vartiainen E, Pallonen U, McAlister A, Koskela K, Puska P. 1983. Effect of two years of educational intervention on adolescent smoking (the North Karelia Youth Project). *Bulletin of the World Health Organization* 61(3):529-532.

Vartiainen E, Pallonen U, McAlister A, Koskela K, Puska P. 1986. Four-year follow-up results of the smoking prevention program in the North Karelia Youth Project. *Preventive Medicine* 15(6):692-698.

Vokes NI, Bailey JM, Rhodes KV. 2006. "Should I give you my smoking lecture now or later?" Characterizing emergency physician smoking discussions and cessation counseling. *Annals of Emergency Medicine* 48(4):406-414, 414-417.

Wakefield M, Chaloupka F. 2000. Effectiveness of comprehensive tobacco control programmes in reducing teenage smoking in the USA. *Tobacco Control* 9(2):177-186.

Wakefield MA, Chaloupka FJ, Kaufman NJ, Orleans CT, Barker DC, Ruel EE. 2000. Effect of restrictions on smoking at home, at school, and in public places on teenage smoking: cross sectional study. *BMJ* 321(7257):333-337.

Wallack L, Dorfman L, Jernigan D, Mekani T. 1993. *Media Advocacy and Public Health.* Newbury Park, CA: Sage Publications.

Waller BJ, Cohen JE, Ferrence R, Bull S, Adlaf EM. 2003. The early 1990s cigarette price decrease and trends in youth smoking in Ontario. *Canadian Journal of Public Health* 94(1):31-35.

Warner KE. 1977. The effects of the anti-smoking campaign on cigarette consumption. *American Journal of Public Health* 67(7):645-650.

Warner K. 2000. The deed for, and value of, a multi-level approach to disease prevention: the case of tobacco control. IOM. *Promoting Health: Intervention Strategies From Social and Behavioral Research.* Washington, DC: National Academy Press. Pp. 417-449.

Warner KE. 1979. Clearing the airwaves: the cigarette ad ban revisited. *Policy Analysis* 5:435-450.

Warner KE. 1985. Cigarette advertising and media coverage of smoking and health. *New England Journal of Medicine* 312(6):384-388.

Warner KE, Mendez D, Smith DG. 2004. The financial implications of coverage of smoking cessation treatment by managed care organizations. *Inquiry* 41(1):57-69.

Washington State Department of Revenue. 2005. *Major Tribal Internet Cigarette Seller Agrees to Provider Customer Lists.* Web Page. Available at: http://dor.wa.gov/Docs/Pubs/News/2005/NR_Smoke signals_settles.pdf, accessed July 11, 2006.

Wechsler H, Kelley K, Seibring M, Kuo M, Rigotti NA. 2001. College smoking policies and smoking cessation programs: results of a survey of college health center directors. *Journal of American College Health* 49(5):205-213.

Weintraub JM, Hamilton WL. 2002. Trends in prevalence of current smoking, Massachusetts and states without tobacco control programmes, 1990 to 1999. *Tobacco Control* 11(Suppl 2)ii8 ii13.

White J, Bero LA. 2004. Public health under attack: the American Stop Smoking Intervention Study (ASSIST) and the tobacco industry. *American Journal of Public Health* 94(2):240-250.

Wiehe SE, Garrison MM, Christakis DA, Ebel BE, Rivara FP. 2005. A systematic review of school-based smoking prevention trials with long-term follow-up. *Journal of Adolescent Health* 36(3):162-169.

Wilcox GJ. 2005, April 14. Apartment smoking bans may widen. *Daily News.*

Worden JK, Flynn BS, Geller BM, Chen M, Shelton LG, Secker-Walker RH, Solomon DS, Solomon LJ, Couchey S, Costanza MC. 1988. Development of a smoking prevention mass media program using diagnostic and formative research. *Preventive Medicine.* 17(5):531-558.

Yolton K, Dietrich K, Auinger P, Lanphear BP, Hornung R. 2005. Exposure to environmental tobacco smoke and cognitive abilities among U.S. children and adolescents. *Environmental Health Perspectives* 113(1):98-103.

Yong HH, Borland R, Siahpush M. 2005. Quitting-related beliefs, intentions, and motivations of older smokers in four countries: findings from the International Tobacco Control Policy Evaluation Survey. *Addictive Behavior* 30(4):777-788.

Yurekli AA, Zhang P. 2000. The impact of clean indoor-air laws and cigarette smuggling on demand for cigarettes: an empirical model. *Health Economics* 9(2):159-170.

Zhu S, Melcer T, Sun J, Rosbrook B, Pierce JP. 2000. Smoking cessation with and without assistance: a population-based analysis. *American Journal of Preventive Medicine* 18(4):305-311.

Zollinger TW, Saywell RM Jr, Muegge CM, Wooldridge JS, Cummings SF, Caine VA. 2003. Impact of the life skills training curriculum on middle school students tobacco use in Marion County, Indiana, 1997–2000. *Journal of School Health* 73(9):338-346.

Zucker D, Hopkins RS, Sly DF, Ulrich J, Kershaw JM, Solari S. 2000. Florida's "truth" campaign: a counter-marketing, anti-tobacco media campaign. *Journal of Public Health Management and Practice* 6(3):1-6.

6

Changing the Regulatory Landscape

The first prong of the committee's blueprint for reducing tobacco use, set forth in Chapter 5, envisions strengthening traditional tobacco control measures. If the plan set forth in Chapter 5 is successfully implemented and sustained, it could have a significant impact on tobacco use; but even an optimistic projection leaves prevalence at 10 percent in 2025, and a more realistic projection might be 15 percent. The main argument presented in this chapter is that a more substantial long-term impact requires a change in the current legal framework of tobacco control to a new, innovative regulatory approach that takes into account the unique history and characteristics of tobacco.

Over the past two decades, tobacco control policy has developed incrementally as the nation has moved step-by-step from a laissez-faire legal system embedded in a smoking culture to a system with coherent antismoking policy grounded in public health. Incremental reforms, however, will not end the nation's tobacco problem. A more fundamental shift must occur. It is time for Congress and other policy makers to change the legal structure of tobacco policy, thereby laying the foundation for a strategic initiative to end the nation's tobacco problem, that is, reducing tobacco use to a level that is insignificant from a public health standpoint. In this chapter, the committee sets forth the blueprint for a new regulatory approach.

Currently (and under the interventions of the blueprint outlined in Chapter 5), the implicit model of tobacco control is demand reduction combined with reactive efforts to prevent the tobacco industry from impeding demand-reducing policies. This leaves in place the supply side (the product and its existing channels of distribution) as well as all the existing incentives for attracting more consumers and selling more cigarettes. A more ambitious strategy would ask these questions: Can anything be done to substantially curtail the availability of tobacco products? Can anything be done to change tobacco products to make them less hazardous? Is it possible to bring the industry's incentives into closer alignment with the public health goals of tobacco control? No existing regulatory statute provides a model for tobacco products because there is no other lawful product for which the declared public goal is to suppress its use altogether. A new legal regime, new models, and new policy paradigms are needed.

The challenge, then, is to craft a policy framework that is aligned with the unique aim of tobacco control policy: to substantially reduce, if not eliminate, the use of this unusually damaging product without replicating the problems associated with the prohibition of alcohol in the 1920s and with the contemporary prohibitions of illegal drugs (e.g., widespread noncompliance, violent black markets, corruption, and high rates of arrest). In this chapter and Chapter 7, the committee offers several ideas for more fundamental change.

FEDERAL REGULATORY AUTHORITY IS NEEDED

It is clear that the U.S. Congress has the constitutional authority to enact national legislation bearing on all domains of tobacco control, including banning the distribution and use of tobacco products, analogous to the authority that it exercises over controlled substances such as peyote and marijuana. The pertinent policy questions are (1) whether Congress should exercise its constitutional authority (by prescribing national rules or by delegating the authority to do so to a federal agency, such as the Food and Drug Administration [FDA]), or, conversely, whether it should allow the states to exercise primary authority to regulate the production, distribution, marketing, and use of tobacco; and (2) if Congress does exercise federal regulatory authority in any of these domains, whether it should leave any room for supplemental state regulation and, if so, within what constraints. The committee believes that the time has come for Congress to exercise its acknowledged authority to regulate the production, marketing, and distribution of tobacco products while freeing the states to supplement federal action with their own measures that aim to suppress tobacco use and that are compatible with federal law.

Relationship Between Federal and State Tobacco Regulation

Setting aside the complexities of a complicated body of federal law, Congress has essentially three options: (1) state control, in which the federal government leaves regulation in a particular domain to the states (and, depending on state law, to localities); (2) federal preemption, in which the federal government has complete regulatory control and precludes any state regulation in the area; and (3) complementary regulation, in which the federal government establishes regulations on a particular subject but does not exclude the states from also establishing regulations. Under the third approach, the federal action typically establishes minimum requirements for the whole country (the basic requirements) while allowing the states to adopt more stringent regulations. Familiar examples of these three approaches include the state regulation of the retail distribution of alcohol, federal preemption of the state regulation of employee benefit plans under the Employee Retirement and Income Security Act, and complementary regulation of controlled substances.

At present, tobacco regulation in the United States is characterized by plenary state control except in the federally preempted domain of information or warnings "based on smoking and health," as defined in the 1969 Cigarette Labeling Act. The preemption language adopted by the Congress has been construed broadly by the U.S. Supreme Court to preempt "failure to warn" product liability suits under state tort law and direct state or local regulation of tobacco advertising, as well as the obviously preempted area of mandated warnings on packages or in advertisements (Cipollone v. Liggett Group I1992;505 U.S. 504; Lorillard Tobacco Company v. Reilly 2001;533 U.S. 525).

Whether federal regulation is needed and, if so, whether and to what extent the federal regulatory statute should preempt compatible state regulation are complex inquiries involving highly contextual judgments. However, the general contours of the analysis can be summarized succinctly. On the one hand, a decision to preempt state regulation in favor of exclusive federal authority may impose an overly rigid and inefficient uniform nationwide approach that is contrary to public preferences in many jurisdictions, especially when the benefits and costs from regulation vary considerably across jurisdictions. For example, a state with no tobacco farmers to protect may want to impose stricter regulations than a tobacco-growing state, or a state with a large Hispanic population might want to insist on labels in both English and Spanish. As another example, because the prevalence of smoking varies by as much as threefold among the states, the voters in a state with more smokers may find public smoking regulations more oppressive than the voters in another state with fewer smokers.

Nationwide rules can be especially inefficient when it comes to regulatory matters that fall almost exclusively within a state's geographic boundaries. Thus the regulation of smoking in public places is primarily a local matter, with individual business establishments and local governments bearing the brunt of the compliance costs. The same might also be said for restrictions on point of sale advertising, including the in-store placement of placards and the proximity of external store window signs to schoolyards. Consider in this respect a hypothetical national ban on certain activity (such as the sale of alcohol) within a certain radius of a school. What seems like a perfectly reasonable distance, say, 1,000 yards, would have a very different impact on lawful access to alcohol in a dense urban area, where the ban might cover an entire city, than it would in a less densely populated suburban or rural area. Finally, the imposition of a nationwide approach can increase the costs of a regulatory error, especially when there is uncertainty over the most appropriate form of regulation and when the scientific evidence and business environment are changing.

As these observations suggest, there are many reasons why regulation of retail distribution, marketing, and use of tobacco should presumptively be left to state regulation and, to the extent that federal regulation is adopted in these domains, that supplementary state regulation should be permitted as long as it is compatible with the federal regulatory objectives.

However, in some contexts, there are strong arguments for a national regulatory approach, and perhaps for national uniformity. One such context is the regulation of commercial products for which there is a national market and where the regulated products are easily transported across state lines. For example, if there are substantial differences in regulatory standards from one state to another, strong incentives would exist for people to purchase less heavily regulated products in one state and sell them in a state with more demanding regulatory requirements, thereby potentially undermining the latter state's regulatory objectives, creating a black market, and possibly attracting the participation of criminal syndicates. Another concern that sometimes arises in situations involving diverse state regulation of product characteristics is inefficiency attributable to the need for manufacturers to comply with 50 different requirements. A third consideration is the need for continuing oversight and research by experts, as is often the case in environmental protection.

Regulation of pharmaceutical products, where national standards have prevailed since adoption of the Pure Food and Drugs Act of 1906, is pertinent illustration of a strong national regulatory interest, potentially high costs to state-by-state variations, and need for ongoing regulatory oversight. Over time, the Congress has tended to both increase the scope of federal regulatory authority and precluded additional state regulation in areas in which the FDA has acted. Explicit statutory preemption has been adopted in connection with FDA regulation of medical devices, over-the-counter drugs, and cosmetics.

As will be explained below, the committee favors strong regulation of tobacco product characteristics, packaging, labeling, and promotion and distribution. The colossal failure of the tobacco market to produce accurate information regarding the health effects of tobacco products and to produce adequate incentives for companies to develop less hazardous products, the national scope of the problem, and the need for creating and sustaining regulatory expertise argue strongly for national regulation. The residual question is whether supplemental, compatible state regulation should be permitted. In the committee's view, a uniform national approach preempting state regulation altogether makes the most sense in relation to regulations governing tobacco product design and labeling, as well as in relation to marketing through national media. A uniform national approach makes the least sense in relation to the retail distribution, local marketing, and consumption of tobacco. Federal regulation may not be needed in some of these areas at all, but even if federal regulations are adopted, the federal rules should set the floor, and supplemental state regulation should be permitted. In this latter respect, the current federal preemption provision unduly constrains the prerogatives of the states in regulating the local marketing of tobacco products.

> **Recommendation 23:** Congress should repeal the existing statute preempting state tobacco regulation of advertising and promotion "based on smoking and health" and should enact a new provision that precludes all direct state regulation only in relation to tobacco product characteristics and packaging while allowing complementary state regulation in all other domains of tobacco regulation, including marketing and distribution. Under this approach, federal regulation sets a floor while allowing states to be more restrictive.

This approach was embodied in the proposed "Family Smoking Prevention and Tobacco Control Act" (S. 625 and HR 1008), introduced on February 15, 2007, by Senators Kennedy and Cornyn with 29 other Senators and Congressmen Waxman, Davis, and Palone. This will be referred to as the proposed Tobacco Control legislation in this report.

Any federal statute preempting direct state regulation of the product and its packaging should not preempt any private or public causes of action, in state or federal courts, based on a failure to warn consumers about any risks (of which the company was aware) not covered by the federally prescribed warnings or based on claims of fraud or conspiracy. Congress should make its intentions regarding the narrow scope of preemption clear in the legislative record.

EMPOWERING FDA TO REGULATE TOBACCO

In 1994, the Institute of Medicine (IOM) report *Growing Up Tobacco Free* urged Congress to adopt a regulatory framework for tobacco products and to empower a federal regulatory agency to implement it:

Congress should confer upon an administrative agency the authority to regulate the design and constituents of tobacco products whenever it determines that such regulation would reduce the prevalence of dependence or disease associated with use of the product or would otherwise promote the public health. The agency should be specifically authorized to prescribe ceilings on the yields of tar, nicotine, or any other harmful constituent of a tobacco product (IOM 1994, p. 246-247).

Soon after the IOM report was released, the FDA surprised many observers by claiming that Congress had already given the agency the authority to regulate cigarettes as nicotine delivery devices under the Food, Drug, and Cosmetic Act (FDCA) and by issuing a rule regulating the marketing and distribution of cigarettes to youth. Eventually, the U.S. Supreme Court rejected the FDA's position, ruling that the FDCA did not authorize the FDA to regulate tobacco products and striking down the 1996 FDA Tobacco Rule (FDA v. Brown & Williamson Tobacco Corp., 529 U.S. 120, 2000).

Since the U.S. Supreme Court's decision, proposals have been pending in the Congress to authorize the FDA to regulate tobacco products. The version pending at the time of the final version of the committee's report is the proposed Tobacco Control legislation, which would give the FDA wide-ranging authority over the manufacture, distribution, and promotion of tobacco products with a few exceptions, which will be described below. The power granted to FDA in the proposed Tobacco Control legislation is even more extensive than that envisioned in Chapter 8 of Growing Up Tobacco Free (IOM 1994).

Under the proposed Tobacco Control legislation:

- The 1996 FDA Tobacco Rule relating to youth access and marketing to youth would be revived.
- FDA would have broad authority to promulgate tobacco product standards whenever such a standard is found to be "appropriate for protection of the public health," taking into consideration "the risks and benefits to the population as a whole, including users and non-users of tobacco products." (The bill embodies the principles relating to products purporting to reduce exposure to toxins and to reduce disease risk developed by the IOM in Clearing the Smoke [2001].)
- Legally required package warnings would be strengthened immediately and FDA would have the authority to revise these requirements upon finding "that such a change would promote greater public understanding of the risks associated with tobacco."

- FDA would have authority to "restrict . . . the sale and distribution of a tobacco product if the Secretary [of the U.S. Department of Health and Human Services] determines that such regulation would be appropriate for the protection of the public health."
- FDA would be empowered to restrict the advertising and promotion of tobacco products "to the full extent permitted by the First Amendment" upon finding "that such regulation would be appropriate for the protection of the public health."

Each of these topics is discussed below. Overall, however, the committee reiterates the view taken by two previous IOM committees (IOM 1994, 2001): broad federal regulatory authority over the manufacture, distribution, marketing, and use of tobacco products is an essential element of a comprehensive public health approach to tobacco control.[1] Congress does not have the institutional capacity to monitor and respond to ongoing innovations in product design (especially those purporting to reduce exposure to tobacco-related toxins), or to changes in marketing or patterns of consumption, whereas FDA personnel are well-positioned to gather the necessary information and to make evidence-based scientific judgments about the likely public health consequences of alternative regulatory approaches. Overall, the potential benefits of agency regulation in this context seem to far outweigh its potential costs. Specifically, the committee does not agree with the view expressed by some tobacco control advocates that empowering FDA to regulate the manufacture, distribution, promotion, and use of tobacco products necessarily "legitimizes" these products or that it will unavoidably lead to the "regulatory capture" of the agency by the tobacco industry. Other objections to the federal regulation and to particular features of the proposed Tobacco Control legislation are discussed below in the specific contexts in which they arise.

Recommendation 24: Congress should confer upon the FDA broad regulatory authority over the manufacture, distribution, marketing, and use of tobacco products.

A REGULATORY PHILOSOPHY

The ultimate regulatory goal is to reduce smoking-related mortality and morbidity to a level that is acceptable to a well-informed American public.

---

[1] The committee assumes that the FDA will be the agency empowered to regulate tobacco products. If Congress decides to confer regulatory authority on another agency, recommendations addressed to FDA should be understood to refer to whatever agency has regulatory authority.

Under the present circumstances, given what is known about the health consequences of tobacco use, reducing the prevalence of smoking and the level of per-capita cigarette consumption are reasonable proxies for reducing harm. In the context of other health and safety regulations, the goal of reducing cigarette consumption to a socially acceptable level might mean reducing it to the lowest feasible level or the level at which the social costs of trying to reduce it further exceed the public health benefits of doing so. Either way, feasibility is a significant constraint on the regulatory measures that can sensibly be adopted. Most importantly, a total prohibition against tobacco manufacture and distribution is not a realistic option at present or for the foreseeable future.

The United States now has 44.5 million adult smokers (CDC 2005), the vast majority of whom are addicted to the nicotine in cigarette smoke. If it were possible to prevent smoking initiation altogether, it might be feasible to embrace a nicotine maintenance approach, under which tobacco products would be lawfully available only by prescription to people who are addicted to nicotine. However, the experience with marijuana and other illegal drugs demonstrates that prohibition does not eliminate initiation even when there is no lawful market for a psychoactive drug, and it is implausible to expect that tobacco products lawfully available to more than 40 million addicts would not spill over into a large "gray" market that would sustain ongoing initiation, especially by young people. Nor is it plausible that the billions of cigarettes produced for the international market would not find their way into the United States.[2]

The challenge, then, is to frame a policy for tobacco production and distribution within the context of a regulated market. What should be the aims of the regulatory agency over the short term? In the committee's view, the following aims should guide tobacco policy for the foreseeable future:

- Undertake significant and sustained efforts to reduce the rate of initiation of smoking
- Maximize the options available to addicted smokers to help them quit or reduce their risk
- Prevent people from becoming addicted to tobacco products if they use them
- Reduce the risks of using tobacco products to the users and to others

---

[2]Although prohibition accompanied by prescription-only cigarettes for already addicted smokers might reduce smoking initiation, the committee anticipates that the costs of enforcing such an approach would be substantial and would exceed the potential public health gains. However, such an approach may be worthy of consideration at some future time, especially if it is combined with the nicotine reduction concept sketched in Chapter 7. Innovative strategies of this kind should be explored by the tobacco policy research office recommended in that chapter.

Policies designed to achieve these aims must be formulated and implemented on the basis of a careful consideration of their potential effectiveness and potential costs. A key factor is the need to avoid creating a substantial black market and its associated costs.

The remainder of this chapter sets forth several elements of the comprehensive regulatory strategy that should supplement the traditional tobacco control approaches described in Chapter 5. Specifically:

- Tobacco product characteristics should be regulated to protect the public health.
- Messages on tobacco packages should promote health.
- The retail environment for tobacco sales should be transformed to promote the public health.
- New models for regulating the retail market should be explored.
- The federal government should mandate industry payments for tobacco control and should support and coordinate state funding.
- Tobacco advertising should be further restricted.
- Targeting of youth by tobacco manufacturers for any purpose should be banned.
- Youth exposure to smoking in movies and other media should be reduced.
- Surveillance and evaluation should be enhanced.

TOBACCO PRODUCT CHARACTERISTICS
SHOULD BE REGULATED

As noted above, the proposed Tobacco Control legislation would grant FDA the authority to regulate tobacco products. FDA was selected because it is the only existing regulatory agency with expertise both in scientific and health issues and in product regulation. The authority that would be conferred on FDA for tobacco regulation in the proposed Tobacco Control Legislation parallels in many ways current FDA authority for the regulation of drugs, although different regulatory criteria are needed. Requiring tobacco products to be "safe" is not an available option, of course, and prohibition of the existing products is not a feasible regulatory strategy. Overall, the regulatory standard should be to "protect the public health" by reducing initiation, promoting cessation, preventing relapse, reducing consumption, and reducing product hazards. This standard incorporates its own limitation because it will require the agency to evaluate the likely consumer responses to any proposed regulation, including the likelihood of product substitution and the creation of black markets that could nullify the anticipated public health benefits of the regulation.

FDA regulates many consumer products, including drugs and foods, and the agency has many tools at its disposal that can be deployed in to-bacco regulation. FDA regulation serves to inform consumers about the constituents of the products that they consume and to enhance the safety of these products. FDA can require existing and new products to meet toxicant exposure standards and can promote new standards and make products less hazardous. FDA can also ensure that the claims made about products are truthful and are not misleading. If FDA is authorized to regulate tobacco products, the task should be undertaken in the context of a comprehensive framework that includes the regulation of novel tobacco products and other nicotine delivery products, the delivery of tobacco smoke constituents, and the regulation of medications used to treat tobacco addiction.

The need for a tobacco regulatory authority is illustrated by the history of the low yield cigarette, which has been described in detail in a recent IOM report and in National Cancer Institute (NCI) Monograph 13 (IOM 2001; NCI 2001). In brief, low-yield cigarettes were developed after sci-entific evidence indicated that cigarette tar contributed to cancer. Low-tar cigarettes were implicitly promoted by the tobacco industry as a way to reduce the health risks of smoking. A large majority of smokers believe that low-yield cigarettes were less harmful, and many have switched to low-yield cigarettes rather than quit smoking (Kozlowski et al. 1998). However, because of the engineering characteristics of the cigarettes and the tendency of the smokers to maintain their desired levels of nicotine in their bodies, smokers easily compensate for low-yield cigarettes by smoking more inten-sively and by smoking more cigarettes (NCI 2001). One strategy used to decrease cigarette tar delivery was to change tobacco blends. However the tobacco contained higher levels of nitrogenous chemicals that resulted in the generation of larger amounts of NNK, a tobacco-derived substance that is known to be a pulmonary carcinogen. The ultimate result of the shift to low-yield cigarettes was no reduction of toxic exposures and no impact on smoking-related disease risks. Unfortunately, however, low yield cigarettes were promoted for more than 30 years before it was publicly understood that they have no beneficial effect on smoking-related risk (NCI 2001).

Evidence introduced in the U.S. Department of Justice Racketeering Influenced and Corrupt Organization (RICO) suit against the tobacco manu-facturers indicated that for many years company scientists and company officials had internal information indicating that "light" cigarettes might not deliver lower doses of toxicants and that such cigarettes delivered lower dos-ages to machines than they did to human smokers (NCI 2001). Moreover, tobacco company researchers had information that the tar from a "light" cigarette might be qualitatively more toxic on a milligram-per-milligram basis than the tar from a regular filtered cigarette. However, public health professionals and officials in other government agencies failed to appreciate the seriousness of the problem for several reasons. First, lacking the information possessed by tobacco manufacturers, they mistakenly assumed that smoking machines could accurately gauge the relative toxicity of cigarettes. They underestimated the complexity of the cigarette product and the ability of manufacturers to change the product in ways not reflected in the machine-based measurements. Second, lacking complete information about smoker compensation possessed by tobacco manufacturers, they underestimated the behavioral inclination of smokers to maintain their desired levels of nicotine intake. As a result of industry deception, there was a massive regulatory failure, as nothing was done to control how these products were marketed.

The best way to prevent such a sequence of events from occurring again is to have a regulatory body that can systematically assess toxic exposures, make judgments about potential risks from tobacco products, regulate industry claims about the products to ensure that they are accurate and not misleading, set minimum standards, and provide relevant surveillance to determine actual human exposures and risks. This is particularly important because a number of tobacco companies are developing and marketing tobacco products that are intended to reduce the harm from smoking and presumably will be promoted as such.

Goals of Tobacco Product Regulation

The regulation of tobacco product characteristics can be seen as having two primary goals (IOM 2001). One is to reduce the harm from the continued use of tobacco products. This might be achieved by reducing the toxic emissions from cigarettes or the toxic constituents of smokeless tobacco. Reducing toxic exposures would potentially lower the risk and severity of disease in people who continue to smoke. It is essential, however, that the federal government assure that consumers are informed about what is and what is not known about the risks of using products that result in reduced toxic exposures (reduced exposure products). Moreover, regulators must take steps to reduce the likelihood that the availability of reduced-exposure products will increase initiation or reduce the number of users who quit. The danger that the marketing of reduced-exposure products could lead to an increase in smoking prevalence by altering risk perceptions about smoking is one of the greatest challenges that the FDA will need to address.

The second goal of regulating tobacco product characteristics is to reduce consumption. The most promising way of reducing consumption through product regulation would be to make cigarettes less addictive, thereby making quitting easier and preventing initiating smokers from becoming addicted. Another promising strategy is the development of new medications for the treatment of nicotine addiction. To the extent that harm reduction policies are pursued, it would be desirable to bring modified tobacco products and medications for smoking cessation within a common regulatory framework.

Reducing Harm from Continued Use

The regulation of tobacco products could potentially reduce the harm of tobacco use in smokers who continue to use these products. The approaches to and the pitfalls associated with harm reduction have been reviewed extensively in a recent IOM report (IOM 2001). Some of the ways in which the harm of tobacco products might be reduced include (1) setting performance standards to reduce toxic emissions from cigarettes, (2) evaluating novel and potential reduced exposure products (PREPs), (3) educating users about the risks and benefits of novel products, and (4) encouraging the development of medication that can substantially reduce cigarette consumption (for example, maintaining abstinence through the use of medications). In addition, a national regulatory program would conduct ongoing surveillance of the use of novel and traditional tobacco products.

Making Tobacco Products Less Addictive

The manufacture of cigarettes allows for the control of the nicotine content of the tobacco. Nicotine can be extracted from tobacco and then added back to tobacco to achieve any desired level of nicotine. Although nicotine-free cigarettes were marketed in the past, they were not commercially successful.

For people addicted to controlled substances or alcohol, a common approach to reducing their drug use and minimizing withdrawal symptoms is to gradually taper the use of an addictive drug over time. Such gradual tapering allows a gradual reduction of the dose, a decrease in the level of tolerance, and minimization of the severity of withdrawal symptoms. This type of treatment has been used to treat heroin addicts by gradually increasing the doses of methadone that they receive and to treat alcohol and sedative drug addicts by using drugs such as phenobarbital and benzodiazepines.

An analogous approach could be the basis for a regulatory strategy to reduce the addictiveness of cigarettes (Benowitz and Henningfield 1994; Henningfield et al. 1998). The idea would be to reduce the nicotine content of cigarette tobacco gradually over time. This would result in a lowering of the level of nicotine intake and, presumably, a lowering of the level of nicotine dependence. As nicotine levels become very low, cigarettes would become much less addicting. As a consequence, fewer novice smokers would become regular lifelong smokers. For previously addicted smokers, a reduction of nicotine dependence would be expected to facilitate quitting. This approach is discussed in more detail in Chapter 7.

Another proposed approach to making tobacco products less addictive includes removing flavorants and additives that enhance the sensory characteristics of cigarettes, as sensory characteristics are thought to contribute to the reinforcing qualities and the addictiveness of cigarettes.

Increasing Medicinal Nicotine Alternatives

Another way to deal with potential compensation would be to make medicinal nicotine more readily available. Currently, nicotine-containing medications are available both over the counter and by prescription, but they tend to be more expensive than cigarettes and are more difficult to obtain. With the ready availability of nicotine-containing medications, smokers could obtain supplemental nicotine to compensate for reduced nicotine intake from low-nicotine–content cigarettes (Henningfield et al. 1998). After complete smoking cessation, the nicotine dose in the medication could be tapered down over time to finally eliminate all dependence on the drug.

The Proposed Tobacco Control Legislation Provisions for FDA Product Regulation

The proposed Tobacco Control legislation would give the FDA authority to "restrict the sale and distribution of a tobacco product if the Secretary determines that such regulation would be appropriate for the protection of the public health." This broad authority is limited only in the following ways: the FDA (1) may not prohibit the sale of tobacco products altogether, (2) may not require a prescription for tobacco products, (3) may not adopt a minimum purchase age higher than 18 years, and (4) may not ban any particular category of retail outlet from selling tobacco products. As general principles guiding FDA authority, decisions would be based on sound science; the goals would be both to reduce consumption and to reduce the mortality and morbidity caused by tobacco use, and the FDA efforts are expected to complement (and not replace) proven prevention and cessation efforts. The proposed Tobacco Control legislation provisions for FDA product regulation has the key elements described in the following sections.

Disclosure

The bill would require tobacco companies to disclose to the FDA all chemical compounds found in both their tobacco products and the products' smoke, whether these compounds are added or occur naturally, by quantity. Tobacco companies would be required to disclose the content and form a delivery based on standards established by the FDA, to disclose research on their product as well as behavioral aspects of its use, and to notify the FDA whenever there is a change in a product.

Testing

The bill would grant the FDA the authority to promulgate regulations on cigarette testing methods, including how the cigarettes are tested and which smoke constituents must be measured. The FDA would also determine what product test data are disclosed to the public to inform consumers, without misleading them, about the risks of tobacco-related disease.

Product Standards

The FDA would be given broad authority to promulgate tobacco product standards whenever such a standard is found to be "appropriate for protection of the public health," taking into consideration the risks and benefits to the population as a whole, including users and nonusers of tobacco products. The FDA is specifically directed to take into account the increased or decreased likelihood that existing users of tobacco products would stop using such products and the increased or decreased likelihood that those that do not use tobacco products would start using such products. As indicated earlier, the proposed Tobacco Control legislation reflects a statutory formulation of the principles developed by the IOM in Clearing the Smoke. The FDA is specifically authorized to promulgate standards requiring "reduction of nicotine yields of the product" as long as it does not require that nicotine be reduced "to zero." (The bill stipulates that only an act of Congress can require that nicotine yields be reduced to zero.) The agency is also empowered to promulgate standards "for reduction or elimination of other constituents, including smoke constituents or harmful components of the product." In short, the FDA is empowered to embrace a harm reduction approach by reducing the toxicity of tobacco products.

Potential Reduced-Exposure Products

The bill would authorize the FDA to develop specific standards for evaluating novel products that companies intend to promote as reduced-exposure or reduced-risk products. Such products would be those, as indicated by the manufacturer explicitly or implicitly, that present a lower risk of tobacco-related diseases or that are less harmful than other commercially-marketed tobacco products; tobacco products or their smoke that contain a reduced level of a substance or whose use results in a reduced exposure to a substance; or tobacco products that, when smoked, do not contain or are free of a particular substance. The FDA would be granted the authority to regulate reduced-exposure and reduced-risk health claims and to ensure that there is a scientific basis for the claims that are permitted.

Public Health Concerns Regarding Federal Tobacco Product Regulation

Proposed FDA regulation has received mixed support from the public health community and from the tobacco industry. Some public health groups, such as the Campaign for Tobacco-Free Kids, have worked with members of Congress in developing the proposed legislation and have been highly supportive of its content. Other public health groups have also endorsed the proposal (Tobacco Free Kids 2007a, 2007b). However, some tobacco control advocates have opposed the bill (AAPHP 2007). They have done so on two quite different grounds. Some opposed the product regulation features of the bill because adoption of a regulatory approach will, in some sense, legitimize a product that should be banned outright. For these opponents, the goal is prohibition, and the most likely political path to prohibition is state-by-state action. Others have argued that the proposed regulatory framework for PREPs, based on the recommendations in Clearing the Smoke, is too demanding and may impede the development of reduced-exposure products by stifling innovation and retarding competition with safer products, especially by small companies and new entrants into the market. For these opponents, the goal is harm reduction, and the federal government should be giving companies incentives to develop PREPs rather than putting regulatory obstacles in their paths.

A third line of objection to federal tobacco product regulation arises out of a deep-seated skepticism about the ultimate utility of federal tobacco regulation. Tobacco control advocates are mindful of the tobacco industry's past successes in using federal legislation to obstruct tobacco control efforts, and their concerns are reinforced by general skepticism about the natural history of regulation. Under this view, regulatory agencies rarely have as much information as the regulated companies and therefore are prone to regulatory mistakes. Eventually, regulatory agencies tend to be captured by the industry that they are regulating, performance standards tend to be set by the industry itself, and consumers are often worse off than they would have been without regulation.

For some of the critics who hold this perspective, the main problem with the tobacco industry is not under-regulation, but, rather, oligopolistic concentration, which tends to encourage collusion and suppress competition. These critics believe that the industry has engaged in collusive activity throughout the century—even since the political and legal tide turned against it—and there is no reason to think that this will change. As long as this is true, the argument continues, there is a need to be realistic about the poor prognosis for getting positive results through federal regulation. Rather, ways should be found to break up the industry. From this perspective, competition, not regulation, is the answer.

Committee Response to Public Health Concerns

The committee has given careful consideration to the concerns raised by some public health advocates about the proposed Tobacco Control legislation's product regulation features. In the end, we think the fears are overstated and that federal tobacco product regulation is an essential element of a long-term strategy for achieving substantial reductions in tobacco use and in tobacco-related morbidity and mortality. One of the major reasons for this conclusion is that active federal monitoring and regulation of the tobacco market is needed to prevent, curtail, and counteract industry efforts to undermine tobacco control policies. A second reason is that the market for reduced-risk products is likely to replicate the "light" cigarette experience in the absence of aggressive regulation of claims about these products.

Reducing use and reducing harm Although harm reduction might be a useful adjunct to a comprehensive tobacco control strategy, it is not at the center of the committee's charge, which is to propose a blueprint for reducing tobacco use in the United States. Reduced-exposure cigarette products may not reduce the prevalence of tobacco use and may have little public health payoff in the short term; moreover, given the numerous uncertainties identified in Clearing the Smoke, even an optimist would have to be reserved about the long-term payoff. A recent simulation study by Tengs and colleagues reinforces the cautious perspective enunciated in Clearing the Smoke (Tengs et al. 2004). They conclude that even if the new products do reduce harm to smokers by as much as 20 percent, the long-term consequences are highly likely to be negative if the rate of cessation drops by 20 to 40 percent.

Whatever the long-term prospects for harm reduction as a tobacco control strategy, however, industry efforts to develop and market reduced-risk or reduced-exposure products must not be left unattended, because their promotion and use could interfere with efforts to reduce tobacco use. This was the sad lesson of so-called "light" cigarettes. From this standpoint, it is imperative that Congress empower the FDA to regulate the claims that may be made regarding PREPs. In this respect, the FDA's regulatory jurisdiction over PREPs is an essential component of the blueprint.

Risks and Benefits of Regulation

The general arguments against product regulation enunciated by opponents of the proposed Tobacco Control legislation strike the committee as overstated in the specific context of tobacco regulation. First, the committee believes that the FDA, a public health agency, is unlikely to become allied with, much less captured by, the tobacco industry. Admittedly, the tobacco industry's successful efforts to fend off regulatory action in the 1970s and 1980s give one pause. For example, the NCI's harm reduction program (the Tobacco Working Group [TWG]), which operated from 1968 to 1977, failed because many of its key members were scientists with direct ties to tobacco manufacturers. The NCI did not assemble a working group of independent scientists in great part because there was insufficient expertise in cigarette design and evaluation outside the industry. As documents produced in litigation have revealed, industry scientists, notwithstanding their pronouncements that they were participating solely as individuals rather than as company representatives, repeatedly informed their companies' legal counsel of any contemplated action by the TWG that might threaten the industry's interests. Company scientists, acting on instructions from counsel, successfully blocked promising research projects that had been proposed to the TWG. Once the TWG was disbanded, the tobacco companies retained two of its government representatives as consultants. In particular, the director of NCI's program, Gio Gori, went on to represent the Brown and Williamson Corporation in various regulatory proceedings.

Likewise, the Federal Trade Commission (FTC) has been criticized for its failure to stand up to the tobacco manufacturers. As documents produced in litigation reveal, the FTC passively allowed the industry to obscure the fact that the machine-tested tar and nicotine testing bore little relationship to human exposure. The FTC had no independent knowledge of cigarette design, and the FTC did not regulate the amounts of tar and nicotine delivered. However, its perpetuation of the testing regime merely served as an instrument for disciplining firms that threatened the industry-wide agreement to stick to machine-measured tar and nicotine numbers and avoid any suggestion that the machines did not accurately gauge human exposure. Moreover, the fact that the Master Settlement Agreement (MSA) had to include a variety of restrictions on misleading and youth-oriented advertising provides evidence of regulatory default by the FTC. Finally, the fact that Judge Gladys Kessler, in her final judgment and order in the government's RICO suit, enjoined the major tobacco manufacturers from using such words as "low tar," "light," "ultra-light," "mild," and "natural" provides even further evidence that the FTC has failed to carry out its legislative mandate (Tobacco Free Kids 2006).

The committee acknowledges the regrettable history of federal regulatory default. However, the committee believes that the widespread condemnation of the tobacco industry's deceit during the 1970s and 1980s, most recently documented in Judge Kessler's opinion in the federal government's RICO suit, makes it less likely that any federal regulatory agency, especially an agency charged with protecting the public health such as the FDA, will be captured by the tobacco industry. There is no doubt that the agency could still be misled, but the proposed Tobacco Control legislation's disclosure requirements are designed to reduce the informational disparity between the industry and the regulators, and the FDA scientists can be expected to be highly skeptical of the data and the interpretations of those data provided by the tobacco industry.

Aside from regulatory capture, the other major criticism of the proposed Tobacco Control legislation is that the agency might retard innovation in the development of PREPs by insisting on high standards of proof regarding the effects of reduced exposure to tobacco toxins. In the committee's view, however, even if the regulatory criteria for permitting reduced-exposure and reduced-risk claims might be applied too cautiously, the dangers of unregulated competition over safety are greater than the dangers of retarding safety innovation. The underlying question regarding harm reduction is whether it is better to err in one direction or the other. In the committee's view, the highest priority is to prevent another "light" cigarette disaster.

The committee concludes that product regulation by the FDA will advance tobacco control efforts in the United States and around the world. The proposed Tobacco Control legislation embodies the principles that should govern the regulation of tobacco products in the coming years. The disclosure and testing requirements are needed to correct massive information failures in the tobacco market. The IOM's approach to reduced-exposure products, which is embodied in the bill, strikes the right balance between encouraging innovation and protecting the public from misleading claims. Empowering FDA to reduce the nicotine content of tobacco products has great potential (see Chapter 7).

Recommendation 25: Congress should empower FDA to regulate the design and characteristics of tobacco products to promote the public health. Specific authority should be conferred

- to require tobacco manufacturers to disclose to the agency all chemical compounds found in both product and the product's smoke, whether added or occurring naturally, by quantity; to disclose to the public the amount of nicotine in the product and the amount delivered to the consumer based on standards established by the agency; to disclose to the pubic research on their product, as well as behavioral aspects of its use; and to notify the agency whenever there is a change in a product;
- to prescribe cigarette testing methods, including how the cigarettes are tested and which smoke constituents must be measured;
- to promulgate tobacco product standards, including reduction of

nicotine yields and reduction or elimination of other constituents, wherever such a standard is found to be appropriate for protection of the public health, taking into consideration the risks and benefits to the population as a whole, including users and non-users of tobacco products; and

- to develop specific standards for evaluating novel products that companies intend to promote as reduced-exposure or reduced-risk products, and to regulate reduced-exposure and reduced-risk health claims, assuring that there is a scientific basis for claims that are permitted.

These recommendations are generally compatible with Articles 9-11 of the WHO Framework Convention on Tobacco Control (WHO 2003).

MESSAGES ON TOBACCO PACKAGES SHOULD PROMOTE HEALTH

The tobacco industry has long used cigarette packaging to identify and market its products, and governments have long used cigarette packaging to convey messages about tobacco risk and exposure. As legal restrictions have increasingly reduced or eliminated media advertising, the importance of the package as a vehicle for promotion has increased (Slade 1997). The packages carried by smokers serve as mobile advertisements for particular products. Promotional displays of packages in retail outlets are also key marketing tools. In response to the increasing importance of the package in promotion, governments have begun to exert more control over packaging characteristics for the dual purposes of reducing this form of marketing and communicating directly with consumers.

Among the reasons for regulatory interest in tobacco packaging are

- communicating product information to consumers and potential consumers,
- warning consumers about hazards and thereby discouraging consumption,
- communicating other health information (e.g., cessation hotline numbers),
- preventing smuggling (by requiring documentation of excise tax payment),
- preventing misleading messages by tobacco companies and providing corrective information to counteract previous deceptions,
- preventing promotional messages by tobacco companies as other avenues of advertising are curtailed, and
- "denormalizing" tobacco products.

The use of packages to convey tobacco-related health risks has a number of potential advantages over other forms of communication. The frequency of exposure is high. The messages are delivered at the moment a smoker desires another cigarette. The messages on packages also communicate information to the public at large, and not merely the consumer.

Package Warnings Regarding Tobacco-Related Health Risks

Congress first required health warnings on cigarette packages in 1966 and in advertisements in 1972. By 1985, four rotating warnings were required on both packages and in advertisements. However, U.S. package warnings are still not prominent and are located on the side of the package in small print (see Figure 6-1). In 1994, a previous IOM committee made the following observation about this country's tobacco health warnings:

> The adequacy of the current cigarette warnings has been repeatedly questioned by public health specialists. Moreover, in the committee's view federal cigarette labeling legislation has reflected an unsatisfactory compromise between the public's health and the tobacco industry's desire to avoid concurrent state regulation and to reduce its exposure to tort liability. Negotiations in the legislative process have tended to favor the industry. . . . The inadequacy of current labeling policy is clearly revealed in the declaration of congressional purpose in the Comprehensive Smoking Education Act of 1984: It is the purpose of this Act to provide a

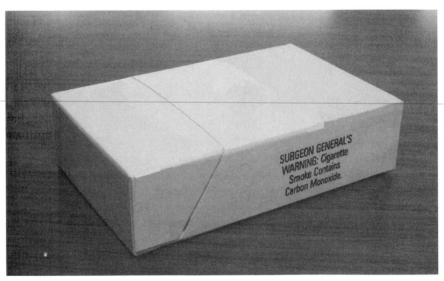

FIGURE 6-1 An example of U.S. government's warning on cigarette packages.

new strategy of making Americans more aware of any adverse health effects of smoking, to assure the timely and widespread dissemination of research findings, and to enable individuals to make informed decisions about smoking. It is time to state unequivocally that the primary objective of tobacco regulation is not to promote informed choice but rather to discourage consumption of tobacco products, especially by children and youths, as a means of reducing tobacco-related death and disease. Even though tobacco products are legally available to adults, the paramount public health aim is to reduce the number of people who use and become addicted to these products, through a focus on children and youths. The warnings must be designed to promote this objective. In the committee's view, the current warnings are inadequate even when measured against an informed choice standard, but they are woefully deficient when evaluated in terms of proper public health criteria" (IOM 1994, p. 236-237).

This committee agrees. Although federal law has remained unchanged for more than 20 years, evidence regarding the ineffectiveness of the prescribed warnings has continued to accumulate. As Krugman and colleagues note, the U.S. package warnings have served the tobacco industry well by reducing their liability exposure while communicating ineffectively with smokers and potential smokers (Krugman et al. 1999). The basic problems with the U.S. warnings are that they are unnoticed and stale, and they fail to convey relevant information in an effective way. In contrast to the messages used in other countries, the United States requires one of four text messages in black and white that occupy only 50 percent of the side of a pack. These messages have not changed in 20 years. They therefore have little effect on decision making or behavior (see Ferrence, Appendix C).

In contrast to the experience with such warnings in the United States, the experiences with these warnings in Canada and other countries have been more promising.

The Canadian Experience

Voluntary health package warnings were introduced in Canada in 1972 but were first imposed by federal law in 1989. Initially, they included four text messages. Five years later, eight stronger messages were introduced, and these messages occupied the top 35 percent of the front and back panels of the pack. These messages clearly specified the diseases and conditions caused by smoking and confirmed that "cigarettes are addictive." These messages were soon adopted in Australia, Thailand, and Poland.

The most important innovation in package regulation is requiring companies to print graphic messages with pictorial content. Graphic warnings were first introduced in Canada in 2001. The manufacturers of cigarettes for sale in Canada are now required to print 1 of 16 health warnings on each pack of

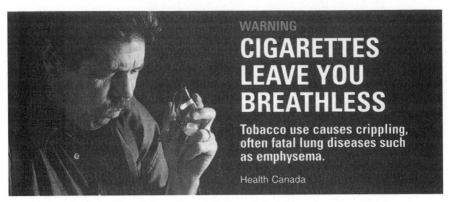

FIGURE 6-2 Example of one of Health Canada's 16 graphic warnings.
SOURCE: (Health Canada 2005) *http://www.hc-sc.gc.ca/ahc-asc/media/photogal/
label-etiquette/img0010_e.html*. Licensed under Health Canada copyright.

cigarettes (see Figure 6-2 for an example of such a warning). The new warning
system extends to carton wrappers, which now include a warning on each of
their six surfaces. The top 50 percent of each main panel on the package (as
opposed to the side panel) must be used for the outside warning. These warnings include a photograph or other illustration, a marker word "Warning," a
short summary statement of the warning, and a brief explanation. Inside each
pack, there must be 1 of 16 other detailed messages that provide information
about quitting or health damage. Warning labels also include information
on damage to nonsmokers exposed to smoke from cigarettes. Other tobacco
products have similar requirements for warning labels.

Other Countries

Since 2001, several other countries have adopted graphic package
warnings including Brazil, Singapore, Thailand, Australia, and Venezuela.
Members of the European Union are now permitted, but not required, to
prescribe graphic warnings, and the European Union has also developed a
standard set of pictorial warnings for consideration by its members. Several
other countries (Bangladesh, Hong Kong, India, Malaysia, New Zealand,
South Africa, and Taiwan) are currently considering graphic warnings. The
World Health Organization Framework Convention for Tobacco Control
(FCTC) requires that warnings cover 30 percent of the front and the back
of the package and recommends package coverage of 50 percent or more.
A series of messages must be rotated. Graphic warnings are permitted but
are not required.

Package warning size and placement vary considerably by country. The front of the package is considered the most prominent location

(Cunningham 2005), and it is probably important to have some health message on all sides, since retailers may position packages to hide the warnings if all sides are not covered.

There are considerable variations in the types of graphics used and in potential emotional impacts of particular graphics. In Brazil, for example, the warnings are more colorful and more dramatic than the Canadian warnings, most showing smokers with obvious health conditions (see Figure 6-3).

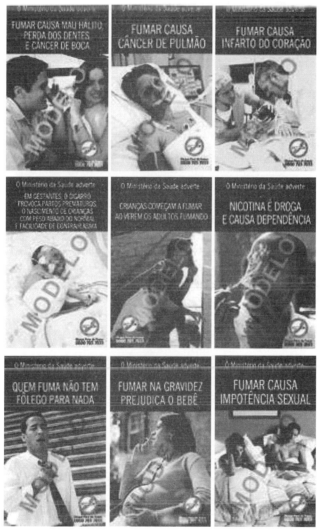

FIGURE 6-3 Examples of Brazil's graphic warnings.
SOURCE: See *www.anvisa.gov.br/eng/informs/news/281003.htm.*

Evidence Regarding Effectiveness

Ferrence and colleagues (Appendix C) have reviewed the scientific evidence regarding the effectiveness of tobacco package warnings in getting the attention of consumers and potential consumers (salience), influencing their awareness of tobacco-related health risks (risk perception), and affecting their self-reported smoking intentions and behaviors. In general, the evidence shows that the salience of warnings is affected by their placement, sizes, and other design features, and that salient warnings affect the consumer's awareness of risks. Although few studies have been able to parse out the effects of warnings on smoking behavior, the available data suggest a beneficial effect on consumption and cessation.

For the committee's present purposes, the question of greatest importance is what is known about the effects of pictorial warnings. Given that Canada was the first country to introduce pictorial warnings, all of the available evidence derives from Canadian smokers. A study conducted with Canadian smokers in 2001 found that more than half reported that the pictorial warnings have made them more likely to think about the health risks of smoking (Hammond et al. 2004). National surveys conducted on behalf of Health Canada also indicate that approximately 95 percent of youth smokers and 75 percent of adult smokers report that the pictorial warnings have been effective in providing them with important health information (Health Canada 2005a; Health Canada 2005b).

The International Tobacco Control Policy Evaluation Survey—a cohort survey of a representative sample of more than 8,000 adult smokers from Canada, Australia, the United States, and the United Kingdom—also provides suggestive findings. When smokers were asked to cite the sources of smoking-related health information, approximately two-thirds of all smokers cited cigarette packages; this proportion was more than radio, print, and electronic sources, and cigarette packages were the second most common source after television (Hammond et al. 2005) However, the results varied substantially by country: respondents living in countries with more comprehensive warnings were more likely to cite packages as a source of health information. For example, 85 percent of Canadian respondents cited packages as a source of health information; in contrast, 47 percent of U.S. smokers cited packages as a source of health information. In addition, specific health warnings were associated with knowledge about specific diseases. For example, in Canada, where package warnings include information about the risks of impotence, smokers were more than twice as likely as smokers from the other three countries to agree that smoking causes impotence. Overall, the study found that warnings that are graphic, larger, and more comprehensive in content were associated with greater health knowledge.

Finally, there is evidence that smokers with less education are less likely to recall health information in text-based messages than people with more education (Millar 1996). Given the inverse association between smoking and educational status, pictorial warnings may be particularly important for communicating with those most at risk. Indeed, preliminary evidence suggests that countries with pictorial warnings demonstrate fewer disparities in health knowledge across educational levels (Siahpush et al. 2006). Pictorial warnings may also be particularly effective in educating people who are illiterate, and could have a significant population impact in developing countries with low literacy rates, as well as regions where numerous languages and dialects are used.

In a series of papers, Hammond and colleagues (2004) have examined the impact of Canadian graphic warning labels on smoking behavior. Smokers who had read, thought about, and discussed the new labels were more likely to have quit, tried to quit, or reduced their smoking at the 3-month follow-up, after adjustment for intention to quit and smoking status at baseline (Hammond et al. 2004). One-fifth of Canadian smokers said that they smoked less because of the labels, whereas only 1 percent said that they smoked more and one-third said that they were more likely to quit because of the warnings. In addition, former smokers identified the pictorial warnings as important factors in their quitting and in subsequently maintaining abstinence (Hammond et al. 2004). Results from the International Tobacco Control Policy Evaluation Survey are consistent with these findings: at least one quarter of respondents from Canada, Australia, the United Kingdom, and the United States reported that package warnings have made them more likely to quit, although Canadian smokers were significantly more likely to report cessation benefits from the warnings than smokers in the other three countries that have text-only warnings (Fong et al. 2004).

As recommended in Growing Up Tobacco Free (IOM 1994) the proposed Tobacco Control legislation would strengthen the required package warnings immediately and would confer authority on the FDA to revise these requirements upon finding "that such a change would promote greater public understanding of the risks associated with tobacco." (The 1994 committee stated that the agency should also be authorized to modify the warnings upon finding that so doing would reduce consumption, such as by making the risks more salient or strengthening the resolve of smokers to quit, and this committee agrees.) The bill would specifically authorize the agency to increase the required label area up to 50 percent of the package and to require color graphics. On the basis of the evidence accumulated thus far, graphic warnings of the kind required in Canada, Brazil, and Thailand "would promote greater public understanding of the risks" of using tobacco and would help reduce consumption.

Recommendation 26: Congress should strengthen the federally mandated warning labels for tobacco products immediately and should
delegate authority to the FDA to update and revise these warnings
on a regular basis upon finding that doing so would promote greater
public understanding of the risks of using tobacco products or reduce
tobacco consumption. Congress should require or authorize the FDA
to require rotating color graphic warnings covering 50 percent of the
package equivalent to those required in Canada.

Using Packages to Convey Other Health Information

Aside from printed health warnings, regulatory authorities can use the
tobacco package to convey health-related information in other ways. For
example, so-called package onserts (printed matter that is affixed to the
package, and that is equivalent to inserts in drug product packaging) provide an appropriate vehicle for supplementing the health warnings printed
on the package with information on ingredients and details regarding
specific health hazards. In addition, the package can be used creatively to
promote smoking cessation by displaying a quitline number and by including coupons for nicotine replacement products (e.g., patches and gum).

Recommendation 27: Congress should empower the FDA to require
manufacturers to include in or on tobacco packages information about
the health effects of tobacco use and about products that can be used
to help people quit.

Restricting Misleading Messages on Tobacco Packages

Tobacco manufacturers have traditionally used the words and trade-
marks on the package as a channel for conveying messages about product
characteristics. Some of these messages are misleading and are not protected
by the First Amendment, because they falsely imply that smoking a particular brand of cigarette is less harmful than smoking other brands.

As Wakefield and colleagues (Wakefield et al. 2004) have noted, package design can help to shape perceptions of a tobacco product's performance and its sensory attributes, even among experienced smokers. This
phenomenon is best illustrated by the use of brand descriptors and colors
to promote perceptions that the tobacco product is safer than other tobacco products. Tobacco manufacturers commonly pair brand descriptors
such as "light" and "mild" with cigarettes that generate low tar yields
under the machine testing protocols. Although the industry has argued
that these terms refer only to the "taste" of a product, these descriptors
help to promote these brands as "healthier" products (Pollay 2001; Pollay

and Dewhirst 2002). Indeed, surveys of smokers in the United States and Canada indicate that a substantial proportion of "light" cigarette smokers believe that their cigarettes are less hazardous (Kozlowski et al. 1998; Shiffman et al. 2001). Adolescents have also been found to have similar misconceptions that "light" cigarettes are less hazardous (Borland et al. 2004; Kropp and Halpern-Felsher 2004; see also Chapter 2).

Ashley and colleagues (2001) reported that in Ontario, Canada, in 1996, one in five smokers of "light" cigarettes incorrectly believed that smoking "light" and "mild" cigarettes lowered the risk of cancer and heart disease. In 2000, 27 percent of Ontario smokers said that they smoked "light" cigarettes to reduce health risks, 40 percent as a step toward quitting, and 41 percent said that they would be more likely to quit if they knew that "light" cigarettes provided the same amount of tar and nicotine as regular cigarettes (Ashley et al. 2001). In a study of smokers' responses to advertisements for potentially reduced-exposure tobacco products, "light" cigarettes, and regular cigarettes, Hamilton and colleagues found that the respondents incorrectly perceived "light" cigarettes as having significantly lower health risks and carcinogen levels than regular cigarettes (Hamilton et al. 2004).

Article 11 of the FCTC calls for the removal of brand descriptors that "directly or indirectly create the false impression that a particular tobacco product is less harmful than other tobacco products," including terms such as "low tar," "light," or "mild." Several jurisdictions have already banned deceptive descriptors. For example, in September 2003, the European Union banned the use of a number of brand descriptors, such as "low-tar," "light," "ultra-light," and "mild," in accordance with Directive 2001/37/EC. Findings from the International Tobacco Control Policy Evaluation Survey suggest that this ban has been effective in reducing misconceptions about the health benefits of brands labeled "light" and "mild" (Fong 2005). However, as the experience in the United Kingdom has demonstrated, tobacco manufacturers have proven adept at substituting numbers and colors for the banned descriptors. For example, pale blue and the number "one" are now being used to indicate a "light" or "mild" cigarette. In Brazil and the United Kingdom, manufacturers openly provided translation guides for this substitution. Because the evidence clearly shows that terms such as "mild," "light," "ultra-light," and similar words are interpreted by consumers to imply reduced risk, the use of these terms should be barred.

In her recent remedial order in the federal government's RICO suit against the big U.S. tobacco manufacturers, Judge Kessler permanently enjoined the companies from "conveying any express or implied health message or health descriptor for any cigarette brand either in the brand name or on any packaging, advertising or other promotional, informational or other material." She specifically enjoined use of the words "low tar," "light," "ultra-light," "mild," "natural," and "any other words which reasonably could be expected to result in a consumer believing that smoking the cigarette brand using that descriptor may result in a lower risk of disease or be less hazardous to health than smoking other brands of cigarettes." Judge Kessler's order is very important, but it has two limitations: it does not apply to all manufacturers and it will require continuing interpretation regarding its application to words and images other than the ones specifically banned in the order.

The committee believes that Congress should supplement Judge Kessler's order with a statutory restriction banning the use of these specific terms and should empower the regulatory agency to ban any other descriptors, signals, or practices that the companies may subsequently use that have the purpose or effect of leading consumers to believe believing that smoking the cigarette brand with that descriptor may result in a lower risk of disease or may be less hazardous to their health than smoking other brands of cigarettes.

> **Recommendation 28: Congress should ban, or empower the FDA to ban, terms such as "mild," "lights," "ultra-lights," and other misleading terms mistakenly interpreted by consumers to imply reduced risk, as well as other techniques, such as color codes, that have the purpose or effect of conveying false or misleading impressions about the relative harmfulness of the product.**

Using Packages to Convey Corrective Communications

Judge Kessler's remedial order in the RICO suit also requires the defendant manufacturers to make various "corrective communications" on their websites, at the point of sale and on package inserts (Tobacco Free Kids 2006). These messages would address the adverse health effects of smoking, the addictiveness of smoking and nicotine, the effects of so-called low-tar cigarettes, the adverse effects of exposure to secondhand smoke, and the impact of marketing on youth smoking. Some of these proposed messages would be substantially equivalent to the health warnings contained in the proposed Tobacco Control legislation, although they would sometimes be more lengthy than package warnings. Some of the messages embody admissions of past deception by the manufacturers.

> **Recommendation 29: Whenever a court or administrative agency has found that a tobacco company has made false or misleading communications regarding the effects of tobacco products, or has engaged in conduct promoting tobacco use among youth or discouraging cessation**

by tobacco users of any age, the court or agency should consider using its remedial authority to require manufacturers to include corrective communications on or with the tobacco package as well as at the point of sale.

THE RETAIL ENVIRONMENT FOR TOBACCO SALES SHOULD BE TRANSFORMED TO PROMOTE THE PUBLIC HEALTH

At present, tobacco use is actively promoted in retail outlets, with little regard to the public interest in discouraging smoking initiation (aside from the occasional warning sign that sale to a minor is prohibited) or in helping people quit. In the committee's view, the retail environment for tobacco should be radically transformed. Effective measures of restricting the commercial distribution of tobacco products to youth are only a starting point. Tobacco is not an ordinary consumer product and should not be treated as such. Although the sale of tobacco products to adults is permitted, it is disfavored as a matter of public policy. The retail environment should be designed to effectuate the public health goals of discouraging tobacco use and reducing tobacco-related disease.

Current Retail Promotional Activities

With the adoption of the MSA in 1998, there was a dramatic shift in the tobacco industry's advertising and promotion budgets, and retail marketing became the dominant strategy (Pierce and Gilpin 2004). The categories of promotional expenditures by tobacco manufacturers since 1980, as reported to the FTC, are presented in Box 6-1 (see also Figure 6-4 and Table 6-1).

Point-of-Sale Advertising

In 2003, tobacco manufacturers spent $165.6 million in payments for the purchase of point-of-sale advertising (FTC 2005). The main venues of such advertising are convenience stores, small grocery stores (often in tandem with the sale of gas), liquor stores, chain supermarkets, and chain pharmacies, with youth exposure especially concentrated at the first two of these locations. The amount spent on point-of-sale advertising in 2003 represents a 41.7 percent decline from that in 2001, when companies spent $284.3 million on point-of-sale advertising, and a decline of 58.6 percent since their peak in 1993 at $400.9 million (FTC 2005). The prime advertising space within most retail stores is the radius around the checkout counter. A study conducted in California found nearly 90 percent of tobacco marketing materials within 4 feet of store checkout counters (Feighery et

BOX 6-1 Domestic Cigarette Advertising and Promotional Expenditures for 2003 (Dollars in Thousands)

ALL MEDIA	2003	
-Newspaper	$8,251	(0.1%)
-Magazines	$156,394	(1.0%)
-Outdoor	$32,599	(0.2%)
-Transit	$0	(0.0%)
-Point-of-Sale	$165,573	(1.1%)
-Sponorships	$31,371	(0.2%)
-Endorsements & Testimonials	$0	(0.0%)
-Direct Mail	$92,978	(0.6%)
-Company Website	$2,851	(0.0%)
-Internet—Other	$0	(0.0%)
-Telephone	$760	(0.0%)
DISCOUNTS		
-Price Discounts	$10,808,239	(71.4%)
-Promotional Allowances—Retailers	$1,229,327	(8.1%)
-Promotional Allowances—Wholesalers	$683,067	(4.5%)
-Promotional Allowances—Other	$2,786	(4.5%)
-Speciality Item Distribution—Branded	$9,195	(0.1%)
-Speciality Item Distribution—Non-Branded	$254,956	(1.7%)
-Public Entertainment—Adult Only	$150,889	(1.0%)
-Public Entertainment—General Audience	$32,849	(0.2%)
PROMOTIONS		
-Sampling Distribution	$17,853	(0.1%)
-Coupons	$650,653	(4.3%)
-Retail-Value-Added—Bonus Cigarettes	$677,308	(4.5%)
-Retail-Value-Added—Non-Cigarette Bonus	$20,535	(0.1%)
OTHER		
-Other	$117,563	(0.8%)
TOTAL	$15,145,998	

NOTE: The twenty-four spending categories are listed as they appear in the Federal Trade Commission's Cigarette Report for 2003. The Committee designated the four main expenditure groups and which spending categories were included in each.

al. 2001). A similar study found that nearly 50 percent of the California retailers surveyed posted tobacco product advertisements 3 feet or lower in height, which is easy eye-level for young children.

Under current law, state restriction of tobacco advertising ("based on smoking and health") at the point of sale is preempted by the 1969 Ciga-

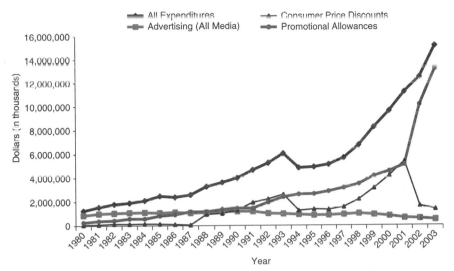

FIGURE 6-4 Domestic cigarette advertising and promotional expenditures for 1980–2003.

rette Labeling Act. However, the committee believes that the states should be free to regulate advertising at the point of sale as long as the regulation is no less restrictive than whatever federal regulation may have been adopted. In fact, this is the approach taken in the proposed Tobacco Control legislation, which would allow the states to ban point-of-sale advertising and other restrictions that would have been preempted under the Cigarette Labeling Act.

Retail Promotional Allowances

Promotional allowances paid to retailers now constitute the lion's share of manufacturers' marketing expenditures (see Figure 6-4 and Table 6-1). They are broadly defined by the FTC to include all payments or allowances to retailers "in order to facilitate the sale of any cigarette." So defined, they include so-called slotting fees, which are industry fees paid to retailers—in the form of discounts—linked to advantageous placement and promotion vis-à-vis competing brands. In addition to product placement itself, these merchandising strategies address an array of product accessories: signage (e.g., regarding discount deals), logos, banners, display racks, and window posters. Another type of retail allowance involves pricing policies. So-called buy-downs feature inventory clearance deals, which are time-constrained discounts. To participate in the buy-down, a retailer must agree to erect special product displays and other promotional signs. In addition to buy-

TABLE 6-1 Promotional Expenditures by Tobacco Manufacturers

Year	All Expenditures	Advertising (All Media)	Consumer Price Discounts	Promotional Allowances	Other
1980	1,242,289	869,880	50,459	265,256	56,694
1981	1,547,658	998,303	81,522	381,607	86,226
1982	1,793,814	1,040,140	141,178	430,683	181,813
1983	1,900,771	1,080,865	125,968	569,987	123,951
1984	2,095,231	1,097,454	148,031	563,666	286,035
1985	2,476,441	1,074,946	140,565	817,887	443,043
1986	2,382,357	1,119,318	98,866	911,603	252,570
1987	2,580,504	1,060,959	55,020	1,165,170	299,355
1988	3,274,853	1,090,125	948,638	1,157,778	78,366
1989	3,616,993	1,155,570	1,017,736	1,354,395	89,290
1990	3,992,008	1,190,923	1,284,691	1,453,558	62,917
1991	4,650,114	1,182,232	1,939,875	1,459,250	68,758
1992	5,231,917	1,021,859	2,224,688	1,943,762	41,608
1993	6,035,437	974,477	2,599,589	2,397,691	63,680
1994	4,833,532	918,971	1,255,870	2,611,019	47,672
1995	4,895,223	857,830	1,362,214	2,641,499	33,680
1996	5,107,700	869,993	1,324,653	2,866,360	46,696
1997	5,660,014	918,556	1,544,978	3,146,273	50,207
1998	6,733,157	994,255	2,194,026	3,483,290	61,584
1999	8,237,631	912,366	3,124,598	4,146,009	54,658
2000	9,592,627	796,732	4,181,075	4,551,433	63,395
2001	11,216,220	631,877	5,381,077	5,098,469	104,797
2002	12,466,358	584,669	1,636,054	10,132,755	112,879
2003	15,145,998	490,777	1,366,349	13,171,308	117,563

NOTE: Dollar amount given in thousands. The Committee designated the four main expenditure groups and which spending categories (24 spending categories are listed in the Federal Trade Commission's Cigarette Report for 2003 [FTC 2005]) were included in each.

downs, there is the most basic of pricing strategies: straight volume discounts for retailers.

Although these practices are common marketing practices for other retail goods, such as food and soft drinks, they are problematic from a tobacco control standpoint for two reasons. First, when the manufacturers purchase display space or other promotional services from the retailer, they are promoting smoking as well as the use of the particular brands displayed or advertised. As discussed below, the committee believes that, aside from properly restrained black-and-white–text only price advertising, all promotional displays should be prohibited, including so-called power walls (large displays of packages of a single brand).

Second, the purchase of space through the payment of slotting fees could reduce or even eliminate the space available for smaller manufacturers who are producing PREPs and who cannot afford to pay the same fees or give similar discounts as the major manufacturers. Even if this practice does not amount to an antitrust violation, it certainly tends to reduce the available shelf space for brands with the smallest market share, such as PREPs introduced by new entrant firms. In the committee's view, the overall public health objective of reducing tobacco use justifies the more aggressive regulation of retail marketing and sales practices. Instead of allowing market forces to give prioritized access to ordinary tobacco products, society should direct retailers who choose to sell tobacco products to give prioritized display space to products that tend to reduce tobacco-related disease, including smoking cessation products and, as they are introduced, to tobacco products that have been found to have genuine potential for reducing tobacco-related disease.

> Recommendation 30: Congress and state legislatures should enact legislation regulating the retail point of sale of tobacco products for the purpose of discouraging consumption of these products and encouraging cessation. Specifically:

- All retail outlets choosing to carry tobacco products should be licensed and monitored (see also youth access section in Chapter 5).
- Commercial displays or other activity promoting tobacco use by or in retail outlets should be banned, although text-only informational displays (e.g., price or health-related product characteristics) may be permitted within prescribed regulatory constraints.
- Retail outlets choosing to carry tobacco products should be required to display and distribute prescribed warnings about the health consequences of tobacco use, information regarding products and services for cessation, and corrective messages designed to offset misstatements or implied claims regarding the health effects of tobacco use (e.g., that "light" cigarettes are less harmful than other cigarettes).
- Retail outlets choosing to carry tobacco products should be required to allocate a proportionate amount of space to cessation aids and nicotine replacement products and, after regulatory clearance by the FDA or a designated state agency, to "qualifying" exposure-reduction products. (The FDA or a suitable state health agency should promulgate a list of "qualifying" exposure-reducing products.)

States are now preempted from implementing some aspects of these recommendations. However, as explained above, the committee believes that the federal preemption should be repealed. In addition, as explained below, the committee also believes that the proposed recommendation is compatible with the First Amendment.

Retail Sales on Indian Reservations

From a tobacco control standpoint, the main concern about retail ciga-rette outlets on Indian reservations is that the marketing and the distribu-tion of tobacco products by tribes could impinge upon or undermine state efforts to increase the price (and collect its revenues) through excise taxes and to reduce the promotion and availability of tobacco.

> **Recommendation 31: Congress should explicitly and unmistakably in-clude production, marketing, and distribution of tobacco products on Indian reservations by Indian tribes within the regulatory jurisdiction of FDA. Authority to investigate and enforce the Jenkins Act should be transferred to the Bureau of Alcohol, Tobacco, Firearms and Ex-plosives. State restrictions on retail outlets should apply to all outlets on Indian reservations.**

New Models for Regulating the Retail Market Should Be Explored

The recommendations just presented aim to inject public health into the existing retail market structure, which comprises a diverse array of privately owned businesses selling tobacco as one of many products in numerous locations. Two additional tools for transforming the retail environment for tobacco sales should also be explored. One is restricting the number and location of the retail outlets, and the other is shifting retail ownership to public control through direct public operation or through a chartered non-profit monopoly. Because state-level regulation of retail distribution of alco-hol after repeal of the 19th Amendment provides the most analogous policy experience, the effects of the alternative models developed by states after Prohibition are briefly reviewed before tobacco outlets are addressed.

The Alcohol Experience

Following the passage of the 21st Amendment, which repealed Prohibi-tion, 17 states adopted a public monopoly system for alcohol distribution. Monopoly methods applied primarily to the retail sales of distilled spirits, considered to be the "primary root of social abuse," whereas wine and beer, thought to be "nonintoxicating," were often excluded from monopoly con-trol (Munshi 1997; Shipman 1940). In addition to retail sales, most state systems included wholesale businesses in distilled liquors, and Wyoming operated only a wholesale monopoly (Munshi 1997; Shipman 1940). The alternative to a monopoly system was a licensing system in which the state granted licenses for a fee to individuals or companies to dispense liquor under government supervision. Both systems were intended primarily to re-duce organized crime and prevent the reemergence of the saloon; however, another objective was to contain consumption and reduce its associated harms (Shankar 1999; Woeste 2004).

Proponents of the monopoly system advocated it in preference to the licensing system for its ability to remove the private profit motive, which, it was feared, "might defeat effective public control" (Munshi 1997; Shipman 1940). In short, a driving insight was to erase at the retail level the vested private interests that tend to increase consumption. Under the monopoly arrangements, "sales promotion is neither necessary nor socially desirable, the products sold are standardized and do not require diversified handling, and the strategy of customer appeal in store premises and equipment is unnecessary" (Shipman 1940). In addition, price controls would be easier to implement under a monopoly system, as most products would be under direct state control (Munshi 1997; Rutledge 1989). Finally, advocates of the monopoly approach believed that because the state would be more concerned with social welfare than with profit—in contrast to the interests of privately licensed bodies—the state would be better positioned to manage the appearance and location of its stores (Munshi 1997).

Although both the public monopoly and the licensing systems were initially intended to contain the number of liquor outlets and promote temperance, these objectives shifted over the course of the 20th century as states saw opportunities to leverage liquor distribution systems to boost state revenues (Spaeth 1991). Furthermore, as public opposition to heavily regulated liquor sales grew, state officials responded by advocating liberalization of stringent control systems. For example, in a debate regarding the future of Pennsylvania's state liquor stores, a state senator cited "poor selection, inconvenience, and high prices" as justification for privatization of the state monopoly system (Munshi 1997). Expressing similar distaste with his state's restrictive licensing scheme, Governor John Carlin of Kansas lobbied for reforming the state's liquor laws out of concern that the state's reputation for radical temperance was thwarting efforts to bring new business to the state (Swain 1996).

Although the recent trend of liberalizing retail access to alcohol, even in the states with monopolies on retail sales, has tended to obscure the differences between the two legal regimes, there is a body of research on the relationship between alcohol consumption and the type of regulation and the number of outlets. Several studies have found that privatization of wine sales and the elimination of a state monopoly on retail sales of distilled spirits led to an increase in overall consumption (Holder and Wagenaar 1990; Wagenaar and Holder 1995).

Reducing the convenience of retail alcohol accessibility typically increases the opportunity cost to the drinker, (i.e., the cost in time and money to actually obtain alcohol from retail sources). Specifically, the number and concentration of alcohol retail outlets affect the convenience of obtaining alcohol, and the distance between outlets increases the cost of doing so. Gruenewald and colleagues (1993) conducted a time series cross-sectional analysis of alcohol consumption and the density of alcohol outlets over the 50 U.S. states. The results indicated that a 10 percent reduction in the density of alcohol outlets would reduce the consumption of spirits from 1 percent to 3 percent and the consumption of wine by 4 percent.

Licensing of alcohol outlets can be used to restrict the number or density of outlets in a given area, as well as the hours of sale, the types of beverages, and the size of beverage containers. Reducing the days and times of alcohol sales restricts the opportunities for alcohol purchasing and can reduce heavy consumption. Licensing is thus a common strategy for reducing drinking-related problems, although the trend in recent years has been to liberalize such restrictions in many countries (Drummond 2000). In general, it appears that changes in licensing provisions that substantially reduce hours of service can have a significant impact on drinking and drinking-related problems overall (Holder 2004).

Options for Restructuring Retail Tobacco Sales

A state retail monopoly for tobacco sales would have advantages and disadvantages. Although it would have the advantage of exerting direct and complete control over the retail environment, it could have the undesirable effect of giving the state a vested economic interest in increased tobacco sales, a concern that would be accentuated if tobacco sales were combined with liquor sales in states that retain retail monopolies over some aspect of alcohol sales. Because states have gradually liberalized (and even encouraged) alcohol sales in recent years, the inclusion of tobacco sales (which should be discouraged) in a consumption-promoting retail alcohol monopoly would send the wrong message altogether. A better option would be to establish a retail monopoly of tobacco-only outlets operated either by the state or by a state-chartered nonprofit corporation. The chartered-nonprofit approach would have the additional advantage of distancing the state from direct participation in tobacco sales. Under either approach, the legislated retail system would have to be carefully structured so that it would have no incentive to engage in marketing and promotional activities. It would be absolutely necessary for the legislature to declare that the sole statutory purpose of the retail outlets would be to facilitate smoking cessation.

Many public health experts will be skeptical about the likelihood that a publicly chartered retail monopoly for tobacco sales could be successfully operated to promote the public health. An alternative to a retail monopoly would be to license private outlets according to a population-based formula. Under this approach, it would be important to structure the system to enable the regulatory authority to reduce the number of outlets when it determines that doing so would promote the public health. The key would be to restrict the license to a reasonably short term, say, 5 years, without any legal presumption of renewal. If it were commercially feasible, licensure could be restricted to outlets that sell only tobacco. Outlets that sell only tobacco would have the additional advantage of being able to facilitate the enforcement of youth-access restrictions.

Under any of the approaches (public monopoly, chartered non-profit monopoly, or a private licensing system), the decisions regarding number and location of outlets should be made by a public health agency, taking into account the potential benefits (in reducing tobacco use) and the possible costs, including the risk of stimulating a black market. Concerns about black-market supply can be reduced by narrowing the wide variation in state tobacco excise taxes. This problem is addressed below.

> **Recommendation 32: State governments should develop and, if feasible, implement and evaluate legal mechanisms for restructuring retail tobacco sales and restricting the number of tobacco outlets.**

The Federal Role

The committee believes the states should take the lead in exploring innovation in tobacco retail regulation. However, the federal government should play a facilitative role in the near term and should be empowered to take a more directive role over the long term.

The proposed Tobacco Control legislation would permit state innovations in retail sale regulation while restricting FDA authority. Although the bill would give the FDA the authority to restrict "the sale and distribution of a tobacco product . . . if the Secretary determines that such regulation would be appropriate for the protection of the public health," it would specifically deny FDA the authority to require a prescription for tobacco products or to ban any particular category of retail outlet from selling tobacco products. The latter limitation would effectively prevent the FDA from adopting a strategy of curtailing the sales of tobacco at retail outlets. However, under the preemption provision, the bill would explicitly leave the states free to adopt restrictions "in addition to or more stringent than" the federal requirements in connection with the sale and distribution of tobacco products. Accordingly, a state could prohibit tobacco products altogether or, more to the point for the present purposes, could require prescriptions or limit the number of retail outlets that sell tobacco.

> **Recommendation 33: Congress should empower FDA to restrict outlets in order to limit access and facilitate regulation of the retail environment, and thereby protect the public health.**

FDA should have the authority to ban categories of retail outlets if it determines that doing so is necessary to implement the regulatory policy, and the proposed Tobacco Control legislation should be modified accordingly. However, the immediate implementation of a federal regulatory scheme would be premature. The first step is to enable and encourage state and local innovation.

THE FEDERAL GOVERNMENT SHOULD MANDATE INDUSTRY PAYMENTS FOR TOBACCO CONTROL AND SHOULD SUPPORT AND COORDINATE STATE FUNDING

This section addresses two distinct problems with current state tobacco control policies as described in Chapter 5: inadequate funding of tobacco control programs and substantial variations in the per-pack rate of state tobacco excise taxes. These problems could be corrected by the states themselves if they were to implement the policies proposed in Recommendations 1 and 2. This section presents a plan for solving both of these problems through federal coordination of state tobacco control policies if the states fail to do so on their own.

As discussed in Chapter 5, substantial state excise taxes on tobacco are an essential component of a comprehensive state tobacco control program, not only as a tool for raising the price and reducing consumption but also as a way of raising revenues that can be used to fund tobacco control programs. Most states allocate insufficient funding for tobacco control programs. Table 6-2 shows each state's proposed tobacco prevention spending for FY 2006, as well as the Centers for Disease Control and Prevention's (CDC) minimum spending targets for prevention programs. With the exception of Delaware, Maine, and Mississippi, the states do not spend up to the CDC minimum target for tobacco prevention programs. The District of Columbia, Michigan, Missouri, New Hampshire, South Carolina, and Tennessee did not allocate any state funds for tobacco control in FY 2006. When each state's actual spending on tobacco use prevention is expressed as a percentage of the CDC's minimum target, the median is 31.2 percent. Accordingly, Recommendation 1 emphasizes the need for states to fund tobacco control programs at the level recommended by the CDC, earmarking funds generated by state tobacco excises as a way of assuring continued funding if doing so is permissible under the state constitution. If this recommendation were fully implemented by the states, the federal role in tobacco control funding could be limited to those programs that are national in scope (such as the youth-oriented national media campaign proposed in Recommendation 15). However, the plan outlined in this section is designed to give states an additional incentive to fund tobacco control programs.

TABLE 6-2 Recommended and Proposed Tobacco Control Program Spending

State	CDC Minimum Prevention Spending Target ($ in millions)	FY 2006 Tobacco Prevention Proposed Spending ($ in millions)
Alabama	26.7	
Alaska	8.1	5.7
Arizona	27.8	23.1
Arkansas	17.9	17.7
California	165.1	79.7
Colorado	24.5	27
Connecticut	21.2	0.04
Delaware	8.6	9.2
District of Columbia	7.5	0
Florida	78.4	1
Georgia	42.6	3.1
Hawaii	10.8	5.8
Idaho	11	
Illinois	64.9	11
Indiana	34.8	10.8
Iowa	19.3	5.6
Kansas	18.1	1
Kentucky	25.1	2.7
Louisiana	27.1	8
Maine	11.2	14.2
Maryland	30.3	9.2
Massachusetts	35.2	4.3
Michigan	54.8	0
Minnesota	28.6	22.1
Mississippi	18.8	20
Missouri	32.8	0
Montana	9.4	6.8
Nebraska	13.3	3
Nevada	13.5	4.2
New Hampshire	10.9	0
New Jersey	45.1	11.5
New Mexico	13.7	6
New York	95.8	43.4
North Carolina	42.6	15
North Dakota	8.2	3.1
Ohio	61.7	47.2
Oklahoma	21.8	8.9
Oregon	21.1	3.5
Pennsylvania	65.6	32.9
Rhode Island	9.9	2.1
South Carolina	23.9	0
South Dakota	8.7	

continued

TABLE 6-2 continued

State	CDC Minimum Prevention Spending Target ($ in millions)	FY 2006 Tobacco Prevention Proposed Spending ($ in millions)
Tennessee	32.2	0
Texas	103.2	7
Utah	15.2	7.2
Vermont	7.9	4.9
Virginia	38.9	12.8
Washington	33.3	27.2
West Virginia	14.2	5.9
Wisconsin	31.2	10
Wyoming	7.4	5.9

NOTE: Federal Tax rate is $0.39 per pack.
SOURCE: Adapted from Campaign for Tobacco Free Kids.
http://www.tobaccofreekids.org/reports/settlements/2006/fullreport.pdf.

A second problem identified in Chapter 5 is that the wide variation in tobacco excise tax rates among the states tends to encourage tax evasion and smuggling through interstate shipments. Table 6-3 shows state cigarette excise tax rates as of January 1, 2006, and reveals a wide disparity in tax rates, ranging from 7 cents to $2.46 per pack, with a median tax of 80 cents per pack. The absolute wide range of state excise tax rates has been increasing over time. Figure 6-5 shows vertical box plots of state excise tax rates in 1998 and 2006.[3] The plots show the extreme values as well as the quartile ranges. The median excise tax rate rose from 34 to 80 cents per pack over this period, while the spread between the 25th and the 75th percentiles rose from 40 cents in 1998 to 82.5 cents in 2006. In Recommendation 2, the committee urges the low-tax states to raise their excise taxes to what is now the upper quintile of state tax rates. If that recommendation were implemented by all the states, it would substantially decrease, if not eliminate, the incentive for cross-state smuggling. However, if the states do not deal successfully with this problem on their own, the increasing variation in state tobacco excise taxes should be addressed by the federal government.

In this section, the committee offers a new federal funding scheme (the National Tobacco Control Funding Plan, described below) as a backup plan to support and coordinate state tobacco control programs, while giving the states with low tobacco excise taxes the incentive to raise them. The basic outline of such a scheme is as follows: the Congress would levy a supplementary remedial assessment on tobacco manufacturers through a per-pack fee, much like the current federal excise tax. The federal gov-

---

[3]The source of the excise tax data for 1998 is Tax Burden on Tobacco.

TABLE 6-3 State Cigarette Excise Tax Rates

State	State Cigarette Excise Tax Rates (in cents per pack)—Updated January 1, 2006	State	State Cigarette Excise Tax Rates (in cents per pack) Updated January 1, 2006
Rhode Island	246	Kansas	79
New Jersey	240	Wisconsin	77
Washington	202.5	Utah	69.5
Maine	200	Nebraska	64
Michigan	200	Wyoming	60
Montana	170	Arkansas (2)	59
Alaska	160	Idaho	57
Connecticut	151	Indiana	55.5
Massachusetts	151	Delaware	55
New York (1)	150	West Virginia	55
Hawaii	140	South Dakota	53
Pennsylvania	135	North Dakota	44
Ohio	125	Alabama (1)	42.5
Minnesota (3)	123	Texas	41
Vermont	119	Georgia	37
Arizona	118	Iowa	36
Oregon	118	Louisiana	36
Oklahoma	103	North Carolina	35
District of Columbia	100	Florida	33.9
Maryland	100	Kentucky (2)	30
Illinois (1)	98	Virginia (1)	30
New Mexico	91	Tennessee (1,2)	20
California	87	Mississippi	18
Colorado	84	Missouri (1)	17
Nevada	80	South Carolina	7
New Hampshire	80		

NOTES: *Counties and cities may impose an additional tax on a pack of cigarettes in AL, 1¢ to 6¢; IL, 10¢ to 15¢; MO, 4¢ to 7¢; NYC $1.50; TN, 1¢; and VA, 2¢ to 15¢.
*Dealers pay an additional enforcement and administrative fee of 0.1¢ per pack in KY and 0.05¢ in TN. In AR, a $1.25/1,000 cigarette fee is imposed.
*Plus an additional 25.5 cent sales tax is added to the wholesale price of a tax stamp (total $1.485).
SOURCE: Adapted from Federation of Tax Administration (http://www.taxadmin.org/fta/rate/cigarett.html)

ernment would use a portion of these funds to support national tobacco control programs (for example, a national media-based educational and prevention program and a national quitline and cessation services network, as recommended in Chapter 5). The remainder of the funds would be distributed to the states based on a formula that rewards states with high excise taxes or high levels of tobacco control spending. This would give states

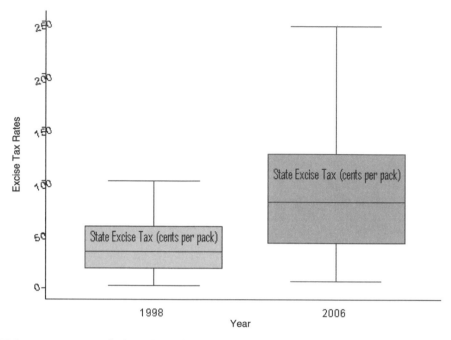

FIGURE 6-5 Box-whisker plots of state cigarette excise tax rates, 1998–2006.

an incentive to increase their spending on tobacco prevention and would give states with low excise taxes an incentive to raise them, thereby narrowing the current wide variation in excise tax rates among the states. The precise details of the formula would have to be based on further research, but the committee has developed an illustrative formula to demonstrate the principles that it has in mind.

Federal Remedial Assessment

Under the committee's proposed National Tobacco Control Funding Plan, the federal government would raise funds for tobacco control on a nationwide basis through a per-pack remedial assessment on cigarettes sold in the United States. These assessments would be based on congressional findings that cigarettes are unreasonably hazardous products, that most smokers are addicted to nicotine, that most addicted smokers began smoking as adolescents, that most adult smokers desire to quit, and that the promotional activities of the tobacco companies have created and sustained addiction to cigarettes.

The precise amount of the assessment would be selected by the Congress to yield a target amount of overall funding for tobacco control, whereas it would produce the optimal incentives for the states to raise tobacco excise taxes and spend state funds on tobacco control.

It will be recalled that the committee recommended a substantial increase in the federal tobacco excise tax rate in Chapter 5 (Recommendation 3). It would be compatible with the committee's recommendation to regard a portion of a new federal excise tax increase as the source of funds for the new tobacco control funding plan. However, the committee has conceptualized the levy as a "remedial assessment" rather than simply as an increase in the excise tax in order to provide a strong rationale for directing the proceeds to tobacco control funding. In addition, it is worth noting that, despite the impact of current federal and state taxes and the regular payments mandated by the MSA, the major U.S. cigarette manufacturers remain highly profitable and still have a substantial ability to help finance the prevention and cessation programs recommended in this report. Table 6-4 shows the pretax domestic operating profits of the three largest U.S.-based tobacco manufacturers for calendar year 2005, as derived from Forms 10-K submitted to the U.S. Securities and Exchange Commission. Their combined pretax operating profits from the sale of cigarettes within the United States exceeded $7 billion in 2005.

An Illustrative Allocation Formula

An example of a formula that would determine the federal funds that would be distributed to the states and that would achieve the committee's basic objectives is $G = aS\sqrt{T}$, where G represents the annual grant to a particular state (in millions of dollars); a is a constant that depends on the total funds available for distribution nationwide; S is the state's annual spending on tobacco prevention (in millions of dollars); and T is the state's excise tax rate on cigarettes (in cents per pack), exclusive of sales taxes. The symbol $\sqrt{T}$ refers to the square root of the excise tax rate.

The formula implies that the state will receive $a\sqrt{T}$ dollars in federal payments for each dollar spent on tobacco control activities. This means

TABLE 6-4 Pre-Tax Domestic Tobacco Operating Profits of the Three Largest U.S.-Based Cigarette Manufacturers, 2004–2005 (in $millions)

Parent Company (Division)	2004	2005
Altria (Philip Morris USA)	4,405	4,581
Reynolds American (RJ Reynolds)	882	1,459
Loews (Lorillard)	1,040	1,151
Total	6,327	7,191

that states with high tobacco excise tax rates receive a higher federal matching rate for tobacco control spending. Moreover, the formula implies that each state would have an incentive to raise its cigarette excise tax, but states with low taxes have the greatest incentive. If a state with a baseline excise tax of 25 cents per pack raised its cigarette tax by 25 cents to 50 cents per pack, it would receive a 41.4 percent increase in federal payments. By contrast, if a state with a baseline excise tax of $1 per pack raised its cigarette tax by 25 cents to $1.25 per pack, it would receive an 11.8 percent increase in federal payments. There is precedent for the use of nonlinear formulas in the distribution of federal funds to the states. For example, the federal medical assistance percentage rates in the Medicaid program are based on the square of each state's per capita income (see Section 1905(b) of the Social Security Act).[4]

Table 6-5 shows how the formula would be used to distribute $500 million (an arbitrarily designated amount), based on the values of S (in Table 6-3) and T (in Table 6-4). At current cigarette prices, an additional federal levy of about 2.75 cents per pack would be required to generate such revenue.[5] The last column of Table 6-5 shows the effective federal matching rate per dollar of state tobacco prevention spending. Thus the state of Georgia has a relatively low tax rate of 37 cents per pack (Table 6-3) and will spend $3.1 million on tobacco prevention in FY 2006. Under a federal incentive scheme that awards a total of $500 million to the states, Georgia would receive a payment of $0.56 per dollar of tobacco control spending, which comes to a grant of $1.72 million for the year (Table 6-5). By contrast, the state of Minnesota has a relatively high tax rate of $1.23 per pack (Table 6-3) and plans on spending $22.1 million on tobacco prevention in FY 2006 (Table 6-5). Under the same federal scheme, Minnesota would receive a payment of $1.01 per dollar of tobacco control spending, which comes to a grant of $22.37 million for the year (Table 6-5). In effect, the federal grant would subsidize all of Minnesota's tobacco control spending. Finally, consider the state of Michigan, which has a much higher tax rate of $2.00 per pack (Table 6-3), but will have made no expenditures on tobacco prevention in FY 2006 (Table 6-5). Under the same federal scheme, Michigan would be eligible to receive a payment of $1.29 per dollar spent

[4]For the most recent rates, see Federal Register Vol. 70, No. 229, p. 71856, November 30, 2005.

[5]According to the USDA Tobacco Situation, total federal taxable removals for 2005 were an estimated 366.7 billion pieces or, equivalently, 18.335 billion packs. The estimated average retail price of a pack of cigarettes in 2005 was $4.32. (See Campaign for Tobacco-Free Kids: http://www.tobaccofreekids.org/research/factsheets/pdf/0207.pdf.) If the short-run price elasticity of demand is -0.4, then a federal levy of about 2.75 cents per pack would generate an additional $500 million in revenue.

TABLE 6-5 State Grants and Matching Payment Rates Under Proposed Federal Scheme[a]

State	FY 2006 Tobacco Prevention Proposed Spending (in $ millions)	State Grant Under Proposed Federal Plan (in $ millions)	Matching Payment per Dollar of State Tobacco Control Spending (in $)
Alabama	0.5	0.19	0.6
Alaska	5.7	6.58	1.15
Arizona	23.1	22.91	0.99
Arkansas	17.7	12.41	0.7
California	79.732	67.86	0.85
Colorado	27	22.59	0.84
Connecticut	0.04	0.04	1.12
Delaware	9.2	6.23	0.68
District of Columbia	0	0	0.91
Florida	1	0.53	0.53
Georgia	3.1	1.72	0.56
Hawaii	5.8	6.26	1.08
Idaho	0.544	0.37	0.69
Illinois	11	9.94	0.9
Indiana	10.8	7.34	0.68
Iowa	5.6	3.07	0.55
Kansas	1	0.81	0.81
Kentucky	2.7	1.35	0.5
Louisiana	8	4.38	0.55
Maine	14.2	18.33	1.29
Maryland	9.2	8.4	0.91
Massachusetts	4.3	4.82	1.12
Michigan	0	0	1.29
Minnesota	22.1	22.37	1.01
Mississippi	20	7.75	0.39
Missouri	0	0	0.38
Montana	6.8	8.09	1.19
Nebraska	3	2.19	0.73
Nevada	4.2	3.43	0.82
New Hampshire	0	0	0.82
New Jersey	11.5	16.26	1.41
New Mexico	6	5.22	0.87
New York	43.4	48.52	1.12
North Carolina	15	7.5	0.5
North Dakota	3.1	1.88	0.61
Ohio	47.2	48.17	1.02
Oklahoma	8.9	8.25	0.93
Oregon	3.5	3.47	0.99
Pennsylvania	32.9	34.9	1.06
Rhode Island	2.1	3.01	1.43
South Carolina	0	0	0.24

continued

TABLE 6-5 continued

State	FY 2006 Tobacco Prevention Proposed Spending (in $ millions)	State Grant Under Proposed Federal Plan (in $ millions)	Matching Payment per Dollar of State Tobacco Control Spending (in $)
South Dakota	0.707	0.47	0.66
Tennessee	0	0	0.41
Texas	7	4.09	0.58
Utah	7.2	5.48	0.76
Vermont	4.9	4.88	1
Virginia	12.8	6.4	0.5
Washington	27.2	35.33	1.3
West Virginia	5.9	3.99	0.68
Wisconsin	10	8.01	0.8
Wyoming	5.9	4.17	0.71

[a]Based on the grant formula $G = aS\sqrt{T}$, where $a = 0.09129$ is calculated so that total federal grants equal $500 million.

on tobacco control activities, but because it has no current tobacco control spending, it would receive no federal grant.

To illustrate how this federal allocation program would work, we consider three separate cases: (1) Georgia raises its cigarette excise tax by 25 cents per pack, (2) Minnesota raises its cigarette excise tax by 25 cents per pack, and (3) Michigan raises its cigarette excise tax by 25 cents per pack and spends $10 million on tobacco control activities.

If Georgia raised its cigarette tax by 25 cents to 62 cents per pack but did not increase its spending on tobacco control activities, its federal matching rate would still increase from $.56 to $.72 cents per dollar of tobacco prevention spending. As a result, Georgia's enactment of an increase in its cigarette excise tax would result in an increase in its federal grant from $1.72 million to $2.23 million. By contrast, if Minnesota raised its cigarette tax by 25 cents to $1.48 per pack but did not increase its spending on tobacco control activities, its federal matching rate would still increase from $1.01 to $1.11 per dollar of tobacco prevention spending. As a result, Minnesota's enactment of an increase in its cigarette excise tax would result in an increase in its federal grant from $22.37 million to $24.54 million. In these two cases, Georgia receives an incentive bonus of approximately $0.5 million for raising its excise tax by 25 cents, whereas Minnesota receives an incentive bonus of more than $2 million for raising its excise tax by the same amount. The explanation is that states with high rates of spending on tobacco prevention get a greater reward for raising their cigarette excise taxes.

Finally, consider the consequences of Michigan's raising its excise tax by 25 cents and, at the same time, increasing its spending on tobacco control activities by $10 million. As a consequence of the excise tax increase, its federal matching rate would increase from $1.29 to $1.37 per dollar of spending on tobacco prevention. Accordingly, the state's newly increased spending of $10 million on tobacco prevention would result in a federal grant of $13.7 million, a grant that entirely subsidizes its tobacco control spending and adds additional funds to the state's coffers. This example illustrates an important feature of the federal allocation formula, namely, that states with higher excise tax rates receive a greater reward for increasing their tobacco prevention spending.

Possible Criticisms of Proposed Allocation Formula

It is arguable that the proposed incentive scheme may not provide sufficient incentives for states with low excise taxes and low spending on tobacco prevention to alter their policies. Thus, consider a state such as South Carolina, which has a very low cigarette excise tax of 7 cents per pack (Table 6-3) and will spend no state funds on tobacco prevention in FY 2006 (Table 6-2). South Carolina would essentially receive a federal subsidy of 24 percent for each dollar that it devoted to tobacco prevention spending, which may not be enough to induce the state to allocate funds for tobacco prevention. However, the size of the effective federal matching rate depends on the amount of funds to be allocated. In a program that allocated $2 billion in federal incentive funds, South Carolina would receive a 97 cent match for every dollar that it decided to invest in tobacco control. Its effective subsidy would be 97 percent for each new dollar of spending on tobacco control. That is, although South Carolina has no current tobacco use prevention program, the federal government would essentially be paying the state to establish a tobacco use prevention program.

Alternatively, one might argue that the incentive system outlined above provides too much reward for past good behavior and too little incentive for future increases in cigarette taxes or tobacco use prevention spending. This is a matter of equity. The grant formula could be modified so that only prospective changes in spending S or cigarette taxes T are rewarded. On the other hand, the formula could be modified to take into account a combination of past and prospective changes in taxes or spending on prevention.

Finally, it could be argued that the nonlinear square root formula does not offer sufficiently strong incentives to equalize tax rates. In that case, the formula could be modified to provide greater incentives to states with lower cigarette excise taxes. For example, if the formula were changed to $G = aS\sqrt[3]{T}$, a scheme to allocate $500 million would give Georgia a higher subsidy rate of 66 cents per dollar of tobacco control spending, whereas

Minnesota would receive a lower subsidy rate of 98 cents per dollar of tobacco control spending.

> **Recommendation 34:** If most states fail to increase tobacco control funding and reduce variations in tobacco excise tax rates as proposed in Recommendations 1 and 2, Congress should enact a National Tobacco Control Funding Plan raising funds through a per-pack remedial assessment on cigarettes sold in the United States. Part of the proceeds should be used to support national tobacco control programs and the remainder of the funds should be distributed to the states to subsidize state tobacco control programs according to a formula based on the level of state tobacco control expenditures and state tobacco excise rates. The plan should be designed to give states an incentive not only to increase state spending on tobacco control, but also to raise cigarette taxes, especially in low-tax states. Congress should assure that any federal coordination mechanism affecting the coverage and collection of state tobacco excise taxes applies to Indian tribes.

Prevalence-Based Penalties

The committee's proposed National Tobacco Control Funding Plan is not the only approach that could be used to tap tobacco industry revenues for the purpose of funding tobacco control activities. For example, various financial formulas have been proposed as devices for penalizing tobacco manufacturers for failing to take steps to reduce the prevalence of smoking among youth. In the proposed final judgment in its RICO suit, the U.S. Department of Justice recommended that the court set specified targets for each defendant on the basis of the 2003 baseline rate of smoking their brands and to reduce the prevalence of smoking among youth by 6 percent each year for 7 years. Under the government's proposed judgment, a manufacturer failing to reach its target in any given year would be assessed $3,000 (adjusted for inflation) for each young person by which the target was missed. According to the U.S. Department of Justice, these penalties would be justified by the specific finding that the companies intentionally marketed cigarettes to youth while denying that they were doing so. Eighty percent of the recommended assessments would have been used to support the National Cessation Quitline Network, which would have been established under the proposed order, and 20 percent would have been used to support prevention activities. Although Judge Kessler found the tobacco company defendants liable under the RICO Act, she declined to order these proposed remedies on the ground that they are precluded by an earlier ruling by the Court of Appeals for the District of Columbia.

In any case, the committee's proposed National Tobacco Control Funding Plan is not meant to be an alternative to other plans that are based on prevalence-based penalties; it is meant to stand on its own and can be used to complement a penalty-based approach if such an approach were to be ordered by a court or embraced by Congress. Accordingly, if the Court of Appeals for the District of Columbia were to take a broader view of the district court's remedial authority under the RICO Act, and the district court were to enter an order similar to that recommended by the federal government, Congress could use the funds raised under the committee's proposed plan to supplement these funds as needed to carry out the national cessation and prevention programs established by the court's order.

TOBACCO ADVERTISING SHOULD BE FURTHER RESTRICTED

The Cigarette Smoking Act of 1969 banned the advertising of cigarettes on television and radio. The FDA's 1996 Tobacco Rule would have limited magazine advertising to a black-and-white–text only format, restricted the use of the trade or brand name of certain tobacco products; prohibited the sale or distribution of promotional brand-identified non-tobacco items, such as hats and tee shirts; and prohibited the use of the brand name of a tobacco product when a tobacco company sponsors entries, teams, and sporting and other events. These restrictions never went into effect. Under the MSA, the participating manufacturers agreed to eliminate billboard advertising, significantly limit brand item advertising, and sharply restrict public advertising in entertainment forms. However, other types of advertising and promotion were not affected. Efforts by the states to restrict point-of-sale advertising have been found to be preempted by the 1969 Cigarette Labeling Act (Lorillard Tobacco Company v. Reilly 2001;533 U.S. 525).

As noted earlier, the proposed Tobacco Control legislation would revive the 1996 FDA Tobacco Rule and would empower the FDA to restrict the advertising and promotion of tobacco products "to the full extent permitted by the First Amendment" upon finding "that such regulation would be appropriate for the protection of the public health." The questions raised are whether restrictions on tobacco advertising and other forms of marketing would reduce the level of smoking in the population, thereby promoting the public health, and whether these restrictions would be constitutionally permissible.

Current Advertising

As noted above, the tobacco industry's advertising and promotion budgets shifted dramatically after the MSA was executed in 1998. Retail marketing became the dominant strategy (Pierce and Gilpin 2004), and traditional forms of advertising in mass media have declined. Magazine advertising has not been abandoned, however, and the industry still spends $107 million per year to produce advertisements containing colorful, attractive, and prominently placed imagery that appeals to both youth and adult consumers (King and Siegel 2001). Expenditures for magazine advertisements have declined dramatically since their peak in 1984, however, when tobacco companies reported spending $425.9 million on advertising in this medium, which then represented more than 20 percent of their marketing and promotion budgets. Magazine advertisements now represent a much smaller percentage of total spending: less than 1 percent, if retail consumer price discounting is included (FTC 2005).

The amount of cigarette advertising in magazines with high youth readership has declined since tobacco companies agreed to avoid targeting youth as a condition of the MSA (Hamilton et al. 2002). Researchers credit this trend to public pressure from advocacy groups and the popular press, as the proportion of advertising expenditures in magazines with at least 15 percent youth readership declined more after public pressure was applied than immediately following the execution of the MSA (Hamilton et al. 2002). Nevertheless, a recent court decision may make tobacco companies take greater care in adhering to the MSA advertising requirements; in 2004, a California court of appeals affirmed a trial court ruling that the R.J. Reynolds Company violated the agreement by placing cigarette advertisements in magazines with high youth readerships (People of the State of California ex reI. Lockyer v. R.J. Reynolds Tobacco Company, 116 CalAppAth 1253, 1291, 2004).

Notwithstanding the decline in industry expenditures on advertising in youth-oriented publications, however, youth exposure to cigarette advertisements remains high. One study found that magazine advertisements for brands of cigarettes preferred by youth (those smoked by more than 5 percent of the smokers in the 8th, 10th, and 12th grades) reached more than 80 percent of young people in the United States an average of 17 times each in 2000 (King and Siegel 2001). Moreover, studies have shown that the MSA itself had little, if any, effect on the exposure of young people to magazine advertisements in the years following the agreement (Hamilton et al. 2002; King and Siegel 2001; Krugman et al. 2005). Cigarette companies continue to promote their products in magazines that reach high percentages and numbers of youth readers (Krugman et al. 2005).

Like magazine advertising, point-of-sale advertising (advertisements at the retail location, excluding outdoor signs on retailer property) also represents a smaller percentage of the promotional spending for tobacco companies than it did in years past. In 2003, tobacco companies reported spending $165.8 million on point-of-sale promotions. This amount represents a 41.7 percent decline from that in 2001, when companies spent $284.3 million on point-of-sale advertising. Current expenditures on point-of-sale advertising have declined 58.6 percent since their peak in 1993 at $400.9 million (FTC 2005).

In this section, the committee addresses advertising (in magazines and at the point of sale). The committee does not address price discounting to either consumers or retailers. The pricing of cigarettes is addressed in connection with cigarette excise taxes in Chapter 5.

Effects of Advertising and Other Promotional Exposures

No one doubts the government's powerful interest in preventing the initiation of tobacco use by youth. A core element of the tobacco control policy agenda for decades has been the elimination of youth exposure to tobacco advertising. However, the long-standing industry position has been that advertising does not create new demand but rather affects the market share among existing smokers. This general position has also long been accompanied by an industry-wide insistence that advertising did not "target" youth and that exposure to advertising by youth was the incidental consequence of a spillover effect of targeting young adult smokers.

In 1994, the IOM reached the following conclusions after reviewing the available scientific literature:

> The images typically associated with advertising and promotion convey the message that tobacco use is a desirable, socially approved, safe and healthful, and widely practiced behavior among young adults, whom children and youths want to emulate. As a result, tobacco advertising and promotion undoubtedly contribute to the multiple and convergent psychosocial influences that lead children and youths to begin using these products and to become addicted to them (IOM 1994, p. 131).

Since 1994, the available literature has been augmented in two important ways. First, internal industry documents disclosed in the course of litigation have yielded substantial evidence that tobacco companies did, in fact, target youth, including teenagers, to create new demand. Second, scientific evidence documenting the relationship between advertising exposure and consumption has accumulated.

Econometric studies examining the link between advertising and demand for tobacco products have provided mixed results, with a majority finding that cigarette advertising is an insignificant determinant of demand and others concluding that cigarette advertising had a positive and significant impact on consumption (Chaloupka and Warner 1999; Tauras et al. 2005). However, a recent review of these studies by Saffer and Chaloupka demonstrated that the study results depended on which of three alternative empirical measures of advertising was used (Saffer and Chaloupka 2000). Most of the studies finding that advertising was not an important predictor of cigarette demand used annual or quarterly national aggregate expenditure data. The investigators argue that these studies lacked statistical power and were thus likely to find insignificant results because national expenditures lose variance because of aggregation effects and measure advertising where the marginal effect of advertising is near zero. In contrast, studies using cross-sectional data (typically measured at the local level for periods of less than a year) have greater variation in the advertising data and greater statistical power and thus are more likely to identify a positive relationship between advertising and consumption. Finally, studies that measure advertising on the basis of advertising bans produced various results that depended on the scope of advertising restrictions, leading the investigators to conclude that comprehensive advertising bans can reduce tobacco consumption but that a limited set of advertising bans will have little or no effect.

Saffer and Chaloupka caution that attempts to restrict advertising must be sufficiently comprehensive to eliminate the possibility that tobacco companies will simply substitute the remaining legal forms of advertising and promotion (Saffer and Chaloupka 2000). Advertising bans achieve the greatest success when they eliminate a wide range of media outlets, which diminishes opportunities for substitution, and which defeats industry efforts to replace advertising in the banned media with advertising in alternative channels. For example, the ban on outdoor advertising required by the MSA may have little effect on consumption because other forms of promotion, including print advertising, point-of-sale advertising, sponsorships, and other forms of retail promotion, will not be prohibited.

From the standpoint of the initiation of smoking by youth, the most important feature of tobacco advertising is its noninformational characteristics. The most compelling data are those that link positive feelings toward smoking with exposure to tobacco advertising and to ownership of commodities with tobacco company logos and paraphernalia.

The very purpose of noninformational tobacco advertising is to associate smoking with positive attributes and consequences and to create a positive affect toward smoking and people who smoke. In addition, advertising in magazines and retail displays creates the impression that smoking is a widespread and normal social practice and that tobacco is a normal consumer product. The images used in tobacco marketing associate smoking with lifestyles and experiences that appeal to young people, and these positive associations tend to displace or override risk information in adolescent decision making. The evidence clearly shows that youth exposure to images that create a positive association with smoking is associated with a higher likelihood of smoking. Although it is difficult to isolate the effect of any particular strand in the web of influences that encourage adolescents to smoke, prevailing scientific opinion regards the relationship between promotional exposures and smoking to be a causal one.

Cigarette advertising also affects demand by current and former smokers. Tobacco advertisements and promotional campaigns may reduce current smokers' willingness to quit smoking and may induce former smokers to resume their habit by reinforcing the attractions of smoking (Chaloupka and Warner 1999; Warner 1986). A review of tobacco industry documents confirmed that the companies have actively researched the determinants of cessation, and based upon their findings, they engaged in marketing efforts expressly designed to discourage current smokers from quitting and to encourage former smokers to relapse (Ling and Glantz 2004; Pollay and Dewhirst 2002). For example, upon discovering that health was the most frequently reported reason for quitting, the companies sought to address potential quitters' concerns by developing and promoting more socially acceptable products (Ling and Glantz 2004) and advertising filtered and low-tar cigarettes as alternatives to quitting (Pollay and Dewhirst 2002). The companies have also attempted to encourage former smokers to resume smoking by increasing the number of advertisements appearing in popular magazines during periods when former smokers may be particularly vulnerable. A review of studies on cigarette advertising revealed that since 1984, advertising for cigarettes is more prevalent in January and February than it is in other months (Basil et al. 2000). Researchers believe that this trend likely reflects an attempt to counter New Year's resolutions by targeting recent quitters when their withdrawal symptoms are peaking.

Tobacco Advertising Should Be Limited to Black-and-White–Text Only

A text-only regulatory approach to tobacco advertising, recommended by the IOM in 1994, is suitably tailored to promote the government's interests in reducing the initiation of smoking by youth, and in reducing the level of smoking in general while respecting the industry's interests in communicating product and price information. The government's compelling interest in preventing the initiation of smoking by youth justifies constraints on the use of promotional messages and images that have a unique appeal to youth (such as cartoon characters) and the placement of commercial messages depicting smoking in a positive light in venues attracting substantial numbers of youth. Under the FDA's 1996 Tobacco Rule, the ban applied to magazines with a youth readerships of greater than 15 percent. However, in light of the overt purpose of all non-informational tobacco advertising to make smoking appear to be attractive to smokers and nonsmokers alike, including youngsters and former smokers, the committee believes that all commercial messages promoting smoking should be limited to a black-and-white–text only format, even if the level of youth exposure is less than 15 percent.

> **Recommendation 35: Congress and state legislatures should enact legislation limiting visually displayed tobacco advertising in all venues, including mass media and at the point-of-sale, to a text-only, black-and-white format.**

The proposed restriction on advertising in mass media would apply to magazines and broadcast media (if the current ban were invalidated) and to advertising over the Internet through third parties. However, the committee recognizes that direct communication with customers through the Internet cannot feasibly be restricted.

Is a Black-and-White–Text Only Restriction Constitutional?

It is by no means clear that restrictions on tobacco advertising of the kind recommended above would survive a constitutional challenge.[6] However, the committee believes that the proposed restriction on non-informational advertising is justified not only by the government's powerful interest in suppressing the use of tobacco, an unreasonably dangerous product, but also by the unique history of deception and manipulation by the tobacco industry. Furthermore, allowing informational advertising in a black-and-white–text only format fully respects the genuine constitutional interests of tobacco companies and consumers. Accordingly, the committee believes that there is a reasonable prospect that the U.S. Supreme Court can be persuaded to uphold restrictions for tobacco advertising that would not be constitutionally permissible in other contexts.

The committee acknowledges that smokers have a legitimate interest in receiving accurate information from the manufacturers regarding the characteristics of their product and from the retailers regarding the prices of those products. In addition, the tobacco companies have a correlative interest in supplying such information, subject to appropriate regulation to prevent deception and unfair competition. Indeed, truthful, non-misleading information about tobacco products, including products that reduce exposure to harmful toxicants and purport to reduce the risks of smoking, can promote the public health. However, in the committee's view, the tobacco industry does not have a constitutionally protected interest in encouraging or promoting smoking, recruiting new smokers, or sustaining the demand

---

[6]Committee member Cass Sunstein has serious doubts about the constitutionality of the committee's proposal and does not endorse it.

of existing smokers. As the committee has previously noted, tobacco appears to be the only lawful consumer product for which the acknowledged governmental objective is to suppress all consumption. In this light, it would be constitutionally confusing if the tobacco companies' desire to promote smoking were held to have any constitutional value under the First Amendment in the context of a pubic policy aiming to suppress consumption.

Admittedly, individuals and companies have a First Amendment right to promote public policies that the government opposes, and to promote viewpoints that are strongly objectionable to their fellow citizens. Moreover, tobacco companies have the First Amendment right to express their opposition to laws and policies aiming to suppress tobacco use—in colorful images if they choose to do so. Spending money to promote political viewpoints on issues and candidates is constitutionally protected speech. However, in the committee's view, spending billions of dollars to promote the use of tobacco products should not be regarded as an exercise of political freedom or as its constitutional equivalent.

The federal and state governments have the constitutional authority to ban tobacco products altogether to protect the public health (see Gonzales v. Raich, 545 U.S. 1, 2005). However, no one believes that prohibition is a viable option in a country with 45 million addicted smokers. Under these circumstances, the federal and state governments have a compelling interest in reducing the prevalence of smoking by preventing smoking initiation and encouraging smoking cessation. The underlying issue, in a nutshell, is whether the U.S. constitutional system creates a fundamental contradiction—empowering the government to take aggressive measures to discourage smoking while simultaneously denying it the authority to restrict industry efforts to promote smoking. To put it another way, is the government barred by the First Amendment from restraining the marketing of an inherently harmful, although legal, product?

The U.S. Supreme Court has rejected the idea that the power to prohibit the sale of a product or service necessarily entails the lesser power to prohibit all commercial speech. If the product is lawful, the First Amendment provides some protection to commercial speech. The committee does not dispute that proposition. However, the question is what protection the First Amendment actually provides. On this point, the committee believes that the First Amendment protects the interests of sellers and buyers in conveying information about the product but does not protect the interest of sellers in promoting the use of a product that the government has a compelling interest in suppressing.

The explicit goal of tobacco policy is to reduce the use of this highly hazardous product in order to reduce tobacco-related mortality and morbidity. The powerful governmental interest in suppressing tobacco use should be sufficient to override whatever economic interest the tobacco manufacturers and retailers have in encouraging people to smoke, an interest devoid of constitutional value. At the very least, the government's compelling interest in preventing youth from smoking justifies a black-and-white–text only restriction of tobacco advertising in any venue where substantial numbers of youth would be exposed to the advertising, defined quantitatively (as an absolute number such as 2 million) or as a percentage of the exposed audience (King and Siegel 2001).

The alternative understanding of the First Amendment would allow no distinctions to be drawn among lawful products with respect to commercial advertising by those who sell them. In effect, such a view would leave legislatures with only two choices: banning the product altogether, or allowing it to be aggressively marketed under the shield of the First Amendment. In the committee's opinion, this view is misguided, and tobacco is the test case.

In sum, the committee is drawing a crucial distinction between promoting tobacco use and informing consumers about tobacco use. Manufacturers and retailers do not have a constitutionally protected interest in promoting the use of their products, but they do have a protected interest in communicating truthful, non-misleading information about their products to consumers. Manufacturers and retailers also have a virtually absolute right to criticize the government's policies toward tobacco use. Neither of these interests is infringed by a black-and-white–text only restriction.

Admittedly, a picture can be worth a thousand words, and it is conceivable that a text-only restriction could suppress commercial expression with informational value and therefore be unconstitutional as it is applied to a specific advertisement. However, the committee regards this prospect as a marginal one. In the committee's opinion, few images in contemporary tobacco advertising convey truthful, non-misleading information about tobacco products. A good indication of the challenge that a tobacco company would have to overcome to support a claim that a visual advertisement is constitutionally protected would be to ask the company to describe the nonverbal message in words.

Diagrams depicting specific aspects of cigarette design to promote reduced-exposure products might convey important information to consumers. For example, Philip Morris and the R.J. Reynolds Company have test marketed cigarette-like products that purport to heat rather than burn tobacco. One might expect some advertisements for such products to show a diagram of the heating element, tobacco column, specialized lighter, and other aspects of design. There is a plausible claim for First Amendment protection here, but the constitutionality of the text-only restriction as applied to such an advertisement can be adjudicated on a case-by-case basis. Relevant considerations would include whether the necessary information can be conveyed effectively in words. Moreover, a regulatory agency charged with adopting rules to implement a text-only restriction might well decide to make an exception for depictions of the product design as they relate to the health effects of smoking. Such an exception would be consistent with the committee's intent and could be written into the authorizing legislation (e.g., all advertising would have to be in black-and-white text except depictions of the product itself).

Under the committee's proposal, a company would not be entitled to show a color picture of a cigarette pack on the advertisement, even for the asserted purpose of informing consumers that its particular brand can be distinguished by a specific logo or color. The reason for holding the line on logos and colors is that these logos and colors are selected not only to convey information but also to affect the attitudes and behaviors of consumers toward the product. To allow such displays would threaten to unravel the constitutionally critical distinction between informational advertising and promotional advertising.

Targeting of Youth by Tobacco Manufacturers for Any Purpose Should Be Banned

For more than two decades, tobacco companies have promoted youth smoking education and prevention programs (Davidson 1998; Landman et al. 2002). Early efforts, introduced in the mid-1980s, were aimed at both children and parents; sample themes included "Talk to Your Kids," "Kids Don't Smoke," "Smoking Isn't Cool," and "Wait Until You're Older." The youth programs portrayed smoking as an adult activity that was inappropriate for teenagers, whereas the parent-oriented messages urged adults to be involved in their children's decision making regarding smoking.

Despite touting these programs as being designed to discourage teenagers from smoking, internal industry documents now reveal that, from their inception, these campaigns were developed largely to fend off increased regulation and to deflect public scrutiny of industry marketing practices. Industry representatives hoped that their youth prevention programs (which ignored the health effects of smoking) would displace the educational initiatives developed by public health groups, which frequently presented smoking as distasteful and unhealthy.

In the early 1990s, tobacco companies shifted their youth smoking prevention efforts to retailers, launching promotional efforts that included messages such as "It's the Law," "We Card," and "Support the Law." These campaigns implied that, in addition to age, upholding the law was an important reason not to smoke; moreover, the programs served to shift attention away from the industry's contributions to youth smoking. Through these youth smoking prevention programs, the industry was able to recruit a network of retailers to assist it in detecting and defeating local tobacco control legislation, such as youth-access measures, advertising restrictions,

and clear-indoor-air laws. The industry also used the presence of this retailer network to fight national legislation, arguing that FDA regulation of
tobacco advertising was unnecessary because the We Card program was
making a "measurable difference" (Landman et al. 2002).

By the late 1990s, the tobacco companies sought the assistance of third
parties to disseminate youth smoking prevention messages. By building al-
liances with youth organizations such as 4-H and Boys and Girls Clubs,
tobacco companies sought to gain credibility with the public and create an
aura of legitimacy for their prevention efforts. Industry documents reveal
that the companies expended very little (if any) effort to study the effect
of their campaigns on reducing the rate of smoking among youth; yet, the
industry carefully assessed the public relations outcomes associated with
the third-party programs (Landman et al. 2002).

Industry documents also reveal that the youth smoking prevention
campaigns also enabled the companies to obtain useful data about the
teen market that was otherwise practically inaccessible to them through
standard marketing surveys (Landman et al. 2002). For example, the Philip
Morris company learned that a smoking prevention advertisement directed
at young teens would likely receive little attention from older youth if the
message were delivered by members of the younger age group. Thus the
company chose not to target teens in the 15- to 18-year-old age group—
those at the highest risk for smoking—with their prevention campaigns.
The Lorillard company developed a similarly innovative approach, invit-
ing teenagers to visit the company's website to learn more about its youth
smoking prevention campaign. When these individuals enter personal information to qualify for sweepstakes, the company also obtains potentially
useful data about the youth market.

A company's efforts to disseminate informational materials about its
programs may constitute no more than veiled attempts to promote its corporate identity among children. The California Departments of Education
and Justice confronted such an attempt by Philip Morris in 2000, when the
company distributed book covers promoting its youth prevention campaign
to schools in California (Landman et al. 2002). This fairly blatant commercial ploy aroused opposition among educators statewide who argued
that Philip Morris could have supported existing programs proven to be
effective if it had been sincerely interested in helping to reduce the rate of
smoking among youth (Landman et al. 2002).

Within the last decade, tobacco companies have expanded youth smoking prevention programs worldwide and have increased their financial
commitments to these programs. Philip Morris announced a $100 million
"Think. Don't Smoke." campaign in 1998 (Tobacco Free Kids 2005), and
provided more than $125 million in grants to schools and youth organiza-
tions to support youth smoking prevention, youth development, and youth

smoking cessation programs between 1999 and 2004 (Philip Morris USA 2006). Similarly, Lorillard has contributed more than $80 million to youth smoking prevention programs since 1999 (Lorillard Tobacco Company 2007). As in the United States, international campaigns have frequently sent messages that have focused on decision making rather than on the negative health effects of smoking and that have presented smoking as an adult activity.

When these expenditures are viewed in terms most favorable to the companies, these expenditures are designed to demonstrate good corporate citizenship on the youth smoking issue and, perhaps, to weaken political support for stronger regulation. However, tobacco control advocates have a more skeptical view of the industry's motivation. According to tobacco control advocates, these "youth prevention" programs are not really designed to prevent youth smoking at all. Instead, they are designed to promote smoking by facilitating industry access to young people through marketing surveys, by counteracting the anti-industry message of tobacco control media efforts by portraying the industry as trustworthy, and finally, by beginning to establish brand identification for future smokers.

In the committee's view, it is not necessary to resolve this dispute regarding the industry's motivation. In light of the history of past industry practices, industry messages targeted at children and adolescents should be regarded as presumptively suspect. The only acceptable justification for an industry-sponsored youth-oriented program is to prevent youth smoking. However, there is no evidence that the industry's prevention programs actually do reduce youth smoking, and there is some evidence that they do not (Wakefield et al. 2006). If the tobacco manufacturers are genuinely interested in preventing youth from smoking, they should support programs known to be effective and should contract with an independent nonprofit organization with the necessary expertise to carry out the program (Warner 2002). To the extent that the companies have a legitimate interest in demonstrating good corporate citizenship, this interest can be served by requiring the recipients of company funding to acknowledge company support for its activities.

> Recommendation 36: Congress and state legislatures should prohibit tobacco companies from targeting youth under 18 for any purpose, including dissemination of messages about smoking (whether ostensibly to promote or discourage it) or to survey youth opinions, attitudes and behaviors of any kind. If a tobacco company wishes to support youth prevention programs, the company should contribute funds to an independent non-profit organization with expertise in the prevention field. The independent organization should have exclusive responsibility for designing, executing and evaluating the program.

The constitutionality of the proposed restriction is not free from doubt, since it curtails the freedom of tobacco companies to communicate with young people for any purpose.[7] However, the proposal does not ban all communication with minors, and the mere exposure of minors to advertising would not be a violation of the proposed ban. Instead, the restriction bans "targeting" of young people (conduct that is also banned by the MSA when it is explicitly promotional). The committee's proposal extends the MSA ban to all targeting of youth, based on the presumption that any communications that target young people are highly likely to reflect a promotional motivation. Any legislation seeking to implement this restriction could certainly allow room for a company to prove that a specific communication had a legitimate purpose and did not have the purpose or effect of promoting tobacco use. On the basis of this analysis and on the unique history of tobacco company efforts to promote youth smoking, the committee believes that the proposed restriction would survive a constitutional challenge.

YOUTH EXPOSURE TO SMOKING IN MOVIES AND OTHER MEDIA SHOULD BE REDUCED

One of the biggest challenges of modern life for parents is to minimize the exposure of their children and impressionable teens to images and messages in the media that encourage or even glorify unhealthy and risky behaviors. Although the values of a free and open society preclude strong measures to cleanse the cultural environment of images and messages that are unfit for children, properly tailored legal restrictions on the time, place, and manner of display of such images and messages are permissible. The fact remains, however, that the authority of the state in this area is limited. These observations highlight the heavy responsibility borne by the entertainment media for formulating and enforcing industry regulations to facilitate parental efforts to protect their children from potentially harmful exposures to images and messages that tend to promote unhealthy (indeed, unlawful) behavior. A recent IOM/National Research Council report on underage drinking reviewed the evidence bearing on depictions and messages encouraging or glorifying drinking and urged stronger industry self-regulation backed up by monitoring of media content by the federal government (IOM/NRC 2004). This committee believes that a similar approach is needed regarding youth exposure to smoking in the entertainment media, especially in the movies.

The scientific literature on smoking in the movies is reviewed by Halpern-Felsher and Cornell in Appendix H, and the following material is drawn

---

[7]Committee member Cass Sunstein doubts the constitutionality of the proposed restriction and does not endorse it.

from that review. Depictions of smoking in the movies doubled in the 1990s, bringing exposure rates closer to those observed in the 1950s (Glantz et al. 2004). Although recent data suggest that depictions of smoking in the movies declined from 2000 to 2004 (Worth et al. 2006), youth exposure to smoking in the movies remains high. In addition to its inclusion in R-rated movies, smoking can readily be observed in many movies rated appropriate for youth, including movies rated G, PG, and PG-13 (Charlesworth and Glantz 2005). Studies that have used content analysis have documented that smoking was portrayed in approximately 87 percent of movies produced from 1988 to 1997 (Dalton et al. 2002), in 77 percent of movies in 2004 (Worth et al. 2006), and in more than 66 percent of children's animated movies released between 1937 and 1997 (Goldstein et al. 1999).

Healthcare professionals and tobacco control advocates are concerned that youth exposure to smoking in the movies will have an impact on adolescents' attitudes toward smoking as well as smoking behavior itself (Charlesworth and Glantz 2005; Sargent 2005; Worth et al. 2006). These concerns are consistent with social cognitive theory, which indicates that adolescents are especially vulnerable to social modeling influences on behavior, including risky behaviors such as the use of tobacco and other drugs (Akers and Lee 1996; Bandura 1986).

Research investigating the impact of youth exposure to smoking in movies has yielded three important findings:

- Exposure to depictions of smoking in movies is associated with more favorable attitudes toward smoking and characters who smoke, and these positive views are particularly prevalent among youth who themselves smoke. As the information in the previous section demonstrates, there is little doubt that youth are being exposed to smoking in the media, including movies, television, magazines, and newspapers, and that such exposures influence youth smoking-related perceptions.

- Exposure to smoking in movies increases the risk for smoking initiation. Cross-sectional and longitudinal studies provide clear support that youth report greater susceptibility and intentions to smoke and are more likely to actually try smoking following exposure to smoking in the movies and on television. Furthermore, even after controlling for other factors known to be associated with adolescent smoking intention and tobacco use, studies show a clear dose effect, whereby greater exposure to smoking in the movies is associated with a greater chance of smoking. Studies have not yet been conducted to determine whether such a relationship between viewing smoking in the movies and tobacco use continues after initial tobacco use (Sargent 2005).

- The increased risk for smoking initiation as a result of exposure to smoking in the movies can be reduced by antismoking advertisements and parental restriction of which movies their children watch.

On the basis of these findings, the committee encourages the entertainment industries to formulate and implement a set of strategies to limit and monitor youth exposure to smoking in the movies, television programming, and videos and to combat the effect of tobacco exposure on youth's smoking attitudes and behaviors. These strategies should both guide and educate the movie industry about the evidence linking smoking in the movies and adolescent tobacco use (Dalton et al. 2003; Sargent et al. 2005), as well as spark a cogent discussion within the movie industry and between the movie industry and policymakers.

A ratings board, which is appointed by the president of the Motion Picture Association of America (MPAA), decides on the ratings assigned to each movie. Currently, such ratings are based on the extent to which there is violence, language, nudity, sensuality, and drug abuse in the film. Tobacco use is not considered. Assigning films with tobacco use a mature (R) rating increases the likelihood that parents will restrict their children's access to such films, a strategy that has been shown to reduce the rate of smoking initiation (Dalton et al. 2002; Sargent et al. 2004, 2003).

The effects of youth viewing of smoking in the movies were found to be reduced among youth who first viewed an antismoking advertisement (Edwards et al. 2004; Pechmann and Shih 1999). Investigations of the effectiveness of antismoking advertisements with adolescents indicate strategies that are effective in reducing the influence of the viewing of smoking depictions in the media in general and that can be applied to smoking depictions in the movies as well. Goldman and Glantz (1998) showed that messages that are aggressive, delegitimize the tobacco industry, deglamorize smoking, and portray the negative effects of secondhand smoke were the most effective at changing perceptions about the normality of smoking and reducing cigarette consumption (Goldman and Glantz 1998). The results of a recent study of a specific antismoking advertising campaign (the truth® campaign) echoes those findings. That study found that this counter-industry media campaign was effective in increasing negative beliefs and attitudes about the tobacco industry and were associated with lower receptivity to pro-tobacco advertising and less progression of smoking intention and behavior (Hershey et al. 2005).

Recommendation 37: The Motion Picture Association of America (MPAA) should encourage and facilitate the showing of antismoking advertisements before any film in which smoking is depicted in more than an incidental manner. The film rating board of the MPAA

should consider the use of tobacco in the movies as a factor in assigning mature film ratings (e.g., an R-rating indicating Restricted: no one under age 17 admitted without parent or guardian) to films that depict tobacco use.

This recommendation urges the MPAA to take smoking into account "as a factor" in its rating system; it does not suggest, categorically, that all movies with smoking receive an R-rating. The objective is to encourage directors and producers to take into account the possible impact of displays of smoking on a teenage audience and give serious consideration whether depicting characters smoking contributes to the artistic aims of the film or is needed for historical or cultural accuracy.

Independent oversight of the industry's standards and strategies is warranted. Such oversight of industry accountability should be facilitated through public monitoring and awareness of industry practices. Accordingly, the committee recommends that the U.S. Department of Health and Human Services be authorized and funded to monitor these media practices and report to Congress and the public. This approach echoes a similar recommendation made by the IOM Committee on Preventing and Reducing Underage Drinking in 2004 (IOM/NRC 2004).

Recommendation 38: Congress should appropriate the necessary funds to enable the U.S. Department of Health and Human Services to conduct a periodic review of a representative sample of movies, television programs, and videos that are offered at times or in venues in which there is likely to be a significant youth audience (e.g., 15 percent) in order to ascertain the nature and frequency of images portraying tobacco use. The results of these reviews should be reported to Congress and to the public.

SURVEILLANCE AND EVALUATION SHOULD BE ENHANCED

Central to successful tobacco control is surveillance for antismoking program design and outcomes. An in-depth discussion of the elements of surveillance for tobacco control is included in Clearing the Smoke (IOM 2001). CDC offers the following definition of surveillance: "Public health surveillance is the ongoing, systematic collection, analysis, and interpretation of health data essential to the planning, implementation, and evaluation of public health practice, closely integrated with the timely dissemination of these data to those who need to know" (Thacker and Berkelman 1988). The extent of tobacco control activity surveillance depends on the goals of the program, the breadth of control activities and methods, the size of the geographic area being evaluated, the availability and accuracy of data elements being sought, and the amount of funding available to conduct surveillance procedures.

Surveillance for tobacco use takes several forms. Most frequently, surveillance is underpinned by assessing tobacco use through household surveys. Such surveys, usually conducted by telephone, often include cigarette smoking behaviors; the intensity, amount and patterns of smoking; the brands of cigarettes and other tobacco products consumed; the sources of tobacco purchase or other acquisition; smoking history; personal smoking cessation attempts and the source and methods of such attempts; indicators of tobacco dependence, tobacco-related consultations as part of interactions within the health care system; family and peer use of tobacco; exposure to formal tobacco education programs during schooling; and environmental exposures to tobacco smoke, including venues where smoking occurs and where it is banned. Survey information may be obtained from dedicated tobacco use surveys or at least in part through multipurpose surveys that may contain additional relevant health and behavioral information.

Household surveys have certain limitations, including less than full and possibly biased participation rates, a high respondent time burden, limited access to minors, the recurring need to demonstrate valid responses, and substantial costs. Validation studies are conducted periodically to determine the accuracy of personal reports and may be supplemented by the use of tests for biological markers of tobacco use. More critically, however, many elements of tobacco control programs cannot be comprehensively determined from household information, and information must be derived from other sources. School-based surveys may be required to monitor adolescent tobacco use. Internet-based surveys may also be valuable, as they reduce the time burden for respondents. Tobacco use among special populations, such as prisoners, patients with major mental illnesses, and homeless people, usually require special institutional surveys and sampling procedures and often require the collection of more detailed informed consent. Surveillance of healthcare professional practices pertaining to tobacco-related education and smoking cessation may best be ascertained through reviews of medical records or the presence of institutional clinical guidelines that are themselves periodically evaluated. Data on the commercial distribution and sales of tobacco and tobacco control products often provide considerable insight into control efforts and can also be used to validate population survey information. Monitoring of jurisdictional environmental regulations and compliance with those regulations, tobacco use in the media and countermarketing activities, seizures of illegal tobacco products smuggled into the United States, the delivery of school-based antismoking educational programs, the resources being spent on community-based tobacco control efforts (public and private), the enforcement of youth-access restrictions, and the activities and management of community-based tobacco control programs themselves are all examples of important surveillance activities occurring outside of household surveys.

Yet another important element of a national control program is toxicological assessment of the contents of tobacco products, both in the distributed product and after the product is burned or other tobacco-containing products are used. Finally, although it may be a long-term endeavor, surveillance for tobacco-related disease outcomes is a critical component of evaluations of tobacco control programs. Such surveillance may take many forms, but most jurisdictions are able to conduct surveillance on the occurrence of smoking-related cancers. Nevertheless, a comprehensive discussion of surveillance elements and methods is beyond the scope of this document.

General guidance for constructing a local and state surveillance program can be found in materials prepared by CDC. The basic elements of existing tobacco control efforts, based on best-practice elements (CDC 1999), provide important guidance to the elements of tobacco control surveillance. However, many state and local control programs have surveillance programs in place and have tailored these programs to their special activities, such as surveillance in workplaces, eating, and drinking establishments, college campuses, urban public places and motor vehicles. Most importantly, surveillance programs allow assessment of the progress that tobacco control programs have made. In turn, surveillance findings are used to drive changes in program activities, direction, and intensity.

Recommendation 39: State tobacco control agencies should conduct surveillance of tobacco sales and use and the effects of tobacco control interventions, in order to assess local trends in usage patterns; identify special groups at high risk for tobacco use; determine compliance with state and local tobacco-related laws, policies, and ordinances; and evaluate overall programmatic success.

Recommendation 40: The Secretary of HHS, through FDA or other agencies, should establish a national comprehensive tobacco surveillance system to collect information on a broad range of elements needed to understand and track the population impact of all tobacco products and the effects of national interventions (such as attitudes, beliefs, product characteristics, product distribution and usage patterns, and marketing messages and exposures to them).

SUMMARY

This chapter recommends a fundamental change in the current legal framework of tobacco control: a new, innovative regulatory approach that takes into account the unique history and characteristics of tobacco and its uses. Under the plan envisioned by the committee, the federal government would assume broad regulatory responsibility for tobacco control to augment the traditional state-centered tobacco control approaches described in Chapter 5. Because a total prohibition against the manufacture and distribution of tobacco products is not a realistic option for the foreseeable future, the new legal structure for tobacco control must be framed within the context of a regulated market. Accordingly, Congress should confer upon the FDA broad regulatory authority over the manufacture, distribution, marketing, and use of tobacco products. Such a broad federal regulatory authority would free the states to supplement federal action with their own measures that aim to suppress tobacco use and that are compatible with federal law.

Within this general framework, the committee recommends federal regulation of tobacco product characteristics and product packaging, aggressive state regulation of the retail environment to promote public health objectives, implementation of a federal tobacco control funding plan to coordinate state funding and reduce the wide range of state excise tax rates, and strong state and federal measures to reduce tobacco advertising and promotion and otherwise reduce initiation of tobacco use by youth.

REFERENCES

AAPHP (American Association of Public Health Physicians). 2007. *American Association of Public Health Physicians*. Web Page. Available at: http://www.aaphp.org/WebLinks/stakeholders.html; accessed May 11, 2007.

Akers RL, Lee G. 1996. A longitudinal test of social learning theory: adolescent smoking. *Journal of Drug Issues* 26(2):317-343.

Ashley MJ, Cohen J, Ferrence R. 2001. "Light" and "mild" cigarettes: who smokes them? Are they being misled? *Canadian Journal of Public Health* 92(6):407-411.

Bandura A. 1986. *Social Foundations for Thought and Action: A Social-Cognitive Model.* Englewood Cliffs, NJ: Prentice Hall.

Basil MD, Basil DZ, Schooler C. 2000. Cigarette advertising to counter New Year's resolutions. *Journal of Health Communication* 5(2):161-174.

Benowitz NL, Henningfield JE. 1994. Establishing a nicotine threshold for addiction. The implications for tobacco regulation. *New Engand Journal of Medicine* 331(2):123-125.

Borland R, Yong HH, King B, Cummings KM, Fong GT, Elton-Marshall T, Hammond D, McNeill A. 2004. Use of and beliefs about light cigarettes in four countries: findings from the International Tobacco Control Policy Evaluation Survey. *Nicotine and Tobacco Research* 6(Suppl 3):S311-S321.

CDC (Centers for Disease Control and Prevention). 1999. *Best Practices for Comprehensive Tobacco Control Programs—August 1999*. Atlanta, GA: U.S. Department of Health and Human Services, Centers for Disease Control and Prevention, National Center for Chronic Disease Prevention and Health Promotion, Office on Smoking and Health.

CDC. 2005. Cigarette smoking among adults—United States, 2004. *MMWR (Morbidity and Mortality Weekly Report)* 54(44):1121-1124.

Chaloupka FJ and Warner KE. 1999. *The Economics of Smoking. National Bureau of Economic Research, Working Paper No. W7047.* Web Page. Available at: http://www.nber.org/papers/w7047; accessed September 13, 2006.

Charlesworth A, Glantz SA. 2005. Smoking in the movies increases adolescent smoking: a review. *Pediatrics* 116(6):1516-1528.

Cunningham R. 2005. *Package Warnings: Overview of International Developments.* Ottowa, Ontario: Canadian Cancer Society.

Dalton MA, Ahrens MB, Sargent JD, Mott LA, Beach ML, Tickle JJ, Heatherton TF. 2002. Relation between parental restrictions on movies and adolescent use of tobacco and alcohol. *Effective Clinical Practice* 5(1):1-10.

Dalton MA, Sargent JD, Beach ML, Titus-Ernstoff L, Gibson JJ, Ahrens MB, Tickle JJ, Heatherton TF. 2003. Effect of viewing smoking in movies on adolescent smoking initiation: a cohort study. *Lancet* 362(9380):281-285.

Dalton MA, Tickle JJ, Sargent JD, Beach ML, Ahrens MB, Heatherton TF. 2002. The incidence and context of tobacco use in popular movies from 1988 to 1997. *Preventive Medicine* 34(5):516-523.

Davidson PA. 1998. Tales from the tobacco wars: industry advertising targets teenage girls. *Wisconsin Women's Law Journal* 13(1)

Drummond DC. 2000. UK government announces first major relaxation in the alcohol licensing laws for nearly a century: drinking in the UK goes 24-7. *Addiction* 95(7):997-998.

Edwards CA, Harris WC, Cook DR, Bedford KF, Zuo Y. 2004. Out of the smokescreen: does an anti-smoking advertisement affect young women's perception of smoking in movies and their intention to smoke? *Tobacco Control* 13(3):277-282.

Feighery EC, Ribisl KM, Schleicher N, Lee RE, Halvorson S. 2001. Cigarette advertising and promotional strategies in retail outlets: results of a statewide survey in California. *Tobacco Control* 10(2):184-188.

Fong GT. 2005. *Evaluating the Effects of the September 2003 European Union Policy Banning "Light/Mild" Cigarette Brand Descriptors: Findings from the International Tobacco Control Policy Evaluation Survey.* Health Canada.

Fong GT, Hammond D, Laux FL, Zanna MP, Cummings KM, Borland R, Ross H. 2004. The near-universal experience of regret among smokers in four countries: findings from the International Tobacco Control Policy Evaluation Survey. *Nicotine and Tobacco Research* 6(Suppl 3):S341-S351.

FTC (Federal Trade Commision). 2005. *Cigarette Report for 2003.* Washington, DC: Federal Trade Commission.

Glantz SA, Kacirk KW, McCulloch C. 2004. Back to the future: smoking in movies in 2002 compared with 1950 levels. *American Journal of Public Health* 94(2):261-263.

Goldman LK, Glantz SA. 1998. Evaluation of antismoking advertising campaigns. *Journal of the American Medical Association* 279(10):772-777.

Goldstein AO, Sobel RA, Newman GR. 1999. Tobacco and alcohol use in G-rated children's animated films. *Journal of the American Medical Association* 281(12):1131-1136.

Gruenewald PJ, Ponicki WB, Holder HD. 1993. The relationship of outlet densities to alcohol consumption: a time series cross-sectional analysis. *Alcoholism: Clinical and Experimental Research* 17(1):38-47.

Hamilton WL, Norton G, Ouellette TK, Rhodes WM, Kling R, Connolly GN. 2004. Smokers' responses to advertisements for regular and light cigarettes and potential reduced-exposure tobacco products. *Nicotine and Tobacco Research* 6(Suppl 3):S353-S362.

Hamilton WL, Turner-Bowker DM, Celebucki CC, Connolly GN. 2002. Cigarette advertising in magazines: the tobacco industry response to the Master Settlement Agreement and to public pressure. *Tobacco Control* 11(Suppl 2):ii54-ii58.

Hammond D, Fong GT, McDonald PW, Brown KS, Cameron R. 2004. Graphic Canadian cigarette warning labels and adverse outcomes: evidence from Canadian smokers. *American Journal of Public Health* 94(8):1442-1445.

Hammond D, Fong GT, McNeill A, Borland R, Cummings KM. 2005. *Effectiveness of Cigarettes Warning Labels in Informing Smokers About the Risks of Smoking: Findings From the International Tobacco Control (ITC) Four Country Survey.* Web Page. Available at: http://tc.bmjjournals.com/cgi/content/full/15/suppl_3/iii19; accessed June 21, 2006.

Hammond D, McDonald PW, Fong GT, Brown KS, Cameron R. 2004. The impact of cigarette warning labels and smoke-free bylaws on smoking cessation: evidence from former smokers. *Canadian Journal of Public Health* 95(3):201-204.

Health Canada. 2005a. *The Health Effects of Tobacco and Health Warning Messages on Cigarette Packages—Survey of Adults and Adult Smokers.* Web Page. Available at: http://www.hc-sc.gc.ca/hl-vs/tobac-tabac/research-recherche/por-rop/impact/2003_e.html; accessed June 23, 2007.

Health Canada. 2005b. *The Health Effects of Tobacco and Health Warning Messages on Cigarette Packages—Survey of Youth.* Ottawa, Ontario: Health Canada.

Henningfield JE, Benowitz NL, Slade J, Houston TP, Davis RM, Deitchman SD. 1998. Reducing the addictiveness of cigarettes. *Tobacco Control* 7(3):281-293.

Hershey JC, Niederdeppe J, Evans WD, Nonnemaker J, Blahut S, Holden D, Messeri P, Haviland ML. 2005. The theory of "truth": how counterindustry campaigns affect smoking behavior among teens. *Health Psychology* 24(1):22-31.

Holder HD. 2004. Supply side approaches to reducing underage drinking: an assessment of the scientific evidence. *Reducing Underage Drinking: A Collective Responsibility.* Washington, DC: National Academy Press. Pp. 458-489.

Holder HD, Wagenaar AC. 1990. Effects of the elimination of a state monopoly on distilled spirits' retail sales: a time-series analysis of Iowa. *British Journal of Addiction* 85(12):1615-1625.

IOM (Institue of Medicine). 1994. *Growing Up Tobacco Free: Preventing Nicotine Addiction in Children and Youth.* Washington, DC: National Academy Press.

IOM. 2001. *Clearing the Smoke: Assessing the Science Base for Tobacco Harm Reduction.* Washington, DC: National Academy Press.

IOM/NRC (National Research Council). 2004. *Reducing Underage Drinking: A Collective Responsibility.* Washington, DC: The National Academies Press.

King C, Siegel M. 2001. The Master Settlement Agreement with the tobacco industry and cigarette advertising in magazines. *New England Journal of Medicine* 345(7):504-511.

Kozlowski LT, Goldberg ME, Yost BA, White EL, Sweeney CT, Pillitteri JL. 1998. Smokers' misperceptions of light and ultra-light cigarettes may keep them smoking. *American Journal of Prevtive Medicine* 15(1):9-16.

Kropp RY, Halpern-Felsher BL. 2004. Adolescents' beliefs about the risks involved in smoking "light" cigarettes. *Pediatrics* 114(4):e445-e451.

Krugman DM, Fox RJ, Fischer PM. 1999. Do cigarette warnings warn? Understanding what it will take to develop more effective warnings. *Journal of Health Communication* 4(2):95-104.

Krugman DM, Quinn WH, Sung Y, Morrison M. 2005. Understanding the role of cigarette promotion and youth smoking in a changing marketing environment. *Journal of Health Communication* 10(3):261-278.

Landman A, Ling PM, Glantz SA. 2002. Tobacco industry youth smoking prevention programs: protecting the industry and hurting tobacco control. *American Journal of Public Health* 92(6):917-930.

Ling PM, Glantz SA. 2004. Tobacco industry research on smoking cessation. Recapturing young adults and other recent quitters. *Journal of General Internal Medicine* 19(5 Pt 1):419-426.

Lorillard Tobacco Company. 2007. *Lorillard Tobacco Company: Youth Smoking Prevention.*

Web Page. Available at: http://www.lorillard.com/index.php?id=5; accessed June 15, 2007.

Millar WJ. 1996. Reaching smokers with lower educational attainment. *Health Reports* 8(2):11-19(Eng); 13-22(Fre).

Munshi MA. 1997. Share the wine—liquor control in Pennsylvania: a time for reform. *University of Pittsburgh Law Review* 58(2):507-547.

NCI (National Cancer Institute). 2001. *Risks Associated with Smoking Cigarettes with Low Machine-Measured Yields of Tar and Nicotine (Monograph 13)*. Bethesda, MD: National Institutes of Health.

Pechmann C, Shih CF. 1999. Smoking scenes in movies and antismoking advertisements before movies: effects on youth. *Journal of Marketing* 63(1-13).

Philip Morris USA. 2006. *Youth Smoking Prevention: Grant Programs*. Web Page. Available at: http://www.philipmorrisusa.com/en/our_initiatives/ysp/grant_programs.asp; accessed September 13, 2006.

Pierce JP, Gilpin EA. 2004. How did the Master Settlement Agreement change tobacco industry expenditures for cigarette advertising and promotions? *Health Promotion Practice* 5(3 Suppl):84S-90S.

Pollay RW. 2001. JTI McDonald, Imperial Tobacco Canada Ltd and Rothmans, Bencon & Hedges InC v. Attorney General of Canada and Canadian Cancer Society. *The Role of Packaging Seen Through Industry Documents*. Supreme Court, Province of Quebec, District of Montreal.

Pollay RW, Dewhirst T. 2002. The dark side of marketing seemingly "Light" cigarettes: successful images and failed fact. *Tob Control* 11 (Suppl 1):I18-131.

Rutledge TE. 1989. The questionable viability of the Des Moines warranty in light of Brown-Forman Corp v. New York. *Kentucky Law Journal* 78(1):209-235.

Saffer H, Chaloupka F. 2000. The effect of tobacco advertising bans on tobacco consumption. *Journal of Health Economics* 19(6):1117-1137.

Sargent JD. 2005. Smoking in movies: impact on adolescent smoking. *Adolescent Medicine Clinics* 16(2):345-370, ix.

Sargent JD, Beach ML, Adachi-Mejia AM, Gibson JJ, Titus-Ernstoff LT, Carusi CP, Swain SD, Heatherton TF, Dalton MA. 2005. Exposure to movie smoking: its relation to smoking initiation among U.S. adolescents. *Pediatrics* 116(5):1183-1191.

Sargent JD, Beach ML, Dalton MA, Ernstoff LT, Gibson JJ, Tickle JJ, Heatherton TF. 2004. Effect of parental R-rated movie restriction on adolescent smoking initiation: a prospective study. *Pediatrics* 114(1):149-156.

Sargent JD, Dalton MA, Heatherton T, Beach M. 2003. Modifying exposure to smoking depicted in movies: a novel approach to preventing adolescent smoking. *Archives of Pediatric and Adolescent Medicine* 157(7):643-648.

Shankar V. 1999. Alcohol direct shipment laws, the commerce clause, and the twenty-first ammendment. *The Virginia Law Review* 85(2):353-383.

Shiffman S, Pillitteri JL, Burton SL, Rohay JM, Gitchell JG. 2001. Smokers' beliefs about "Light" and "Ultra Light" cigarettes. *Tobacco Control* 10(Suppl 1):i17-i23.

Shipman GA. 1940. State administrative machinery for liquor control. *Law and Contemporary Problems* 7:600-620.

Siahpush M, McNeill A, Hammond D, Fong GT. 2006. Socioeconomic and country variations in knowledge of health risks of tobacco smoking and toxic constituents of smoke: results from the 2002 International Tobacco Control (ITC) Four Country Survey. *Tobacco Control* 15:65-70.

Slade J. 1997. The pack as advertisement. *Tobacco Control* 6(3):169-170.

Spaeth SJ. 1991. The twenty-first ammendment and state control over intoxicating liquor: accommodating the federal interest. *California Law Review* 79(1):161-204.

Swain KW. 1996. Liquor by the book in Kansas: the ghost of temperance past. *Washburn Law Journal* 35(2):322-345.

Tauras JA, Chaloupka FJ, Emery S. 2005. The impact of advertising on nicotine replacement therapy demand. *Social Science and Medicine* 60(10):2351-2358.

Tengs TO, Ahmad S, Moore R, Gage E. 2004. Federal policy mandating safer cigarettes: a hypothetical simulation of the anticipated population health gains or losses. *Journal of Policy Analysis and Management* 23(4):857-872.

Thacker SB, Berkelman RL. 1988. Public health surveillance in the United States. *Epidemiology Review* 10:164-190.

Tobacco Free Kids. 2005. *A Long History of Empty Promises: The Cigarette Companies' Ineffective Youth Anti-Smoking Programs*. Web Page. Available at: http://www.tobaccofreekids.org/research/factsheets/pdf/0010.pdf; accessed September 13, 2006.

Tobacco Free Kids. 2006. *Tobacco Free Kids Action Fund, American Cancer Society, American Heart Association, American Lung Association, Americans for Nonsmokers' Rights, and National African American Tobacco Prevention Network V. Philip Morris, Inc*. Web Page. Available at: http://tobaccofreekids.org/reports/doj/JudgmentOrder.pdf; accessed May 30, 2007.

Tobacco Free Kids. 2007a. *Congress Has Historic Opportunity to Save Children and Save Lives by Granting FDA Authority Over Tobacco Products*. Web Page. Available at: http://tobaccofreekids.org/Script/DisplayPressRelease.php3?Display=966; accessed May 11, 2007.

Tobacco Free Kids. 2007b. *Letter to Representative*. Web Page. Available at: http://tobaccofreekids.org/organization/letters/092804.pdf; accessed May 11, 2007b.

Wagenaar AC, Holder HD. 1995. Changes in alcohol consumption resulting from the elimination of retail wine monopolies: Results from five U.S. states. *Journal of Studies on Alcohol* 56(5):566-572.

Wakefield M, Kloska DD, O'Malley PM, Johnston LD, Chaloupka F, Pierce J, Giovino G, Ruel E, Flay BR. 2004. The role of smoking intentions in predicting future smoking among youth: findings from Monitoring the Future data. *Addiction* 99(7):914-922.

Wakefield M, Terry-McElrath Y, Emery S, Saffer H, Chaloupka FJ, Szczypka G, Flay B, O'Malley PM, Johnston LD. 2006. Effect of televised, tobacco company-funded smoking prevention advertising on youth smoking-related beliefs, intentions, and behavior. *American Journal of Public Health* 96(12):2154-2160.

Warner KE. 1986. *Selling Smoke: Cigarette Advertising and Public Health*. Washington, DC: American Public Health Association.

Warner KE. 2002. What's a cigarette company to do? *American Journal of Public Health* 92(6):897-900.

WHO (World Health Organization). 2003. *WHO Framework Convention on Tobacco Control*. Geneva, Switzerland: WHO.

Woeste K. 2004. Reds, whites, and roses: the dormant commerce clause, the twenty-first ammendment, and the direct shipment of wine. *University of Cincinnati Law Review* 72(4):1821-1848.

Worth K, Tanski S, Sargent J. 2006. *Trends in Top Box Office Movie Tobacco Use, 1996–2004. First Look Report*. Washington, DC: American Legacy Foundation.

7

New Frontiers of Tobacco Control

E nding the tobacco problem will require creative policymaking. Effective use of the traditional tools of tobacco control, reviewed in
Chapter 5, can move the nation closer to that goal, but is unlikely
to take us all the way. The next big step forward will require a new legal
foundation and a substantial federal presence. The plan outlined in Chapter
6 is designed to lay that foundation and to authorize new approaches to tobacco control, such as adopting pictorial warnings, regulating claims about
products that purport to reduce exposures to toxicants, and restructuring
the retail environment for tobacco products. However, these innovations
require thorough analysis before being implemented and careful monitoring afterward. Such an analysis will require a robust capacity to conduct
tobacco policy analysis, including state-of-the-art modeling of the effects of
new industry initiatives and potential regulatory interventions.

This chapter has two objectives: first, it fleshes out the case for investing in tobacco policy analysis and development and highlights several new
frontiers of tobacco control that merit investigation by the new policy
development office. Second, it discusses in some detail the most promising
of these ideas—gradually reducing the nicotine content of cigarettes. If this
idea proves feasible, its implementation could provide the nation's best
hope for ending the tobacco problem.

TOBACCO POLICY ANALYSIS AND DEVELOPMENT

An investment in tobacco policy analysis and development is an essential component of a comprehensive federal effort to reduce the heavy

public health burden of tobacco use, especially when history so clearly documents the capacity of the tobacco industry to mount effective countermeasures against and to neutralize potentially effective innovations in tobacco control.

> **Recommendation 41: Congress should direct the Centers for Disease Control and Prevention to undertake a major program of tobacco control policy analysis and development and should provide sufficient funding to support the program. This program should develop the next generation of macro-level simulation models to project the likely effects of various policy innovations, taking into account the possible initiatives and responses of the tobacco industry as well as the impacts of the innovations on consumers.**

The proposed tobacco policy development office might sensibly be located in the Food and Drug Administration (FDA) after Congress confers on FDA the necessary authority to regulate tobacco products.

Improving Policy Simulation Models

One of the policy office's first tasks should be to foster improvements in tobacco policy simulation models. The current generation of tobacco policy models has been valuable to the committee, and the committee is confident that the projections provided to the committee represent the best that can be produced with the currently available tools. However, the implications of tobacco policy decision making are of sufficient magnitude to warrant a greater investment to help policy analysts advance the state of the art. The current tobacco policy models could benefit from the following improvements.

Incorporate State-Dependent or Endogenous Transition Rates

Smoking initiation is influenced by peers, particularly peers' rates of smoking. More generally, individuals' decisions to start, stop, or restart smoking may be influenced by the smoking or nonsmoking of others. These feedbacks from current prevalence to various flow rates include personal interaction effects (e.g., when smoking teens encourage their friends to smoke), societal-level effects (e.g., if smoking is rare, it is more likely to be shunned, which might reduce relapse rates), and market-level effects (e.g., if there are fewer smokers, and hence less demand for tobacco, the market equilibrium price for cigarettes might be affected, which in turn can affect smoking rates).

Distinguish Between Different Intensities of Smoking

Policy simulation models of other forms of substance abuse differentiate between light and heavy users. The incorporation of such distinctions in tobacco-use models would be valuable, inasmuch as a nonnegligible proportion of current smokers are not daily smokers, various policy interventions (including tax increases) may affect the frequency of smoking as well as the overall smoking prevalence, and some health outcomes of interest may be state-dependent.

Recognize Behavioral Response on the Part of Industry

The tobacco industry may undertake new innovations in smoking or respond to changes in smoking prevalence, or it may respond to changes in smoking policies in various ways that are not reflected in current models. A simple example is the industry's response to a tax increase. Current tobacco policy models typically assume that excise tax increases are passed along to consumers in the form of dollar-for-dollar increases in the retail prices, but tobacco manufacturing is an oligopolistic industry, so other outcomes are possible, as are other forms of strategic behavior or product innovation. For example, declining sales might trigger the aggressive promotion of new products, such as flavored cigarettes, which might affect smoking initiation rates.

Model Black and Gray Market Behavior

Excise tax increases are a particularly important and appealing policy lever. Yet, various forms of retail tax evasion and other forms of illicit marketing already exist, and one would expect them to become more common as taxes increase further. Modeling of that behavior is essential to determining the best tax policies.

Track Vectors of Health Outcomes in Addition to Smoking Prevalence

Policy is ultimately more concerned with health outcomes than with smoking per se, so it would be useful if tobacco policy models translated smoking rates into various types of health consequences. Some models can do this to some degree, but in many cases the current state of the art is rather limited.

Beyond these structural changes, a range of more pedestrian measures can be taken to improve the modeling infrastructure and to better inform tobacco policy. These include calibration of the models to longer and more age-specific age series, the use of more detailed demographic modeling (e.g., immigration), allowance for more multidimensional parametric sensitivity analysis and associated confidence interval calculation (e.g., through Monte Carlo simulation), and investigation of more scenarios (e.g., advances in lung cancer treatment and the introduction of low-nicotine cigarettes).

Policy Innovations Worthy of Study

Among the interesting ideas that should be studied by a tobacco policy development office are the ideas explored in the previous chapters, including restructuring the retail market and reducing the number of retail outlets (Chapter 6) and implementing a nicotine-reduction strategy (see below). Other suggestions presented in the tobacco policy literature include establishing a wholesale purchasing monopsony (Borland 2003) and creating policy mechanisms for changing the incentives of tobacco companies to align their goals with public health goals.

Tobacco Wholesale Purchasing Monopsony

Borland has proposed an innovative model of tobacco distribution designed to eliminate marketing and to spur competition for reduced-exposure products (Borland 2003). Under the proposal, a new agency, the Tobacco Products Agency (TPA), would be chartered to be the exclusive buyer and distributor of tobacco products. It would purchase the products from domestic manufacturers and importers and distribute them to retailers. The agency's goal would be to promote the public health by reducing tobacco consumption and otherwise reducing harm. It would negotiate with the manufacturers to purchase the least-harmful products, giving them an incentive to compete on the basis of safety and thereby serving a quasi-regulatory function. In turn, the TPA would distribute the products generically, thereby cutting the link between manufacturer and consumer and removing any marketing incentive. Similarly, the TPA would control the marketing at the retail level. The core idea is eliminating any entity with a vested interest in promoting smoking. Only a Borland model or something like it (a retail nonprofit monopoly) will be able to maintain high prices and eliminate the promotions that have been the most important marketing tools used by the companies (Chaloupka et al. 2002). Similarly, the TPA could be expected to use plain packaging, which would eliminate brand identity and the various devices that manufacturers use to signal reduced-harm messages without making explicit claims. The committee believes that the Borland proposal is worthy of serious study by the proposed policy development office.

Changing the Incentives of Tobacco Manufacturers

In the clear light of history, there can be no doubt that the promotion and marketing of cigarettes by tobacco companies have been the vectors of an enormous public health problem. The extent to which industry ef forts to suppress the truth about tobacco's health effects contributed to and sustained the tobacco problem, and whether this conduct persists are factual inquiries that have recently been addressed by federal district Judge Gladys Kessler in the U.S. Justice Department's Racketeering Influenced and Corrupt Organization (RICO) suit, United States v. Philip Morris (2006). Judge Kessler noted in her opinion that she was doubtful that the industry's aims have changed:

> As Defendants' senior executives took the witness stand at trial, one after another, it became exceedingly clear that these Defendants have not, as they claim, ceased their wrongdoing or, as they argued throughout the trial, undertaken fundamental or permanent institutional change (p. 1605). . . . [D]espite Defendants' claims that they have materially altered their management and are now "new" companies, the evidence demonstrates that they have not changed their policies or personnel in any meaningful way (p. 1609).

In the committee's view, even if the industry's misleading and deceptive conduct has ended, it is difficult to see how an industry whose aggressive marketing was the primary vector of a major public health problem and whose profits continue to be generated by selling cigarettes could possibly be an ally of public health efforts to discourage smoking and, eventually, to eliminate it. Indeed, evidence of industry efforts to defeat and curtail the tobacco control measures outlined in Chapter 6 is abundant, as are the industry's current promotional expenditures.

What conduct should now be expected of tobacco companies? Recent efforts by Philip Morris to align the company "with society's evolving expectations of a responsible tobacco company," including support for en-actment of federal legislation that empowers the FDA to regulate tobacco products and support for cessation and prevention programs, are intriguing. However, unless public policies fundamentally transform a tobacco company's economic incentives, the committee knows of no model of corporate responsibility that can reconcile a tobacco company's responsibility to its shareholders with a business plan of discouraging smoking and promoting cessation, that is, with measures designed to put itself out of the tobacco business.

Admittedly, the cause of tobacco control is better off today than it was when the tobacco companies were uniformly denying that smoking was ad-dictive or harmful and when smoking was aggressively promoted in every mass medium and on much of the visual space on highways and in urban centers. However, the emergence of the truth about smoking and about the tobacco industry's efforts to suppress it has not ended the companies' interest in generating profits. Nor has it erased the interests of convenience stores and other retailers in selling as many cigarettes as possible. For this reason, the committee has repeatedly emphasized the need to remove or offset the influences that tend to promote tobacco use or that otherwise impede successful efforts to reduce it.

The only socially useful role for the tobacco industry is to satisfy the residual demand among current smokers for tobacco products while financing compulsory remedial measures to undo the damage caused by the companies' past conduct. To the extent that the tobacco companies want to shift into the "harm reduction" market, these initiatives need to be carefully policed to ensure that consumers are not misled and that the marketing of reduced-exposure products is not actually a disguised effort to deter smoking cessation and to preserve the demand by addicted smokers—and that it does not, in fact, have that effect.

The challenge for policy makers is to develop creative measures for aligning the companies' incentives as closely as possible with public health interests. Specifically, how might incentives be created to deter companies from stimulating new demand for smoking, especially among youth (defined as those younger than 21 years of age); to encourage them to reduce the harmfulness of tobacco products; and, ideally, to help addicted smokers quit?

In its RICO suit against the major domestic manufacturers, the U.S. Department of Justice unsuccessfully urged the district court to set goals for youth smoking and penalize the companies $3,000 for every underage smoker exceeding the annual target (as had been proposed by the state attorneys general in 1997 during negotiations for a so-called global settlement of the state Medicaid reimbursement suits). Targets could also be set for reducing the prevalence of adult smokers based on a finding that smoking prevalence is substantially higher than it would have been in the absence of the manufacturers' illegal behavior.

The committee is not in a position to assess the economic plausibility of different incentive plans. However, responsible agencies of the federal government, including the policy development office, should evaluate the possible effects of different approaches to aligning the incentives of tobacco manufacturers more closely with public health objectives.

REDUCING THE NICOTINE CONTENT OF CIGARETTES

As discussed in Chapter 4, the ethical case for the forceful regulation of cigarettes and other tobacco products is squarely grounded in the addictive property of nicotine. Young people begin using tobacco products without genuinely appreciating the risk and meaning of addiction, and most addicted users experience deep regret and frustration about their inability to quit. One possible long-term strategy for reducing tobacco use and its associated harms is to reduce the addictiveness of tobacco products. For this reason, the committee believes that the responsible federal agencies, including the proposed tobacco policy development office, should give a high priority to exploring the feasibility of a long-term policy of gradually reducing the nicotine content of cigarettes. The goal of such a policy would be to reduce the addictiveness of cigarettes, thereby reducing the likelihood of progression from occasional to regular smoking by adolescents and young adults and making it easier for addicted smokers to quit by reducing their level of nicotine addiction (Benowitz and Henningfield 1994).

The committee acknowledges that the FDA's 1996 Tobacco Rule rejected a nicotine-reduction strategy in the short run. Similarly, recent reports on nicotine and on tobacco ingredients by the World Health Organization's Scientific Advisory Committee on Tobacco Product Regulation (SACTob) conclude that major scientific uncertainties and practical concerns preclude such a strategy, at least in the short term (SACTob 2003a, 2003b).

However, neither the FDA nor the WHO Scientific Advisory Committee has ruled out nicotine reduction as a long-term strategy—implemented over decades, perhaps—as its supporters have envisioned it (Benowitz and Henningfield 1994). In addition, to be implemented successfully, nicotine reduction would have to build on, and be integrated with, other components of the blueprint identified in Chapters 5 and 6, especially innovations in product regulation. Developing knowledge and experience with tobacco product regulation is a necessary precondition for implementing a nicotine-reduction strategy; however, regulation of tobacco product characteristics to make them less addictive could be a first step in the direction of the nicotine-reduction strategy (Henningfield et al. 2004).

With these caveats in mind, the committee elaborates below on the rationale for giving serious consideration to nicotine reduction as a long-term strategy.

Feasibility of a Reduced-Nicotine–Cigarette Strategy

The nicotine content of cigarettes could be lowered independently of changes to other constituents of cigarette tobacco, although the agency authorized to regulate tobacco products could also require manufacturers to reduce or eliminate specific toxic constituents of tobacco smoke, according to the perceived health risks and technical feasibility (see Chapter 6). However, it is unlikely that making cigarettes "safer" will ever be a satisfactory long-term strategy as long as tobacco use is addictive. Furthermore, on the basis of the experience with other addictive drugs, a gradual reduction of the nicotine content of cigarettes is more sensible than an effort to eliminate cigarettes altogether, given the costs of enforcing prohibition. The exact decrements of nicotine content and the rate at which these decrements are mandated would depend both on scientific considerations and on the practicality of changing tobacco manufacturing procedures. For a nicotine reduction strategy to work, it must apply to all manufactured cigarettes, and the extent of nicotine reduction across cigarette brands must be uniform. If not, smokers will simply select higher-nicotine–content cigarettes to sustain their addiction. Most likely, a nicotine-reduction strategy would need to take place in decrements over 10 to 15 years, with decrements of 10 to 15 percent of nicotine content per step. Currently available research suggests that smokers will find a gradual reduction of nicotine content acceptable when the other characteristics of tobacco smoke remain the same (Benowitz et al. 2004).

The ultimate level of nicotine reduction would need to be determined by ongoing scientific research and by the results of surveillance of the smokers of reduced nicotine products over time. Currently, marketed cigarettes contain 10 to 15 milligrams of nicotine per cigarette. The smoker systemically absorbs only about 10 percent of the nicotine in the rod of tobacco (cigarette), so the machine-determined nicotine yields of current cigarettes are approximately 1 milligram. Benowitz and Henningfield estimated that a reduction of the total nicotine content of cigarettes to 0.5 milligrams per rod would be a good initial estimate of what would be necessary to minimize the addictiveness of cigarettes (Benowitz and Henningfield 1994). The estimate was based on a daily intake level of 5 milligrams per day (compared with the 20 milligrams per day currently taken in by the typical addicted smoker) and the possibility that a person smokes up to 30 cigarettes per day very intensively. The nicotine content of tobacco can be reduced either by extracting nicotine from the tobacco or by using tobacco that is genetically engineered to have a lower nicotine content. Both of these methods have been used in the manufacturing of low-nicotine-content cigarettes in the past (for the Next™ brand of cigarettes by extracting nicotine and for the Quest™ brand of cigarettes by using genetically engineered tobacco). The nicotine content of cigarette tobacco can be determined by straightforward and unambiguous chemical analytical methods. It would also be essential that cigarette manufacturers be prohibited from changing the design of cigarettes to make nicotine more bioavailable than it is at present. (Bioavailability could be assessed by smoking machine testing or human bioavailability studies by using biomarkers of nicotine exposure. The details of testing and enforcement would have to be worked out by the regulatory authority.)

One of the consequences of reducing the nicotine available from cigarettes might be that smokers would smoke cigarettes more intensively or
smoke more cigarettes per day, thereby increasing their exposure to other
toxic smoke constituents. This could produce short-term adverse health
consequences. It is well known that when smokers switch from higher- to
lower-yield commercial cigarettes, they adjust their smoking behavior to
maintain the desired levels of nicotine intake (NCI 2001). Smokers take
deeper and more frequent puffs, block ventilation holes, or smoke more
cigarettes to sustain adequate levels of nicotine. It should be recognized,
however, that currently available commercial low-yield cigarettes contain
as much nicotine as high-yield cigarettes (NCI 2001). Therefore, it is quite
easy for a person to adjust his or her smoking behavior to compensate for
low yields. However, these are not the same types of low-nicotine cigarettes
that would be part of a nicotine reduction regulatory strategy.

Recent research with low-nicotine–content cigarettes in which the nicotine content was gradually tapered down (by extracting the nicotine from
the tobacco) suggests that smokers do not increase their toxic exposures,
despite substantial reductions in their nicotine intakes. Benowitz and colleagues conducted a 6-week longitudinal study of 20 smokers who smoked
their usual brand and who then smoked five different types of research
cigarettes with progressively lower nicotine contents (ranging from 10 to
0.6 milligrams), each for 1 week (Benowitz et al. 2004). The intake of nicotine, as measured by determination of the smokers' plasma cotinine con-
centrations, declined progressively as the nicotine content of the cigarettes
was reduced, with little evidence of compensation. The level of cigarette
consumption and biomarkers of exposure to carbon monoxide and poly-
cyclic aromatic hydrocarbons remained stable, whereas the level of urinary
NNAL (tobacco-specific nitrosamine) excretion decreased. These data suggest that the availability of nicotine in tobacco can be lowered without
increasing the level of exposure to the toxins of tobacco smoke.

The reasons for a lack of compensatory smoking are likely to include
the difficulty in obtaining more nicotine (because less nicotine is available in
the tobacco) and the satiating effects of the tar, the levels of which remained
unchanged in these reduced-nicotine cigarettes. Smokers could smoke more
cigarettes per day in the first phases of a gradual reduction strategy, but
for most smokers, compensation for low-yield cigarettes is done primarily
by puffing more intensively. Although there is strong evidence of titration
of nicotine intake from cigarettes, sensory aspects such as the taste and
harshness of cigarette smoke do provide some reinforcement and may
lessen withdrawal symptoms compared with those experienced when both
nicotine and tar deliveries are reduced in combination. Similar findings of
little compensation from the smoking of reduced-nicotine, higher-tar ciga-

rettes have been reported by Rose and Behm (2004), using tobacco that was genetically engineered to be low in nicotine content, and by Benowitz and colleagues using manufactured cigarettes from which nicotine had been extracted (Benowitz, Peyton, and Herrera 2006).

A key element in any regulatory proposal must be careful surveillance of smokers over time. Surveillance would need to include measurement of cigarette consumption, measurement of the smokers' level of exposure to nicotine and tobacco toxins by determining the levels of various biomarkers, and assessment of smoking initiation rates and subsequent cigarette consumption by adolescents and young adults. Surveillance of biomarkers could entail cross-sectional or longitudinal studies of cohorts of smokers. The numbers and characteristics of smokers who would be selected and which biomarkers would be monitored would need to be determined by the regulatory authorities.

Some smokers may not get enough nicotine from reduced-nicotine cigarettes to sustain their addiction and may experience withdrawal symptoms. To deal with such smokers, nicotine-containing medications should be made readily and inexpensively available. Making nicotine-containing medication available could also be done as part of a tobacco regulatory strategy (NCI 2001). Although nicotine in itself is likely to have some intrinsic toxicity, such toxicity is minimal compared with the toxicity of cigarette smoking. Smokers who move from cigarettes to pure nicotine either could continue to take nicotine in pure form over time to sustain their addiction, or could gradually reduce their level of nicotine over time. In any case, the health risks associated with nicotine use is far less than those of continued smoking.

A nicotine-reduction strategy would require considerable education of the public about the goals of the program and the nature of the new cigarettes that will be introduced every year or two. The potential utility of nicotine replacement therapy to deal with insufficient nicotine intake would need to be explained, and resources would need to be available to help those smokers who do decide to quit as their level of addiction is reduced. Vehicles for public education might include media campaigns and information supplied in cigarette package "onserts." The details of the public information program would most logically be coordinated by a central regulatory authority working with local communities to ensure that various populations of smokers are reached.

One concern with a mandatory reduction in the nicotine content of cigarettes is the creation of a demand for contraband or other tobacco products that do not meet the requirements set by the agency of regulatory authority. Such products might include manufactured cigarettes with high levels of nicotine that are illegally imported or manufactured, or loose tobacco which could be rolled into cigarettes by the user. The regulatory agency would need to monitor such activities and products and determine whether intervention is needed to protect the public health. If contraband use is relatively low and if contraband products are used by only a small percentage of smokers who are highly addicted and want to continue to be addicted, then the public health problem would not be great and enforcement may not become a major issue. However, if a substantial market for contraband products arises, the regulatory agency would have to consider alternative approaches, such as raising the authorized level of nicotine for all cigarettes or allowing a higher-level nicotine cigarette to be obtained with a prescription.

If the nicotine reduction approach were successfully implemented, it is anticipated that cigarettes containing very low levels of nicotine would eventually appeal to a very small number of consumers and would be smoked primarily in social situations. The decision to smoke or not to smoke would not be driven by drug addiction and could be exercised more rationally by the smoker. A marked reduction of cigarette consumption and the promotion of quitting by currently addicted smokers would have an enormous impact on the adverse health effects of tobacco use.

Impact of a Reduced-Nicotine–Cigarette Strategy

The committee is in no position to assess the feasibility of a nicotine reduction strategy or to predict the consequences of implementing it. However, the committee believes that this approach has great promise and should be seriously explored by the regulatory agency recommended in Chapter 6 or the tobacco policy research office recommended in this chapter. The potential impact of federally mandated nicotine-reduction strategy was recently examined by an exploratory computer simulation conducted by Tengs and colleagues (2005). They developed a mathematical model based on the U.S. population in 2003, which was divided into cohorts according to age, gender, and smoking status. The smoking behaviors that were modeled included smoking initiation, cessation, and relapse. The model outcome was quality-adjusted life years. In examining the effects of a reduced-nicotine–cigarette strategy, Tengs and colleagues assumed that the nicotine content of cigarettes would be reduced over 6 years and that the reduced addictiveness of the reduced-nicotine–content cigarette after completion of the mandated tapering would result in an 80 percent increase in cessation rates and an 80 percent decrease in relapse and initiation rates over the 6 years. The model also included a 10 percent increase in the annual probability of death among continued smokers because of compensation and the probability that 10 percent of smokers would seek high-nicotine cigarettes from the black market, with both probabilities increasing linearly over 10 years. The simulation projects that the prevalence of smoking among the adult population could decline from 23 to 5 percent over 50 years, with a cumulative gain of 157,000,000 quality-adjusted life years. The investigators also performed a number of sensitivity analyses. All showed a similar gain in quality-adjusted life years. The investigators concluded that "policy makers would be hard-pressed to identify another domestic public health intervention, short of historical sanitation efforts, that has offered this magnitude of benefit to the population." Although the computer simulation by Tengs and colleagues includes too many ungrounded assumptions to serve as a basis for estimating the consequences of a phased-in nicotine reduction strategy, the study does reinforce the committee's view that this approach merits serious consideration by policy makers.

Other Regulatory Approaches to a Reduced-Nicotine–Cigarette Strategy

Although a regulatory strategy that would mandate changes in product characteristics by a central authority is likely to be the most effective in reducing the addictiveness of cigarettes, two other regulatory approaches that could be implemented should be mentioned. One approach would be to mandate warnings on packages describing the nicotine content of the cigarettes and the relative addictiveness of the products. Individuals could choose to smoke less addictive cigarettes if they desired. Reduced-nicotine–content cigarettes are being marketed as the brand Quest™, but their sales are quite low. On the basis of prior experience with cigarette labeling and the compulsion of addicted individuals to continue the use of their addictive drug, if it is available, as well as the lack of public uptake of Quest™ cigarettes, it is unlikely that such an approach would be successful.

Another approach would be the progressive taxation of cigarettes on the basis of their nicotine content. Although highly addicted smokers are likely to accept moderate increases in price, so that they may obtain their desired dose of nicotine, if the tax increases were very high, the high taxes might force some smokers to accept lower-nicotine–content cigarettes. Progressive tax escalation based on the higher nicotine contents of cigarette tobacco over a number of years might result in many smokers switching to less addictive cigarettes. However, a mandated approach for nicotine reduction that is uniform across all cigarette brands might have the biggest payoff at the population level. The advantages and disadvantages of these alternative regulatory approaches should be explored by the regulatory agency.

> **Recommendation 42: Upon being empowered to regulate tobacco products, the FDA should give priority to exploring the potential effectiveness of a long-term strategy for reducing the amount of nicotine in cigarettes and should commission the studies needed to assess the feasibility of implementing such an approach. If such a strategy ap-**

pears to be feasible, the agency should develop a long-term plan for implementing the strategy as part of a comprehensive plan for reducing tobacco use.

CONCLUSION

The new tobacco policy development office should be charged with conducting the necessary research and analysis to advise policy makers on the likely effects of existing policies and of proposed new ones and of measures that can be taken to increase the prospects of the successful implementation of these policies. For example, the aggressive tobacco control measures recommended in Chapter 6 rest on emerging public understanding of the characteristics of tobacco products that warrant such measures, and successful implementation over the long term will entail ongoing educational efforts to reinforce and sustain public understanding. In addition, tobacco use is a worldwide problem, and many other countries have embraced aggressive measures of tobacco control. The policy development office should also study the effects of policies adopted in other countries as well as the effects of free trade policies on tobacco control efforts in the United States and abroad.

In short, even if the aggressive measures recommended in this report were speedily adopted and implemented, ending the tobacco problem will require decades of sustained and careful policymaking, accompanied by vigilant monitoring and flexible response. A robust capacity for policy analysis and development is an essential component of a strategic initiative to end the tobacco problem. The policy development office as well as the FDA should take a long-term view and should initiate serious study of approaches on the frontier of tobacco control.

REFERENCES

Benowitz NL, Hall SM, Dempsey D, Allen F, Peng M, Jacob P. 2004. Safety of a nicotine reduction strategy. Paper presented at Society for Research on Nicotine and Tobacco Research annual meeting.

Benowitz NL, Henningfield JE. 1994. Establishing a nicotine threshold for addiction. The implications for tobacco regulation. *New England Journal of Medicine* 331(2):123-125.

Benowitz NL, Peyton J, Herrera B. 2006. Nicotine intake and dose response when smoking reduced-nicotine content cigarettes. *Clinical Pharmacology Therapy* 80:703-714.

Borland R. 2003. A strategy for controlling the marketing of tobacco products: a regulated market model. *Tobacco Control* 12(4):374-382.

Chaloupka FJ, Cummings KM, Morley CP, Horan JK. 2002. Tax, price and cigarette smoking: evidence from the tobacco documents and implications for tobacco company marketing strategies. *Tobacco Control* 11(Suppl 1): 162-172.

Henningfield JE, Benowitz NL, Connolly GN, Davis RM, Gray N, Myers ML, Zeller M 2004. Reducing tobacco addiction through tobacco product regulation. *Tobacco Control* 13(2):132-135.

NCI (National Cancer Institute). 2001. *Risks Associated with Smoking Cigarettes with Low Machine-Measured Yields of Tar and Nicotine (Monograph 13)*. Bethesda, MD: National Institutes of Health.

Rose JE, Behm FM. 2004. Effects of low nicotine content cigarettes on smoke intake. *Nicotine and Tobacco Research* 6(2):309-319.

SACTob (World Health Organization's Scientific Advisory Committee on Tobacco Product Regulation). 2003a. *Recommendation on Nicotine and the Regulation in Tobacco and Non-Tobacco Products*. Geneva, Switzerland: World Health Organization.

SACTob. 2003b. *Recommendation on Tobacco Product Ingredients and Emissions*. Geneva, Switzerland: World Health Organization.

Tengs TO, Ahmad S, Savage JM, Moore R, Gage E. 2005. The AMA proposal to mandate nicotine reduction in cigarettes: a simulation of the population health impacts. *Preventive Medicine* 40(2):170-180.

Index

A

Abt Associates Inc., 165, 169, 170
Access to tobacco products
  adolescent perceptions of, 167
  community mobilization, 205
  Internet sales, 11-12, 20, 207-210
  minimum age, 206
  price and, 42
  recommendations, 10-11, 20, 205, 210
  youth restrictions, 118-119, 120, 159,
    167, 203-206
Action on Smoking and Health, 110
Addictiveness of tobacco products. *See*
    Nicotine
  adolescents, 89, 118-119
  atypical patterns of smoking and, 93,
    95
  and cessation, 5, 117
  conditioning, 79, 80
  deception by tobacco industry, 7, 33,
    35, 114, 121-122, 125, 127,
    146, 148
  environmental and personal factors,
    80, 81, 201
  flavorants and additives and, 283
  genetic factors, 79, 82, 86-87, 96-97
  industry acknowledgment of, 125
  and litigation, 119, 121-122
  nature of, 77-82

and paternalism issue, 151-152
as "pediatric disease," 119, 148
physiological effects of smoke, 79
public understanding of, 7-8, 33, 35,
  89, 108, 147
risk perception, 90, 91, 93
sensorimotor factors, 81
and tobacco control movement, 111-
  112, 116-118, 119
warning labels, 298
Adolescent tobacco use
  alcohol policy compared, 153
  cessation programs, 21
  effectiveness of programs on, 11, 68,
    124-125, 201
  exposure to advertising, 320, 322-323
  glamorization of smoking in movies
    and, 330-333
  household bans on smoking and,
    201-202
  illegal sales, 164, 203
  initiation rates, 3, 4, 5, 6, 11, 31, 34,
    35, 45-46, 49, 51, 56-57, 70,
    98, 112, 147-148, 149, 150-151,
    167, 200
  invulnerability concept and, 88, 89
  media glamorization of smoking and,
    330-333
  mental illness and, 95

motivation, 92-93, 98, 183
paternalism issue and, 34, 150-151
prevalence, 31, 46, 52-54, 124, 167-
    168, 169, 170-171
prevention interventions, 8, 11, 123
price of cigarettes as deterrent, 9,
    183-184
restricted access to tobacco and, 118-
    119, 120, 159, 167, 203-206
risk perceptions and, 4, 5, 6, 8, 35,
    88-93, 98, 149, 150-151, 187,
    297
and smoking career, 58, 98
targeting by tobacco industry, 50,
    112, 129, 148, 327-330
Adult tobacco use. See also Young adult
    tobacco use
cessation rates, 4, 5, 49, 57, 66-67
ever smoked, 49
never smoked, 45
per capita consumption, 45, 54, 56,
    168
prevalence, 1, 4, 5, 13, 29, 32, 45, 48,
    51-52, 62, 64, 65, 66, 124, 125,
    146, 166, 168, 170-171, 231,
    278
risk perception and, 80, 90, 91, 151
Advertising. See Marketing and advertising
Advocacy. See also Antitobacco activism;
    Community mobilization
grassroots, 119, 147, 189, 196, 241-
    243, 244
African Americans, 60, 61, 62, 63, 64, 94,
    161, 171, 185, 247
Age. See also Adolescent; Adult; Young
    adult tobacco use
and initiation of smoking, 81, 94-95
minimum for tobacco purchases, 206
and nondaily smoking, 94
and prevalence of smoking, 52, 53,
    58-59
Alabama, 174, 309, 311, 315
Alaska, 174, 309, 311, 315
Alcohol
    excise taxes, 193
    policy changes, 153, 241, 242, 273,
        304-306
    shipping restrictions, 210
American Academy of Family Physicians,
    21, 222
American Academy of Pediatrics, 21, 222

American Cancer Society, 109, 110, 120,
    179
American College Health Association, 20,
    198, 199
American College of Emergency Physicians,
    221
American College of Physicians, 21, 222
American Correctional Association, 19,
    194-195, 196
American Heart Association, 109, 179
American Indian and Alaska Natives, 60,
    62, 63, 64
American Jail Association, 194-195
American Legacy Foundation, 2, 123, 124,
    129, 130, 133, 229-231, 243
American Lung Association, 109, 179
American Medical Association, 21, 109,
    117, 120, 222
American Nonsmokers' Rights Foundation,
    198
American Nursing Association, 21, 222
American Psychiatric Association, 117
American Stop Smoking Intervention Study
    (ASSIST), 120, 121, 159, 163,
    172, 241-242, 243, 244, 246
Annenberg Tobacco Survey, 89, 90
Antidepressants, 87
Antitobacco activism, early movements, 34,
    107-108, 109-110, 115
Arizona, 115, 119, 160, 172, 174, 309,
    311, 315
Arkansas, 66, 172, 309, 311, 315
Asians, 60-61, 62, 63, 64, 94, 161, 247
Attention-deficit/hyperactivity disorder, 96
Australia, 83, 201, 291, 292, 295
Austria, 213

B

Ballin, Scott, 117
Bangladesh, 292
Bans on smoking. See Restrictions on
    smoking
Banzhaf, John F., 110
Behavior Risk Factor Surveillance System
    (BRFSS), 46, 65, 93, 164, 165
Botvin, Gil, 212
Brain-derived neurotropic factor, 82
Brandt, Allan, 107
Brazil, 292, 293, 295, 297

Bright Futures, 219
Brown and Williamson Company, 43, 209, 287
Bupropion treatment, 82, 87, 233
Bureau of Alcohol, Tobacco, Firearms, and Explosives, 209, 304
Bush Administration, 123

C

California
    adolescent smoking, 167
    Adult Tobacco Survey, 164
    bans on smoking, 192, 195, 196, 202-203, 214, 245
    cessation rates, 67, 136
    Department of Education, 161
    Department of Health Services, 161, 164
    effectiveness of programs, 166-168, 169, 184, 192, 226, 242-243
    evaluation of programs, 164, 165
    excise taxes, 160, 161, 177, 184, 311
    funding for tobacco control, 161-162, 166, 167, 175, 180, 315
    Healthy Kids Program, 161
    heart disease mortality, 166-167
    marketing violations by industry, 320, 328
    media campaigns, 120, 161, 184, 224-226, 227
    MSA allocations, 178, 180, 320
    nonsmokers' rights movement, 147
    per-capita cigarette consumption, 166, 167
    prevalence of smoking, 66, 67, 94, 136, 165, 166, 167-168, 169, 170, 171
    retail environment, 299-300
    revenues and expenditures for tobacco control, 174, 177, 178, 180, 309
    school-based interventions, 212, 214
    Smokers' Helpline, 161
    Student Tobacco Survey, 168
    Tobacco Control Program, 119, 120, 124-125, 157, 159, 160, 161-162, 163, 164, 165, 174
    Tobacco Survey, 94, 164
    youth access law, 208
    Youth Tobacco Survey, 164
California Apartment Association, 196

Carlin, John, 305
Camel cigarettes, 43
Campaign for Tobacco-Free Kids, 179, 285
Canada
    bans on smoking, 202
    excise taxes, 183
    health warnings on tobacco products, 291-292, 295
    regretful smokers, 83
    risk perceptions, 297
Cancer, 29, 30, 44, 89, 92, 108, 110, 115, 116, 125, 127, 191, 226, 247, 280, 297, 335, 337
Cardiovascular disease, 29, 30, 95, 110, 166-167, 191, 215-216, 247
Catechol-O-methyltransferase gene, 82
Center for Tobacco Prevention and Control, 163
Centers for Disease Control and Prevention, 21, 29, 128, 161, 192, 193, 224, 228, 238, 242, 244
    Best Practices for Comprehensive Tobacco Control Programs, 159, 175, 176, 242, 335
    BRFSS, 46, 65, 93, 164, 165
    goals for tobacco control, 249
    Guidelines for School Health Programs to Prevent Tobacco Use and Addiction, 109
    IMPACT program, 120, 159, 246
    Office on Smoking and Health, 22, 159, 172, 246
    recommended funding level for state programs, 9, 19, 172-173, 175-176, 181-182, 308, 309-310
    YRBSS, 46, 53, 171
Centers for Medicare and Medicaid Services, 126
Cessation attempt fatigue, 86
Cessation of smoking
    abstinence defined, 85
    access to programs, 12-13, 21-22, 84, 126, 129, 185
    addictiveness of nicotine and, 5, 117
    adolescent programs, 21
    age trends, 58, 59
    airway sensory replacement and, 81
    behavioral and counseling interventions, 80, 87, 109, 126, 160, 161, 219, 220, 221, 222, 232, 233, 236, 240

challenges, 84, 235-236
clinical practice guidelines, 87, 126,
    129, 240
community mobilization, 222, 234,
    236-237, 238
components of care management, 232
cost-effectiveness to interventions,
    239-241
delivering services, 238-239
demand for programs, 234, 235-236
disseminating programs, 12, 13, 16,
    17, 21, 22, 24, 87, 234, 235,
    236-238, 303
duration of quit attempts, 85, 86
education about quitting process,
    235-236
effectiveness of programs, 6, 12, 13,
    68, 87, 159, 232-234, 236,
    239-231
environment and, 16, 17, 24, 84, 86,
    160, 192, 193, 201
ethical context for policies, 14, 34,
    149-150
funding programs, 187, 240
gender differences, 62
genetic factors, 82, 97
geographic differences, 64, 65, 66-67
hardcore smokers, 6, 233, 234
health improvements, 231
industry discouragement of, 24, 323
initiation age and, 59
intensity of smoking and, 59, 85, 86-
    87, 97
intensity of treatment and, 232-233,
    234
interventions, 6, 12, 21, 22, 120,
    231-241
"light" cigarettes and, 297
limitations of programs, 234
mental illness and, 68, 69
motivation, 83, 109, 184, 221
nicotine replacement therapies, 17,
    82, 87, 117, 147, 185, 233, 234
nondaily smoking and, 94
paternalism issue and, 149-150
pharmacotherapies, 82, 87, 109,
    119, 126, 147, 233, 234, 240,
    281-282
physician participation in, 83-84, 129,
    219-222

and prevalence of smoking, 232, 235,
    249, 250, 251-252
price of cigarettes and, 182-183, 184
quitlines, 21, 84, 126, 133, 161, 221,
    236, 237
quitting attempts, 5-6, 65, 85-87, 97,
    233, 234
surveillance and monitoring, 239
race/ethnicity and, 61
rates, 4, 5, 12, 45, 49, 57, 58, 62, 66-
    67, 82-83, 193
recommendations, 12, 21, 22, 236, 239
reimbursement for treatment, 12, 13,
    22, 84, 126, 234, 238, 239-241
relapses, 86, 97, 193, 201, 233, 234
and smokeless tobacco use, 2, 3
socioeconomic status and, 63
Stages of Change model, 84-85
stepped-care approach, 232, 233, 234,
    235, 239
trends, 31, 57, 77
warning labels on packages and, 295
Children, exposure to secondhand smoke,
    115, 192, 199, 200-201
Chinese Americans, 61
Cigar smoking, 30, 41, 43, 198
Cigarette Labeling and Advertising Act,
    110, 273, 300-301, 319
Cigarette manufacturing, 41-42, 107, 152
Cigarette Smoking Act of 1969, 110, 319
Cipollone, Rose, 113
Clinician's Handbook of Preventive
    Services, 219
Clinton Administration, 119, 123
Clonidine, 87
Coalition for Tobacco-Free Colorado, 245
Coalition on Smoking OR Health, 109, 117
College, 20, 198, 199. *See also* Young
    adult tobacco use
Colorado, 174, 243, 245, 309, 311, 315
Community Intervention Trial for Smoking
    Cessation (COMMIT), 83, 87,
    192
Community mobilization
    action projects, 213-214
    alcohol policy compared, 241
    cessation programs, 222, 234, 236-
        237, 238
    education programs, 215-216, 230,
        231
    effectiveness, 215, 242, 244, 246

evaluation of programs, 242, 246
expenditures, 175
funding, 159, 163, 244, 246
grassroots advocacy, 119, 147, 189,
    196, 241-243, 244
lobbying challenge from tobacco
    industry, 121, 241, 243-244
local health departments, 161, 163
maintaining momentum, 244-246
recommendations, 246
school programs combined with, 214,
    215-217, 218, 231
smoking bans, 115, 119, 189, 196,
    203, 244-246
state strategy, 120-121, 154, 241-242
youth access restriction, 205
Comprehensive Smoking Education Act of
    1984, 110
Comprehensive state programs. *See also*
    Excise tax rates; Restrictions on
    smoking; *individual states*
    CDC best practices, 159, 175, 176,
        242
    community mobilization strategy, 22,
        120-121, 154, 241-242, 246
    description, 160-163
    effectiveness, 67, 68, 120, 124-125,
        136, 157-158, 159, 160, 161,
        165-172
    elements of, 120, 152, 160
    evaluation of, 120, 159-160, 164-165,
        171-172
    expenditures, 30, 158, 163, 173-176,
        226, 309-310, 315-316
    funding, 120, 128, 157, 158-159,
        172-182, 226-227, 308-319
    intensity of, 160
    interventions, 158, 159
    media campaigns, 119, 120, 159, 160,
        161, 162-163, 224-229
    monitoring and surveillance, 164
    MSA allocations, 128, 178-181
    public health partnerships, 154
    recommendations, 181-182
    revenue sources, 158, 176-181
    youth access restrictions, 120, 159
Conduct disorders, 95
Congress. *See also* Legislation
    authority over states, 188 n.3
    Cigarette Labeling and Advertising
        Act, 110, 273, 300-301, 319

Cigarette Smoking Act of 1969, 110,
    319
Fair Housing Act, 197
Federal Smoking Prevention and
    Tobacco Control Act, 126, 206,
    275
Food, Drug and Cosmetic Act, 117,
    126, 152
proposed legislation, 275, 283-285,
    307
Connecticut, 66, 67, 115, 125, 309, 311, 315
Consumer Product Safety Commission, 111
Consumer sovereignty issue, 7, 8, 32, 111,
    114, 117, 145-146, 150-152. *See
    also* Paternalism issue
Controlled Substances Act, 112, 152
Correctional facilities. *See* Inmates
Council for Tobacco Research, 111, 123
Council of Emergency Medicine Residency
    Directors, 221
Crawford, Victor, 226
Current Population Survey Tobacco Use
    Supplement, 46, 64, 96
Current smokers/smoking
    cessation attempts, 82
    correlates of, 57-68
    decline in, 45
    defined, 47, 166 n.2
    intensity of smoking, 55
    prevalence, 48, 51
CYP2A6 gene, 82
CYP2B6 gene, 97

D

Daily smoking/smokers, 52-53, 54, 55, 65,
    95, 217
Davis, Ronald, 109
Deaths, 1-2, 29, 30, 34, 89, 113, 116, 126,
    130, 166-167, 226, 228, 231
Decarboxylase, 82
Decisional Balance Inventory, 92
Decline in smoking
    health scares and, 44, 109
    Healthy People 2010 goals, 124
    industry response to, 44, 46-51
    maintaining momentum, 6-7, 30-31
    media campaigns and, 124, 160, 184,
        217, 218, 223, 225-226, 227,
        228, 229, 230-231

policy changes and, 130, 145
smoking bans and, 10, 94, 125, 184,
    185, 191-202
trends, 4-5, 45-46, 70
Delaware, 125, 128, 173, 174, 175, 176,
    179, 245, 308, 309, 311, 315
Denmark, 213
DHL, 209
Disabled individuals, 95
Discount brands, 133
Dopamine, 79, 80, 82, 97
Drug Abuse Resistance Education, 211

E

Eclipse cigarette, 127
Economic effects of tobacco use, 2, 30,
    192, 195, 200, 239
Educational attainment
    and nondaily smoking, 94
    and prevalence of smoking, 6, 62-64,
        65, 67, 96, 187
Educational initiatives, 109-110. See also
    Media campaigns; School-based
    interventions
    community mobilization, 215-216,
        230, 231
    effectiveness, 70, 198
Emergency Medicine Residents Association,
    221
Emergency Nurses Association, 221
Employee Retirement and Income Security
    Act, 273
Environmental tobacco smoke. See
    Secondhand smoke
Epidemiology of tobacco use. See also
    Cessation of smoking; Decline in
    smoking; Initiation of smoking;
    Intensity of smoking; Prevalence
    of smoking
    atypical patterns of smoking, 94
    cessation rates, 82
    decline in use, 4-5, 45-51
    growth of problem, 4, 41-44
    recent trends, 51-68
European Union, 292
Excise tax rates
    and adolescent smoking, 183-184
    appropriate level of, 159, 181, 182,
        185-187, 249

avoidance, 9, 177, 184, 185-186, 188,
    207
cessation services funded with, 187,
    240
and cigarette use, 182-184
congressional authority over states,
    188 n.3
disparities among states, 9, 176-
    177, 182, 186, 188-189, 308,
    310-311
and expenditures for tobacco control,
    178
external costs of consumption and,
    186-187
federal, 10, 19, 50, 125, 185, 188,
    189
funding tobacco control with, 9, 19,
    159, 160, 162, 176, 177-178,
    181, 182, 188-189, 218, 224,
    227, 314-317
impacts of, 9, 170, 181, 182, 184,
    185, 249, 250
interaction with other antismoking
    measures, 184-185
Internet retail shipments and, 185,
    186, 207, 209, 210
new measures, 36, 188-189
recommendations, 9, 10, 17-18, 19,
    25, 182, 189, 318
regressivity concerns, 187
revenues, 9, 174-175, 176, 177, 178
state, 9, 19, 119-120, 125, 158, 159,
    160, 162, 170, 176-178, 182-
    189, 310-311
tax-exempt outlet sales and, 185, 207

F

Fair Housing Act, 197
Fairness Doctrine, 110, 113-114, 223-224
Family Smoking Prevention and Tobacco
    Control Act, 126, 206, 275
FDA Tobacco Rule, 126
Federal Acquisition Streamlining Act of
    1994, 243
Federal Bureau of Prisons, 195
Federal Communications Commission,
    110, 223
Federal Express, 209

Federal Food, Drug, and Cosmetic Act,
117, 126, 152
Federal Trade Commission, 47, 110, 112,
113, 287, 299, 301
Fetal growth retardation, 110
Field Institute, 164
Filtered cigarettes, 44, 70, 323
Finland, 215
Firearms policy, 153
Florida
bans on smoking, 245
effectiveness of programs, 171-172,
229
excise tax rates, 311
funding for programs, 227, 315
media campaigns, 120, 224, 227-229
Medicaid litigation, 122-123
revenues and expenditures for tobacco
control, 174, 224, 309
tobacco control program, 125, 128,
160, 174, 227-228
Youth Tobacco Survey, 228
Food and Drug Administration
authority, 17, 25, 36, 117, 118, 119,
122, 123, 126-127, 154, 203,
272, 275-277, 283-285, 307-308
integrity, 287-288
Tobacco Rule, 203, 205, 206, 276,
319, 323, 347
youth-oriented policy, 148, 276
Former smokers, 47, 57 n.7, 65
Framework Convention for Tobacco
Control, 3, 34, 289, 292
Freedom of Information Act, 121, 243
Funding tobacco control. *See also* Excise
tax rates
allocation formula, 311-312, 314-318
American Legacy Foundation, 129
budgetary constraints, 9, 128, 157,
160, 161-162, 165, 166, 167,
171, 172, 180, 224, 226-227
and effectiveness of state programs,
160
federal role, 22, 159, 246, 308-319
MSA allocations, 9, 128, 129, 158,
163, 173, 174, 178-181, 227-
228, 308-319
philanthropic, 22, 120, 246
prevalence-based penalties, 318-319

recommended and proposed spending,
9, 17-18, 19, 25, 172-173, 175
176, 181-182, 308, 309-310
remedial assessment on cigarettes,
312-313
state programs, 120, 128, 157, 158-
159, 172-182, 224, 226-227,
308-319

G

Gallup Organization, 164, 167
Gamblers, 95
Gamma-aminobutyric acid 2 gene, 82
Gender differences. *See also* Women, as
marketing target
cessation of smoking, 62
initiation of smoking, 81
natural history of smoking, 58
motivation to smoke, 183
prevalence of smoking, 51, 58, 60-62
Generic brands, 50
Genetic vulnerability, 79, 82, 86-87, 96-97
Georgia, 174, 309, 311, 314, 315, 316, 317
Germany, 213
Glamorization of smoking, 6, 42, 110,
330-333
Gori, Gio, 287
Grassroots activism, 119, 147, 189,
196, 241-243, 244. *See
also* Antitobacco activism;
Community mobilization
Great Depression, 44
Group Against Smokers' Pollution (GASP),
115
Growing Up Today Study, 183
Guide to Clinical Preventive Services, 219
Guidelines for Adolescent Preventive
Services, 219
Guidelines for Health Supervision
of Infants, Children, and
Adolescents, 219

H

Hard-core smokers, 6, 8, 69, 96-97, 98
Harm reduction policies, 282
Hawaii, 174, 245, 309, 311, 315
Health Belief Model, 88
Health care expenditures, 2, 30

Health Supervision Guidelines, 219
Healthy People 2010, 7, 13, 52, 124, 133, 135, 136, 199, 250, 251
Heavy smokers, 47, 54, 61, 68, 69, 95, 96, 145
Hispanics, 60, 61, 62, 63, 64, 94, 161, 247
History of tobacco use, 107-108
Home production of cigarettes, 185, 186
Homeless individuals, 6, 95, 96, 248
Hong Kong, 292
Hutchinson Project, 211

I

Idaho, 174, 245, 309, 311, 315
Illinois, 174, 309, 311, 315
Impotence, 294
Income
expenditures on cigarettes, 51
and prevalence of smoking, 6, 44, 62-64, 65, 67, 187
Inconsistent preferences, 151
India, 292
Indian reservations, 24, 185, 207
Indiana, 174, 213, 309, 311, 315
Industry. See Tobacco industry
Infant exposure to tobacco smoke, 29
Infectious diseases, 29
Initiation of smoking
adolescents, 3, 4, 5, 6, 11, 31, 34, 35, 45-46, 49, 51, 56-57, 70, 98, 112, 147-148, 149, 150-151, 167, 200
age and, 81, 94-95
defined, 56 n.6
deterrents, 7, 12-13
environment and, 200, 219
gender differences, 81
genetic influences, 81
psychiatric and behavioral comorbidities, 95-97
racial/ethnic differences, 69
regret among smokers, 5, 83, 88, 93, 97, 151
risk perceptions and, 6, 88-93
socioeconomic status and, 63
trends in rates, 13, 31, 45, 46, 49, 56-57, 77, 252
young adults, 5, 6, 45-46, 49, 57, 69, 70, 94-95, 167

Initiatives to Mobilize for the Prevention and Control of Tobacco (IMPACT) program, 120, 159, 246
Inmates, 6, 95, 96, 194-196
Institute of Medicine, 118, 119, 125, 130, 148
Insurance coverage, 12, 13, 22, 84, 126, 234, 238, 239-241
Intensity of smoking
age at initiation and, 98
and cessation, 59, 85, 86-87, 97
gender differences, 61-62
genetic factors, 81
per-capita consumption, 45, 54, 56, 166, 168-169
price of cigarettes and, 182, 183
and risk perception, 90
and smoking career, 59, 85, 98
socioeconomic status and, 69
trends, 5, 6, 45, 54-56
Interagency Committee on Smoking and Health, 126, 129
International Agency for Research on Cancer, 191
International Tobacco Control Policy Evaluation Survey, 294, 295, 297
International comparisons, 3, 34-35, 193, 291-293, 329
Interventions. See Cessation of smoking; Prevention interventions
Iowa, 174, 213, 309, 311, 315
Ireland, 193

J

Jenkins Act, 207, 304
Joe Camel character, 50, 112
Joint Commission on Accreditation of Healthcare Facilities, 194

K

Kansas, 174, 179, 216, 305, 309, 311, 315
Kentucky, 65, 66, 94, 134, 135, 174, 176, 309, 311, 315
Kessler, David, 117, 118, 119, 122, 123, 148
Kessler, Gladys, 127-128, 287, 297-298, 318, 345

Klinger, Richard, 107
Kool cigarettes, 43
Koop, C. Everett, 115, 122
Korean Americans, 61, 247

L

Legacy Media Tracking Surveys, 229
Legislation
    advertising restrictions, 110, 118
    bans on smoking, 36
    exemptions for tobacco industry,
        111-112
    FDA empowerment, 126-127, 279-
        280, 283-285
    proposed, 122, 276, 279-280, 283-
        285, 286-287, 295, 301
    public health gains, 113
    state excise taxes, 119, 210
    warning labels, 110, 113, 126, 154,
        273, 295
    youth access control, 118, 210
Lethality of smoking, beliefs about, 89-90
Leukoplakia, 30
"Light" cigarettes, 89, 91-92, 112, 122,
        123, 127, 280-281, 286, 287,
        288, 296, 297-298, 303, 323,
        325, 329
Light smokers (chippers), 95
Life Skills Training (LST), 211, 212-213
Litigation, 33
    addictiveness of nicotine and, 119,
        121-122
    antilobbying challenge by industry,
        121, 241, 243
    class action suits, 121-122
    common-law lawsuits, 196, 197
    MSA, 50, 56, 122-123, 124, 125,
        128, 129, 157, 178
    Medicaid-related, 7, 122-123, 148,
        157, 178
    punitive damages, 128
    regulatory challenges by industry,
        119, 209
    RICO, 123, 127-128, 157, 280-281,
        287-288, 297-298, 318, 319,
        345, 346
    smokeless tobacco products, 127
    tort claims, 113, 114, 121-122, 147,
        197, 291

Lobbying
    advocacy groups falsely accused of,
        121, 241, 243-244
    by tobacco industry, 111, 122, 157
Lorillard, 329
Louisiana, 174, 245, 309, 311, 315
Low-nicotine cigarettes, 48, 346-353
Low-tar cigarettes, 44, 48, 112, 117, 122,
        280, 287, 296, 297, 298, 323
Low-yield products, 48, 280, 349
Lucky Strike cigarettes, 43
Luxembourg, 213

M

Maine, 124, 125, 128, 160, 173, 174, 208-
        209, 245, 308, 309, 311, 315
Malaysia, 292
Marketing and advertising
    black-and-white text only, 302, 319,
        323-327
    constitutionality issues, 324-327
    current practices, 48, 319-323
    deceptive health claims, 43, 44, 117,
        123, 125, 296-298
    developing countries, 113
    discount prices/coupons, 48, 50-51,
        61, 302
    effects of, 42, 43, 50-51, 61, 152,
        321-323
    expenditures by industry, 47-48, 114,
        129, 299, 300, 302, 319-320
    Fairness Doctrine, 110, 113-114,
        223-224
    in magazines, 300, 320, 321, 322,
        323, 324, 331
    point-of-sale, 16-17, 24, 114, 273-
        274, 299-301, 303, 319, 320-
        321, 322
    promotional activities, 20, 50-51,
        114, 118, 119, 123, 126, 129,
        154, 184, 199, 289, 299-300,
        301-303, 322
    recommendations, 16-17, 18, 24, 25,
        303, 324, 329
    restrictions, 16-17, 18, 20, 24, 25, 48,
        50, 110, 113-114, 119, 120, 123,
        129, 154, 158, 159, 198, 199,
        223-224, 273-275, 277, 287,
        289, 300-301, 303, 324, 319-330

364

ENDING THE TOBACCO PROBLEM

targeting women, 43, 50, 112
targeting youth, 20, 50, 112, 129,
148, 198, 199, 226, 287, 320,
323-324, 327-330
warnings on advertisements, 113
Marlboro Friday, 50
Marlboro Man, 226
Maryland, 174, 309, 311, 315
Massachusetts
Adult Tobacco Survey, 184
bans on smoking, 197, 245
community mobilization, 242
Department of Public Health, 162
effectiveness of programs, 165, 166,
168-171, 184, 227, 242-243
evaluation of programs, 164-165
excise taxes, 160, 162, 170, 177, 184,
311
funding for tobacco control, 162,
163, 172, 177, 315
media campaigns, 120, 133, 162, 184,
224, 226-227
per-capita cigarette smoking, 168-169,
170
prevalence of smoking, 165, 166,
168-171, 172
Prevalence Study, 171
revenues and expenditures for tobacco
control, 163, 174, 224, 309
Smoker's Quitline, 163
Tobacco Control Program, 119, 125,
128, 157, 160, 161, 162-163,
242-243
Tobacco Survey, 164
Try to Stop Resource Center, 163
Master Settlement Agreement (MSA), 9,
50, 56, 122-123, 124, 125, 128,
129, 157, 158, 163, 173, 174,
175, 176, 178-180, 181, 185,
206, 243, 287, 299, 313, 319-
320, 322, 330
McCain, John, 122
McClarren, Wayne, 226
McHugh, John, 210
Media campaigns
American Legacy Foundation's truth®
Campaign, 124, 229-230, 332
effectiveness, 124, 160, 184, 217,
218, 223, 225-226, 227, 228,
229, 230-231, 249

elimination, 133, 223-224
evaluation, 225-226, 229, 231
expenditures, 226, 229, 230
exposure and receptivity, 227
Fairness Doctrine, 223-224, 229
funding, 11-12, 224, 225, 226-227,
238
goals, 225, 226
recommendations, 11-12, 20, 21, 218,
231, 238
school-based programs combined
with, 11-12, 21, 215-218,
230-231
social marketing of cessation
interventions, 237-238
state, 119, 120, 159, 160, 161, 162-
163, 224-229, 241-242
youth-oriented, 11-12, 21, 57, 215-
218, 224, 227, 228, 229
Medicaid, 12, 22, 30, 122-123, 148, 178,
240, 314
Medicare, 12, 22, 236, 240
Mental illness
and cessation therapy, 233, 234, 247
and prevalence of smoking, 6, 68, 69,
70, 95-96, 98
Menthol cigarettes, 43, 44, 48, 61
Michigan, 173, 174, 176, 179, 196-197,
308, 309, 311, 314, 315, 316,
317
Midwestern Prevention Project, 215,
216-217
Military personnel, 95, 107-108, 248
Minnesota, 93, 115, 122-123, 160, 174,
196, 309, 311, 314, 315, 316,
317-318
Class of 1989 project, 215-216
Smoking Prevention Program, 216
Mississippi, 122-123, 128, 160, 174, 308,
309, 311, 315
Missouri, 173, 174, 308, 309, 311, 315
Models. See Policy simulations
Monitoring the Future, 46, 52, 169
Montana, 174, 175, 245, 309, 311, 315
Moore, Michael, 122
Motion Picture Association of America,
25-26, 332-333
MSA. See Master Settlement Agreement

N

National Academy of Sciences, 115
National Action Plan for Tobacco
    Cessation, 126
National Association of State Attorneys
    General, 209-210
National Cancer Institute, 21, 69, 238
    ASSIST program, 120, 121, 159, 163,
        172, 241-242, 243, 244, 246
    Smoking and Tobacco Control
        Program, 109
    Tobacco Working Group, 287
National Cancer Policy Board, 125
National Committee for Quality Assurance,
    239
National Health Interview Survey, 46, 48,
    49, 52, 53, 55, 59, 60, 62, 63,
    82, 85, 94, 95, 199
National Household Survey on Drug
    Abuse, 63
National Institutes of Health, 34, 128,
    182-184, 201-202, 204, 211,
    230, 235, 240
National Quitline Network, 21, 126, 221,
    237, 318
National Research Council, 115, 125
National Survey on Drug Use and Health,
    45, 46, 56, 58, 61, 63
National Survey on Environmental
    Management of Asthma
    and Children's Exposure to
    Environmental Tobacco Smoke,
    199
National Youth Tobacco Survey, 199
Natural history of smoking, 58-59
Nebraska, 174, 309, 311, 315
Nevada, 174, 179-180, 309, 311, 315
New Hampshire, 173, 174, 308, 309, 311,
    315
New Jersey, 174, 176, 189, 245, 309, 311,
    315
New Mexico, 174, 309, 311, 315
New York, 122, 125, 172, 174, 185, 181,
    182, 193, 207, 209, 210, 213,
    245, 309, 311, 315
New Zealand, 292

Nicotine
    addiction/addictiveness, 5, 77-82,
        95, 97, 111-112, 116-118, 119,
        121-122, 125, 146, 147, 148,
        151-152
    drug classification, 152
    FDA regulation, 117-118, 119, 125
    filtered cigarettes, 44
    flue curing and, 42-43
    illegal drugs compared, 58, 153
    industry manipulation of levels, 118,
        152
    "light" cigarettes, 92, 112
    low-level exposures, 95
    maintenance approach to policies, 278
    medicinal alternatives, 281-282, 283
    menthol cigarettes, 61
    neuroadaptation, 80
    priming effect on children of smokers,
        201
    product differences, 43
    and quitting, 4, 5, 97
    reduction strategy, 154, 281, 282-283,
        346-353
    replacement products, 17, 82, 87,
        117, 147, 185, 233, 234
    and smoking career, 59, 97
    tolerance to, 82
    withdrawal, 80
Nicotinic acetylcholine receptor alpha4
    gene, 82
NNK, 280
Nondaily smoking, 93-95, 166
North Carolina, 174, 176, 180, 309, 311,
    315
North Dakota, 174, 175, 245, 309, 311,
    315
North Karelia project, 215
Nortriptyline, 87

O

Ohio, 66, 174, 200, 309, 311, 315
Oklahoma, 66, 174, 309, 311, 315
Oregon, 160, 172, 174, 177, 185, 201,
    242, 309, 311, 315

P

Packaging of tobacco products. *See also*
  Warning labels
    corrective communications, 24,
      298-299
    misleading messages, 24, 289,
      296-298
    other health information, 296
    promotional, 289
    recommendations, 16, 23, 24, 298
    regulation of, 24, 289, 296-298
Parental smoking, 29, 110, 186-187, 200-
  201, 218, 219
Paternalism issue, 7, 111, 149-152, 202.
  See also Consumer sovereignty
  issue
Pennsylvania, 174, 176, 213, 305, 309,
  311, 315
Philip Morris, Inc., 50, 112, 121, 122, 125,
  126-127, 313, 326, 328, 345
Physicians
  antismoking, 111
  prosmoking, 108
  screening, educating, and counseling
    smokers, 83-84, 129, 219-222
Poland, 291
Policy analysis and development. *See also*
  Policy simulations
  incentives for manufacturers, 345-346
  innovations worthy of study, 344-346
  nicotine content reduction, 154,
    346-353
  recommendations, 26, 342
  wholesale purchasing monopsony,
    344-346
Policy framework. *See also* Regulation
  of tobacco; Restrictions on
  smoking; Tobacco control
  measures
  alcohol policy compared, 152
  blueprint outline, 3, 35-36, 154
  charge to committee, 31-35
  consumer sovereignty issue, 7, 8, 146-
    147, 150-152
  context for, 7-8, 146-148
  ethical context, 33-34, 148-150
  federal role, 154, 272-275
  firearm policy compared, 152
  goals, 32, 278-279
  horizon for projections, 32

inherent dangers of tobacco and, 8,
    152-153
  paternalism problem, 7, 33-34, 111,
    146, 147, 149-152
  product safety problem, 8, 145-146
  slippery slope argument, 153
  state role, 154
  youth-oriented, 8, 147-148, 153
Policy simulations
  black and gray market behavior, 343
  health outcomes tracking, 343-344
  industry response element, 343
  intensities of smoking in, 343
  models, 342-344
  reduced-nicotine cigarette, 154,
    351-352
  SimSmoke model, 130-133, 134,
    249-251
  state-dependent or endogenous
    transition rates, 342
  steady-state scenario, 4, 6-7, 131-133,
    136, 249, 250
  strengthened policies (best-case), 4,
    12-13, 137, 249-253
  System Dynamics Model, 130-133,
    134, 135, 136, 251-252
  uncertainty in, 130-131, 133
  worst-case scenario, 4, 6-7, 133-137,
    250
Potential reduced-exposure products
    (PREPs), 15, 23, 282, 284-
    285, 286, 288, 289, 302-303,
    344-346
Pregnancy, smoking during, 29, 110, 187,
    200, 234
Prevalence of smoking. *See also* Decline in
    smoking
  adolescents, 31, 46, 52-54, 124, 167-
    168, 169, 170-171
  adults, 1, 4, 5, 13, 29, 32, 45, 48,
    51-52, 62, 64, 65, 66, 124, 125,
    146, 166, 168, 170-171, 231
  age and, 52, 53, 58-59, 278
  bans on smoking and, 192-193, 198,
    201
  cessation rates and, 232, 234,
    251-252
  defined, 97
  nondaily patterns, 93-94
  educational attainment and, 62-64,
    65, 67, 96, 187

gender and, 51, 52, 53, 61-62
geographic differences, 64-68, 134,
    273
income and, 62-64, 65, 67, 187, 248
initiation rates and, 251-253
goals, 251
Master Settlement Agreement and, 56
media campaigns and, 160
mental illness and, 6, 68, 69, 70, 247
and motivation to quit, 85
penalties based on, 318-319
price of cigarettes and, 56, 170,
    182-184
projections, 12-13, 231, 249-253,
    271; *see also* Policy simulations
race/ethnicity and, 60-61, 62, 64, 247
trends, 6-7, 52-54
surveillance and monitoring, 333-335
young adults, 198
Prevention interventions. *See also* Media
    campaigns; School-based
    interventions
for adolescents, 8, 11, 123
applicable tobacco products, 32
cost-effectiveness, 149
delivery of services, 221-222
expenditures on, 2
health care-based, 20-21, 210,
    219-222
implementation, 32, 214
parent- or family-based, 11, 210, 218-
    219, 222
recommendations, 20-21, 222
synergistic effects, 184-185
for vulnerable populations, 247-248
Price of cigarettes, 5, 7, 9, 10, 16, 24, 42,
    44 n.1, 48, 50, 56, 94, 120, 125,
    129, 132, 133, 136, 170, 182-
    185, 186, 187, 191, 226, 236,
    300, 301, 302, 303, 304, 305,
    311, 314, 320, 321, 323, 324.
    See also Excise tax rates
Project SHOUT, 211, 213-215
Project STAR, 216
Promotions. *See* Marketing and advertising
Public Health Cigarette Smoking Act, 110
Public health remedies
    educational initiatives, 109-110
    secondhand smoke campaign,
        114-116
    tobacco industry response, 110-114

Puerto Ricans, 61
Puerto Rico, 66, 94, 185
Pure Food and Drug Act of 1906, 149, 274
Put Prevention into Practice, 219

Q

Quitlines, 21, 84, 126, 133, 161, 221, 236,
    237
Quitting. *See* Cessation of smoking

R

Rabin, Robert, 122
Race/ethnicity
    and cessation of smoking, 61
    and initiation age, 69
    and intensity of smoking, 69
    and mortality related to smoking, 61,
        247
    and nondaily smoking, 94
    and prevalence of smoking, 60-61, 62,
        63, 64, 247
Racketeer Influenced and Corrupt
    Organizations Act (RICO), 123,
    127-128, 280-281
Reduced-nicotine cigarette strategy
    feasibility, 347-351
    impact, 351-352
    nicotine content warnings, 352
    recommendations, 26, 352-353
    taxation based on nicotine content,
        352-353
Regret, 5, 83, 88, 93, 97, 148, 149, 150,
    151, 153, 187
Regulation of tobacco
    alcohol experience compared,
        304-306
    cigarette testing methods, 15, 23, 281,
        284, 287, 288, 296
    content disclosure, 23, 283-284, 288
    enforcement practices, 10, 203-205,
        207
    exemptions for tobacco industry,
        111-112
    FDA empowerment, 14-15, 22, 119,
        275-277, 288-289
    federal authority, 36, 111, 158, 272-
        275, 283-285, 307-308

federal-state relationship, 158,
        272-275
goals of, 277-279, 281-283
harm reduction from continued use,
        278, 281-282, 286
Internet sales and delivery, 207-210
"legitimization" concerns, 277, 285
nicotine content, 15, 119, 281-283,
        284
packaging characteristics, 276,
        289-299
potential reduced-exposure products,
        15, 23, 282, 284-285, 286, 288,
        289, 302-303
product characteristics, 15, 23, 111,
        279-289
product standards, 15, 23, 276, 284,
        288-289
proposed legislation, 275, 283-285
public health concerns, 277, 285-286
recommendations, 14-18, 22-26, 275,
        288-289
retail environment, 10-11, 20, 203-
        210, 273, 277, 283, 299-308
risks and benefits, 286-289
state authority, 272, 273
warning labels, 110, 113, 126, 154,
        273, 276, 290-296
Respiratory diseases and disorders, 29, 30,
        108, 110, 181-182, 200, 220-
        221, 222
Restrictions on smoking. *See also*
        Secondhand smoke
on airlines, 115, 116, 121-122
in child care facilities, 116, 190
and cigarette consumption by
        smokers, 192-193, 201
on college campuses, 198-199
in correctional facilities, 190, 194-196
constitutionality, 195
coverage of state laws, 189, 190
effects of, 10, 94, 125, 184, 185,
        191-202
grassroots activism, 115, 119, 152,
        189, 196, 244-246
in hospitals and health care facilities,
        19, 190, 194
and initiation of smoking, 201-202
industry response to, 121
legislation, 36

in multiunit residential locations,
        196-197
and nonsmoker health, 191-192
in outdoor spaces, 202-203
in privately owned vehicles, 20, 199-
        202, 222
in public buildings, 147, 184, 189-
        191, 193-194
on public transportation, 115, 116,
        121-122, 189, 190
recommendations, 10, 19, 20, 194,
        196, 197, 199, 202, 203
in residences, 20, 199-202, 219, 220,
        222
in restaurants and bars, 115, 125,
        190, 191, 193-194, 245
statewide, 125
in workplaces, 115, 147, 184, 189-
        194, 201, 245
Retail environment
adult purchases for minors, 206
age verification, 207-209, 327, 328
alcohol experience compared,
        304-306
buydowns, 301-302
on college campuses, 198
federal role, 307-308
on Indian reservations, 24, 304
Internet sales, 11-12, 20, 133, 185,
        186, 207-210
licensing mechanisms, 10, 20, 204,
        206, 304-305, 306-307
models for regulation, 304-307
monitoring compliance, 10, 203-205,
        206
monopoly systems, 304-306
promotional activities, 289, 299-303,
        322; *see also* Marketing and
        advertising
promotional allowances, 50-51,
        301-303
point-of-sale advertising, 114,
        299-301
recommendations, 10-12, 16-17, 20,
        24, 205, 210, 303, 307
restructuring options, 306-307
self-service displays and vending
        machines, 10, 205, 206
slotting fees, 301, 302-303
Rhode Island, 125, 174, 175, 176, 208,
        245, 309, 311, 315

Risk perceptions
    addiction and cessation, 90, 91, 93
    adolescents, 4, 5, 6, 8, 35, 88-93, 98,
        149, 150-151, 187, 297
    adults, 80, 90, 91, 151
    effects of smoking, 89-91
    level and stage of smoking and, 90,
        95
    "light" cigarettes, 91-92, 296-297
    media campaigns and, 160
    optimism bias, 89, 150, 151-152
    and paternalism issue, 150-151
    smokeless tobacco, 2, 31
    warning labels on cigarettes and, 293
R.J. Reynolds Company, 43, 48, 50, 112,
        118, 127, 313, 320, 326
Robert Wood Johnson Foundation, 120,
        159, 161, 164, 243, 244

S

Sackman, Janet, 226
Safe and Drug-Free School Act, 11, 20, 218
School-based interventions. *See also*
        individual programs
    CDC guidelines, 109
    community mobilization component,
        214, 215-217, 218, 231
    effectiveness, 211-217, 249-250
    evaluation of, 212, 213, 216
    funding, 11, 218
    media campaign combined with, 215-
        218, 230-231
    recommendation, 11, 20, 21, 218-219
    school-only programs, 211-215
    social competence approach, 212-213
    social influences approach, 211-212,
        216, 217
Schroeder, Steven, 120
Secondhand smoke, 34. *See also*
        Restrictions on smoking
    campaign against, 35, 114-116, 147,
        159, 163, 226
    children exposed to, 115, 192, 199,
        200-201
    common-law lawsuits, 196, 197
    deaths, 1-2, 29, 88, 116
    economic costs, 30, 192, 195, 200
    effects of smoking bans, 125, 191-202

    and external costs of cigarettes,
        186-187
    harm reduction products, 127
    health hazards, 115, 147, 191, 192,
        200
    monitoring exposure, 165, 229
    and paternalism issue, 147, 149, 150,
        152
    tort litigation, 121-122, 147
    warning labels, 298
Self-Regulation Theory, 88
Serotonin, 79, 82, 97
Singapore, 292
Smokeless cigarette, 117, 325
SmokeLess States program, 120, 159, 161,
        243-244, 246
Smokeless tobacco, 2-3, 30, 31, 41, 127,
        281
Smokers, defined, 47
Smuggling and black markets, 3, 14, 34,
        177, 185, 186, 188, 189, 195,
        278, 279, 289, 350-351
Social costs of smoking, 30, 33-34, 146,
        148-149, 152, 186-187
Social norms
    antismoking, 5, 7-8, 115, 246
    prosmoking, 6, 98, 129
Socioeconomic status. *See also* Educational
        attainment; Income
    and access to interventions, 247-248
Some-day smokers, 65 n.11, 93-94
South Africa, 292
South Carolina, 173, 174, 176, 188 n.3,
        308, 309, 311, 315, 317
South Dakota, 174, 175, 245, 309, 311,
        316
Spain, 213
Stanford University, 164, 167
States. *See also* Comprehensive state
        programs; *individual states*
    early smoking bans, 152
    excise tax revenues by, 177
    MSA allocations by, 179
    nondaily smoking rates, 94
    prevalence of smoking by, 64-68
    tobacco control revenues and
        expenditures by, 174-175
    variation in policies among, 9, 176-
        177, 182, 186, 188-189, 273
Sudden infant death syndrome, 29, 192,
        200

Surgeon General's reports, 4, 35, 45, 70,
    77, 78, 79, 88, 108, 109, 110,
    111, 113, 115, 117, 118, 119,
    122, 147, 148, 151, 158, 242
Survey of Health-Related Behaviors Among
    Active Duty Military Personnel,
    248
Synar Amendment, 118, 203-204

T

Taiwan, 292
Tar, 92. *See also* Low-tar cigarettes
Teen Tobacco Summit, 228
Tennessee, 66, 173, 174, 308, 309, 310,
    311, 316
Terry, Luther, 113
Texas, 122-123, 160, 174, 193, 310, 311,
    316
Thailand, 291, 292, 295
Theory of Planned Behavior, 88
Thompson, Tommy, 126
Tobacco and Alcohol Prevention Project
    (TAPP), 211-212
Tobacco control measures. *See also*
    Community mobilization;
    Comprehensive state programs;
    Excise tax rates; Funding
    tobacco control; Policy
    simulations; Regulation of
    tobacco
campaign against secondhand smoke,
    114-116
effectiveness, 5, 6, 7, 68, 94, 124-128
evaluation of, 6, 333-335
expenditures, 30, 128
future of, 4, 128-136
inherent danger of tobacco products
    and, 152-153
international, 3
legislation, 110, 111-112
litigation strategies, 113-114, 121-123
modern movement, 108, 109-116
nicotine as addictive drug and,
    116-118
political momentum, 2, 124-128, 157
retail shipments, 207-210
smuggling as threat to, 3
special populations, 247-248

state actions, 119-121; *see also*
    Comprehensive state programs
status of, 138-129
status-quo policies, 4, 6-7, 131-133
strengthened policies, 4, 8-12, 249-253
surveillance and monitoring, 26, 120,
    333-335
weakened policies, 4, 6-7, 133-136
youth access restrictions, 118-119,
    203-206
youth exposure restrictions, 330-333
Tobacco industry. *See also* Litigation;
    Marketing and advertising
cigarette mass production, 41-42,
    107, 152, 327-330
deceptive practices, 7, 33, 35, 114,
    121-122, 125, 127, 146, 148,
    225, 226, 228, 274-275, 280-
    281, 285-286, 298, 345-346
discouraging cessation, 24
economic assistance to growers, 126,
    180
mandatory payments for tobacco
    control, 308-319
motivating conduct changes, 345-346
new product development, 46, 48,
    112, 127, 145
nicotine manipulation, 117
political and commercial power, 157
pricing strategies, 46, 48, 50-51
profits, 313
public relations and lobbying
    campaigns, 110-114, 121, 123
response to decline in product use, 44,
    46-51
response to public policy advocacy,
    121, 241, 243-244
transnational companies, 34, 113
youth education and prevention
    programs, 327-330
Tobacco Institute, 111, 115, 123
Tobacco Related Disease Research
    Program, 161
Toxic Substances Control Act, 111, 152
Transtheoretical Model of Change, 88

U

U.S. Department of Defense, 248
U.S. Department of Education, 11, 20, 218

U.S. Department of Health and Human Services, 21, 203-204, 238, 333
    Clinical Practice Guideline for Treating Tobacco Use and Dependence, 87
    Healthy People 2010, 7, 13, 52, 124, 133, 135, 136, 199, 250, 251
    National Quitline Network, 126, 237
U.S. Department of Justice, 280, 318, 346
U.S. Environmental Protection Agency, 116, 147, 199
U.S. Government Accountability Office, 180
U.S. Postal Service, 209-210
U.S. Public Health Service, 240
U.S. Securities and Exchange Commission, 313
United Kingdom, 83, 295, 297
University of California, 161
    San Diego, 164
University of Massachusetts Medical School, 163
University of Southern California, 164, 167
UPS, 209
Utah, 67, 94, 125, 174, 177, 245, 310, 311, 316

V

Varenicline, 87, 233
Venezuela, 292
Vermont, 67, 125, 127, 175, 245, 310, 311, 316
    Mass Media Project, 215, 217
Veterans Health Administration, 248
Vietnamese Americans, 61, 247
Virgin Islands, 66
Virginia, 175, 180, 310, 311, 316
Virginia Slims, 50, 112
Vulnerable populations, 6, 22, 57, 69, 95-97, 98, 247-248, 334

W

Warnings labels. *See also* Packaging of tobacco products
    on advertisements, 113, 154, 290
    black-and-white text, 291, 295
    Canadian experience, 16, 23, 291-292, 295, 296
    on carton wrappers, 292
    current policy, 290-291
    effectiveness, 294-296
    graphic/pictorial, 15-16, 23, 291-293, 294, 295, 296
    health risks, 110, 113, 126, 154, 276, 290-293
    industry endorsement of, 126
    international comparisons, 291-293
    legislation, 110, 113, 273
    recommendations, 15-16, 23, 296
    size and placement, 292-293
    and tort claims, 291
    smuggling, 289
Washington, D.C., 94, 115, 128, 159 n.1, 170, 173, 174, 175, 178, 179, 190, 191, 207, 224, 245, 308, 309, 311, 315, 318, 319
Washington state, 125, 175, 196, 207, 245, 310, 311, 316
We Card program, 327, 328
West Virginia, 65, 94, 175, 310, 311, 316
Winston cigarettes, 48
Wisconsin, 175, 310, 311, 316
Women, as marketing target, 43, 50, 112
Women's liberation movement, 112
World Health Organization, 3, 34, 113, 117, 289, 292, 347
World War I, 43
World War II, 44, 152
Wyoming, 175, 304, 310, 311, 316

Y

Young adult tobacco use
    on college campuses, 198-199
    initiation of smoking, 5, 6, 45-46, 49, 57, 69, 70, 94-95, 98, 167
    prevalence, 46, 58, 70, 167
    prevention interventions, 11
    price of cigarettes as deterrent, 50, 183, 184
    targeting by industry, 50
Youth. *See also* Adolescent tobacco use
    correctional facilities, 195
Youth Behavior Risk Surveillance System (YRBSS), 46, 53, 171